THE DEVELOPMENT OF PSYCHOPATHOLOGY

The Development of Psychopathology

Nature and Nurture

BRUCE F. PENNINGTON

Foreword by
Dante Cicchetti

THE GUILFORD PRESS
New York   London

© 2002 The Guilford Press
A Division of Guilford Publications, Inc.
72 Spring Street, New York, NY 10012
www.guilford.com

Printed in the United States of America

This book is printed on acid-free paper.

Last digit is print number: 9   8   7   6   5   4   3

Library of Congress Cataloging-in-Publication Data

Pennington, Bruce Franklin, 1946–
    The development of psychopathology : nature and nurture / by Bruce F.
Pennington.
        p. cm.
Includes bibliographical references and index.
    ISBN-10: 1-57230-755-2   ISBN-13: 978-1-57230-755-1 (hc)
    ISBN-10: 1-59385-235-5   ISBN-13: 978-1-59385-235-1 (pbk)
    1. Psychology, Pathological. 2. Mental illness—Etiology. 3.
Developmental psychobiology. 4. Cognitive neuroscience. I. Title.
    RC454 .P393 2002
    616.89—dc21   2002003911

For my family—Linda, Amy, and Luke

About the Author

Bruce F. Pennington, PhD, is John Evans Professor of Psychology at the University of Denver, where he heads the Developmental Cognitive Neuroscience program. He received his BA in English at Harvard University in 1968 and his PhD in Clinical Psychology at Duke University in 1977. He has earned an international reputation for his research on dyslexia, autism, and attention-deficit/hyperactivity disorder, and has published over 150 scientific papers on these topics. His honors include Research Scientist, MERIT, and Fogarty awards from the National Institutes of Health.

Dr. Pennington's earlier book, *Diagnosing Learning Disorders* (Guilford Press, 1991), emphasizes a close relation between research and practice. In addition to being a researcher and research mentor, he is also a child clinical neuropsychologist and has been active in clinical practice and training throughout his career.

Foreword

During the latter part of the 20th century, developmental psychopathology emerged as a new science that was the product of an integration of various disciplines, the efforts of which had been previously distinct and separate, including genetics, neuroscience, epidemiology, sociology, psychiatry, and clinical, developmental, and experimental psychology. Since its inception, scientists in the field of developmental psychopathology have striven to ascertain how these multiple levels of analysis may influence individual differences, the continuity or discontinuity of adaptive or maladaptive behavioral patterns, and the pathways by which the same developmental outcomes can be achieved. Advances in our knowledge of the normal course of genetic, biological, social, and psychological processes have played a significant role in facilitating the identification of the mechanisms that contribute to the emergence and course of psychopathological disorders.

For example, multidisciplinary investigations have contributed to the growing understanding that a number of the most severe mental disorders, such as schizophrenia and the pervasive developmental disorders (e.g., autism), arise in part from exogenous or endogenous disturbances in brain development. Likewise, the veritable knowledge explosion that has occurred in developmental neurobiology, the area of neuroscience that focuses on factors regulating the normal and abnormal development of neurons and neural circuitry, has provided insight into the neuropathological wiring that occurs in serious mental disorders. The incorporation of the methods of cognitive psychology into sophisticated neuroscience technologies has enabled the anatomical and physiological imaging of the brain. This interdisciplinary connection opened up new vistas for examining normal and pathological developmental processes. Additionally, multidisciplinary collaborations between molecular geneticists and neurologists have enabled scientists to comprehend for the first time the genetic basis of certain neurological disorders, especially those diseases with a monogenic etiology.

In this compelling volume, *The Development of Psychopathology: Nature and Nurture*, Bruce F. Pennington describes a new paradigm, drawn from work in the fields of developmental psychopathology and cognitive neuroscience, which can elucidate the understanding of normal and abnormal human behavior. In keeping with a dynamic developmental systems theory perspective on normality and psychopathology, Pennington conceptualizes human behavior as emerging from embedded and interacting complex systems. Each of the major systems posited by Pennington defines a level of analysis for comprehending the emergence and course of psychopathology. Within Pennington's framework, these systems include the genome, the mechanisms that cause genes to activate or express themselves in development and in epigenesis, the brain, interacting psychological functions, and the individual in his or her social and cultural contexts. Pennington also demonstrates that virtually all mental disorders are developmental in nature and therefore must be understood in the context of what is known about normal development.

Pennington theorizes that the interacting nature of these multiple systems provides humans with the capacity to adapt to ever-changing contexts and experiential demands. Whereas individuals without any mental disorder are thought to make these adaptations quite readily, persons with psychopathology are thought to have more restricted options for confronting changing contextual challenges.

Pennington's systems viewpoint that brain–behavior relations are multidimensional is consistent with contemporary theoretical conceptualizations of brain–behavior relations in neuroscience. The brain is viewed as operating in a plastic, dynamic, self-organizing fashion and as being less constrained by predetermined "localized" boundaries than previously thought. One outgrowth of systems theorizing has been acceptance of the viewpoint that neurobiological development and experience are mutually influencing. For example, a number of investigations have demonstrated that, just as gene expression alters social behavior, social experience exerts actions on the brain by feeding back on it to modify gene expression, as well as brain structure and function. Furthermore, it also has been discovered that alterations in gene expression induced by learning and by social and psychological experiences produce changes in patterns of neuronal and synaptic connections and, thus, in the function of nerve cells. Such modifications not only contribute to the biological basis of individuality, but also exert a prominent role in initiating and maintaining the behavioral anomalies that are provoked by social and psychological experiences. Relatedly, Pennington states that all psychopathologies emerge in a social and cultural context, which can modify their definition, emergence, maintenance, and developmental course.

In Pennington's neuroscientific perspective on psychopathology, there are four levels of analysis that must be examined: the genetic and environmental mechanisms that cause psychopathology (i.e., etiology); the brain mechanisms that alter the developmental process; the impact that experience exerts on brain development; a specification of which neuropsychological processes are disrupted; and the delineation of the symptom or surface level of the psychopathological condition. Thus, because levels of organization and processes are reciprocally interactive, it is difficult, if not impossible, to reduce psychopathology to any one level. It is essential to consider each level of analysis in order to have a thorough understanding of the genesis and epigenesis of psychopathological disorders.

Pennington reviews and analyzes the extant methods needed to formulate an integrated neuroscience-based understanding of three classes of psychiatric syndromes (disorders of motivation, disorders of action regulation, and disorders of language and cognitive development). In the final section of the volume, Pennington cogently synthesizes what we have learned from these methods about a number of specific mental disorders. Moreover, he points out what remains to be learned about these mental disorders that must be addressed by a multiple-levels-of-analysis approach. I came away from reading the volume with a feeling of optimism that continued research on the genetic, neurobiological, neuropsychological, and psychological processes that take into consideration the individual's social and cultural context throughout the course of development will contribute to important breakthroughs in our understanding of the etiology and course of mental disorders.

Although Pennington has focused on the application of a neuroscientific approach to mental disorders in this volume, I believe that his multiple-levels-of-analysis framework could also be applied to research on resilience. As predicted from general systems theory, not all persons who are exposed to the same adverse biological, social, and psychological experiences are affected in the same manner. Indeed, some individuals develop in a competent fashion despite the magnitude of risk they encounter. A limitation of the resilience literature to date is the paucity of investigations that have included biological and genetic variables as potential protective factors or mechanisms in the development of resilience. In addition, there have been few investigators studying resilience who have conducted their research programs from a multiple-levels-of-analysis perspective. Through examining concurrent genetic, biological, psychological, and social-contextual changes longitudinally in individuals who have undergone significant adversity, as would follow from the approach proffered by Pennington, researchers should be in a stronger position to elucidate the pathways to resilient adaptation. For example, such multilevel investigations may reveal the mechanisms responsible for inhibiting the expression of genes that are probabilistically associated with maladaptive developmental outcomes and psychopathology. Furthermore, interdisciplinary, multiple-levels-of-analysis approaches may reveal mechanisms that activate the expression of genes that may serve a protective function for individuals experiencing adversity.

In summary, Pennington has produced a volume that beautifully integrates neuroscience and developmental psychopathology. His approach not only illuminates an understanding of pathological functioning, but also can serve as a road map to better understanding the avoidance of psychopathological outcomes. Ultimately, this work can inform prevention efforts with populations at risk for the development of psychopathology.

DANTE CICCHETTI, PhD
University of Rochester

Preface

This book is about a new paradigm for understanding human behavior, one that is based on the emerging field of developmental cognitive neuroscience. It explains and then applies this new paradigm to some of the more difficult questions about the human condition: where do mental illnesses come from, how do they develop, why are they so common, how can they be treated, and how might they eventually be prevented? Although some mental illnesses have been recognized since ancient times, scientifically adequate explanations of mental illness have only begun to emerge in the last few decades. For most of history, our explanations of this large source of human misery have been woefully thin. The very real suffering has been denied, or when it cannot be denied, it has been explained by supernatural forces, folk psychology, or cleverly disguised tautologies. Now real scientific explanations are beginning to emerge as a result of hard empirical work at many levels of analysis. This book describes what a scientifically adequate explanation of psychopathology will look like and how close we are to such an explanation for different psychopathologies.

The key ideas in this new paradigm for understanding psychopathology can be expressed fairly simply. Human behavior emerges from embedded and interacting complex systems that include the genome and its expression in epigenesis and development, the brain, interacting psychological functions, and the individual in his or her social and cultural contexts. As a result of these interacting complex systems, behavior is richly pluripotential, allowing humans to adapt quickly to changing contexts. Psychopathology represents a deviation from this adaptive range such that behavior is restricted to a narrower range of options. To understand psychopathology, a framework is needed that incorporates all these complex systems, each of which defines a level of analysis.

Some basic principles emerge from this paradigm. We cannot reduce psychopathology simply to genes, early environmental experiences, neural synapses and networks, psychological processes, or social contexts. Instead, we need *all* these levels of analysis to understand the development of psychopathology for the following reasons: First, it is likely that most, if not all, psychopathologies are caused by an interaction of genetic and environmental risk factors, some of which are social in nature. All psychopathologies are brain disorders in that all behavior is mediated by the brain, but to understand how a change in brain structure or function affects behavior, we need other levels of analysis, in particular a neurocomputational analysis of how interactions among neurons generate behavior. Virtually all psychopathologies are developmental and must be understood in the context of developmental theory. Because all psychopathologies represent deviations from normal human functions, an explanation of any psychopathology requires a specification of which neuropsychological processes are disrupted. All psychopathologies emerge in a social and cultural context, which can modify their definition, initiation, persistence, and course.

This book is organized into three main sections: fundamental issues, methods of syndrome analysis, and reviews of specific disorders. Chapter 1 considers topics that are basic to the study of psychopathology, including the need for an integrated approach, issues in the use and validation of diagnoses, and fallacies that can impede our understanding. Chapter 2 reviews the methods of syndrome analysis that are needed to achieve an integrated neuroscientific understanding of the development of a psychopathology. These methods come from the fields of epidemiology, behavioral and molecular genetics, neurobiology, and psychology. Chapters 3–5 review what we have learned from these methods—about disorders of motivation, disorders of action regulation, and disorders of language and cognitive development—and what we still need to learn. Chapter 6 discusses the main conclusions about our current knowledge of the development of psychopathology, including implications for prevention and treatment, as well as implications for future research.

The organization of the book permits it to be used both as a text for graduate-level students and as a reference for professionals in the field. Thus, the book was designed to be useful and accessible for readers with different levels of expertise and can be read at different levels of depth. Those interested in broad issues and methods for studying psychopathology will find Chapters 1, 2, and 6 most helpful. Those seeking a summary of recent research findings about a particular disorder will be more interested in Chapters 3–5. These summaries strive to be representative of current knowledge and issues but they are by no means exhaustive reviews.

Acknowledgments

Much like a long journey, a book is completed one tiny step at a time. I would not have completed this journey without the help and encouragement of many others, including my good friend Richard Mangen and my dear wife, Linda. The original idea for this book came from teaching a graduate class in developmental psychopathology over the last 13 years. My students, present and former, encouraged the idea of the book. Once I had a draft, I piloted it as a text and the students in that class provided very thoughtful feedback about both the substance and style of the manuscript.

Since the book is based in part on my own research and what I have learned about how to study disorders of development over the past 30 years, I owe a great deal to the funding agencies that have continuously supported my work. These include the National Institute of Mental Health, the National Institute of Child Health and Human Development, the March of Dimes, and the Orton Dyslexia Society.

My colleagues both here in Colorado and around the world have contributed a great deal both to my scientific development and to this book. Richard Boada, Claudia Cardoso-Martins, Uta Frith, Elizabeth Griffith, Marshall Haith, Peter Hobson, Danny McIntosh, Sally Ozonoff, Rob Roberts, Randy Ross, Robbie Rossman, Melissa Rutherford, Michael Rutter, Stephen Shirk, Erik Willcutt, and Piotr Winkielman all read an earlier draft. Their suggestions shaped the final product in innumerable helpful ways and saved me from some of my errors. Once they read the first draft, it was a great relief to hear that, on balance, they liked it.

I also thank my publisher, Seymour Weingarten at The Guilford Press, for the occasional friendly inquiries that help keep an author going. He and the rest of the staff at Guilford have been very helpful through all phases of the book's production.

Eric Olson did a wonderful job of translating my rudimentary drafts of figures into real illustrations. Debbie Porter, my research administrator, helped with the meticulous proofreading of the galleys and taught me that a capital letter does not always follow a colon.

Finally, my deepest thanks go to my administrative assistant, Suzanne Miller, who has provided unflagging assistance with manuscript preparation and assembling the bibliography. She has seen me through two books and knows all too well that not all those tiny steps go forward.

Contents

Chapter 1

Fundamental Issues

This chapter first considers the need for a framework to integrate the various levels of analysis necessary for understanding the development of a psychopathology. Such a framework raises a key issue: the mind–body problem in psychopathology. After examining this issue, we turn to the use and validation of diagnoses, and conclude with fallacies that have impeded understanding of this difficult topic.

ECUMENISM VERSUS INTEGRATION: THE NEED FOR A NEW FRAMEWORK

Despite considerable empirical progress in the field of psychopathology in the last few decades, we lack a satisfactory comprehensive theory. The 20th century began with a comprehensive theory of psychopathology, Freud's psychoanalytic theory, which dominated the field for at least 50 years. Its focus on the importance of early relationships and development are still important insights, and are still being investigated by attachment theorists. Psychoanalysis as a treatment has evolved into interpersonal forms of psychotherapy, some of which are empirically validated. Yet psychoanalytic theory's shortcomings as a scientific explanation of psychopathologies are now well known. Within psychology,

1

psychoanalytic theory was replaced by learning and then by cognitive-behavioral theories of psychopathology. Within psychiatry, Freudian theory has largely been replaced by biological psychiatry. But neither biological psychiatry nor cognitive-behavioral psychology offers a comprehensive theory for understanding psychopathology.

Biological psychiatry has the advantage of placing the brain squarely in the center of the understanding of psychopathology, but it often has been too reductionistic: too focused on single causes (e.g., alterations in a given neurotransmitter) or on a single level of analysis (e.g., synapses).

Current psychological theories have the advantage of dealing with interpersonal and social contexts that shape the development of a psychopathology, but they are weak at explaining individual differences and mostly ignore the brain.

This state of affairs is often reflected in contemporary abnormal psychology or psychiatry books by an uneasy ecumenism. Psychological and physiological theories are laid out side by side but rarely integrated. Some texts speak of a "biopsychosocial" model, but this model is usually an ecumenical umbrella for covering disparate approaches rather than an integration.

So we are at an interesting point in the history of the science of psychopathology. Previous comprehensive theoretical paradigms have failed; new empirical methods are rapidly producing data that need to be accounted for, but current theories of psychopathology are inadequate for the task of integration. At the same time, a new scientific paradigm is emerging in cognitive neuroscience. However, to deal with the development of psychopathology, cognitive neuroscience needs to be broadened in three key ways: (1) It must focus explicitly on individual differences; (2) it must integrate emotion and social influences into the study of cognition; and (3) it must incorporate development. Although this book does not pretend to offer a complete new theory of psychopathology, it does attempt to lay out the conceptual and empirical constraints that a new theory of psychopathology will have to meet, and to show how a cognitive neuroscientific approach can satisfy those constraints.

Hence, a basic message of this book is that we need a way to integrate research on the biological and psychological mechanisms involved in developmental psychopathologies. Consider a child with mild depression, or dysthymia. A biologist might seek the explanation for this clinical condition in differences in receptors for neurotransmitters. But a psychologist might seek the explanation in differences in attachment security. These very different ways of thinking about the same clinical phenomenon are not necessarily competing explanations. Rather, they may be complementary, each operating at a different level of analysis. However, for either the biologist or the psychologist to think about how these two explanations relate to each other is not straightforward because a theoretical framework for integrating these different levels of explanation is only beginning to emerge.

This neuroscientific framework seeks to relate behavior and mind to the brain. It is important to realize that every psychopathology requires us to solve the brain–behavior or mind–body problem. It is not enough to frame an explanation of a psychopathology purely in terms of mental or psychological constructs. To do so ignores the brain. At the same time, to frame an explanation purely in terms of brain variables such as receptor efficiencies or densities is not enough. To do so reveals a naive reductionism, because even if the causal brain variables were known, we would still need to know how these brain differences lead to changes in behavior.

The important overall point of a neuroscientific perspective is that analyses of normal or abnormal function need to be informed by an understanding of the brain structures and processes that implement the function. In other words, "hardware" matters and provides important constraints for developmental theories, whether they are theories of neo-Piagetian cognitive operations or internal working models in attachment theory. So taking a neuroscientific perspective forces us to confront a latent "dualism" in much of developmental psychology, the assumption that analyses of behavioral function can proceed completely independently of analyses of brain. As Patricia Goldman-Rakic (1987a) aptly said in discussing the relation between neuroscience and developmental psychology, "The 'empty organism' has long since been filled with intentionality and information-processing skills, but not necessarily with a central nervous system" (p. 601).

To draw out the implications of this point, let us take as an example a hypothetical developmental psychopathology that is *entirely* determined by the social (i.e., interpersonal) environment—no genetic influence; no traumatic, toxic, or other noninterpersonal environmental alteration of brain development. It is very easy to catch oneself thinking that in such a case the pathogenetic social influences are registered somewhere other than the brain—in the attachment system, in object relations, or what have you. The point of a neuroscientific perspective is that *all* social influences affect brain development in some way or another, and all psychological constructs are implemented by brain mechanisms. For instance, the neuropsychology of traumatic social experiences such as loss, neglect, and abuse is becoming fairly well understood. Such traumas can cause very persistent changes in brain development. Moreover, positive social experiences also affect brain development and function. Humans are social animals and are therefore "open" systems, dependent on social relations. So taking a neuroscientific perspective does not limit the unit of analysis to an individual person (or his or her nervous system). Psychopathology may exist in an individual, a dyad, or a social group; I am simply arguing that a neuroscientific perspective is relevant in each case. For instance, it has been shown that an individual baboon's neurochemistry changes when its position in the dominance hierarchy changes (Sapolsky, 1994).

These considerations mean that the familiar clinical distinction between "functional" and "organic" is misleading and, in a strict sense, fundamentally incorrect. There is no autonomous substrate for functional pathologies, nor does the functional–organic distinction neatly divide disorders either by treatability or mode of treatment. For instance, it is frequently assumed that functional disorders call for behavioral treatments and are more amenable to treatment, whereas organic ones are less treatable and call for biological interventions. However, many counterexamples, such as phenylketonuria (PKU) on the one hand, and multiple personality disorder on the other, can be cited.

One can discern this functional versus organic assumption in contemporary psychopathology textbooks. The most heritable disorders, such as bipolar illness or autism, are thought of as "biological" disorders, whereas less heritable disorders, such as dysthymia or phobias, are thought of as functional disorders produced by socialization or experience. As we will see, there is a striking absence of psychological theories for the development of bipolar disorder and fewer psychological treatments. Also, the success of early psychological treatments for autism questions this assumption. The main point is that as soon as we accept this assumption, we have given up on a universal theory of psychopathology.

It is also important to emphasize that a commitment to a neuroscientific perspective does not commit one to a belief in single, deterministic causes for developmental psychopathology. Developmental psychopathologies are complex behavioral disorders in two senses: The disrupted behaviors are complex, and the multiple developmental pathways that led to the disruption are complex. For most psychopathologies, multiple risk and protective factors, both genetic and environmental, affect outcome in a probabilistic rather than deterministic fashion. Both normal and abnormal development result from the self-organizing properties of complex systems, so single causes are unlikely, and interactions and nonlinearities are to be expected.

So, clearly, my point about the relevance of brain mechanisms for understanding a purely social pathology is not an argument for reductionism. Risk factors will be found at different levels of analysis for different developmental psychopathologies: the molecular level for some, and the attachment system for others. But all risk factors act on the same complex developmental system that cannot be eliminated from an explanation. Thus, no level of analysis is entirely autonomous or encapsulated; interpersonal systems do not exist in some "social ether" outside of human organisms. Learning and using such systems is constrained by the real human brain, which evolved for just that function, among others. Moreover, dynamic principles that describe network properties within a brain may well have some utility in describing the dynamics of social networks.

Our claims about the relevance of neuroscience for purely social pathologies are integrative rather than reductionistic. The point is that neuroscience potentially provides a broad-enough paradigm to encompass *all* of developmental psychopathology. While a complete explanation for some pathologies may emphasize different levels of analysis than the explanation of others, all can (and need to) fit within the same broad paradigm. A pathology that is caused in part by genetic influences will require an explanation that begins at the deepest explanatory level, with an altered DNA sequence, and proceeds across many levels of analysis, up to the level of observable behavior. In contrast, a pathology that is completely caused by aberrant parenting may require fewer levels of analysis, but these levels will overlap with those used in the previous example; we should not have to invoke a totally different paradigm. Moreover, aberrant parenting may change gene expression and brain development.

In summary, the argument is that we need a new framework or paradigm for understanding the development of psychopathology, and cognitive neuroscience provides that framework. As discussed by O'Reilly and Munakata (2000), there are two complementary aspects of a cognitive neuroscience approach: physical reductionism and reconstructionism. *Both* aspects are needed for a comprehensive understanding of psychopathology. Unlike most contemporary psychological theories of psychopathology (e.g., cognitive-behavioral or developmental theories), cognitive neuroscience is explicitly committed to physical reductionism: The components of cognition and behavior must be reduced to their physical substrate, the brain, just as key aspects of living organisms have been reduced to molecular biology. Biological psychiatry has applied physical reductionism to psychopathology with noteworthy success, but physical reductionism alone cannot give us an explanation of complex behavior. Unlike much of biological psychiatry, cognitive neuroscience is also explicitly committed to reconstructionism: an account of how interactions among the elementary units (i.e., neurons) of the nervous system give rise to the phenomena of cognition and behavior. Achieving this reconstruction has been greatly aided by the development of neural network models, which, as we will see, have provided a much deeper functional understanding of how complex cognitive phenomena arise from the interaction of neuron-like elements. (But, unfortunately, there are relatively few neural network models of psychopathology.) In short, current approaches to psychopathology are either functional theories unrelated to the brain or biological reductions that do not attempt to reconstruct function. Although both approaches have made empirical progress and have led to the development of effective treatments, they cannot by themselves be integrated. A different framework is needed to accomplish that, one that includes both physical reductionism *and* reconstructionism.

Applying a cognitive neuroscientific approach to psychopathology will enrich both fields and change the boundaries of what we currently consider to be psychopathology. We have just discussed how the field of psychopathology will be enriched. One benefit to cognitive neuroscience is that it will have to include emotion and arousal in its models. As we will see, there is a notable paucity of neural network models of mood and anxiety disorders. In terms of boundaries, the current artificial division between psychiatric and neurological disorders reflects the misleading functional versus organic distinction discussed earlier. For example, some developmental disorders, such as dyslexia and mental retardation, are not always considered psychopathologies. Some neurological disorders, such as attentional neglect or the alien hand syndrome, are virtually never considered psychopathologies. This artificial division exists in spite of the fact that psychopathology is traditionally defined as an alteration in thought, mood, or behavior that impairs adaptive functioning; clearly, developmental and neurological disorders fit this definition. A cognitive neuroscientific approach aspires to explain all these kinds of disorders—traditional psychopathologies, developmental disorders, and neurological disorders—with similar models. At the same time, how we think about developmental and neurological disorders will be enriched by thinking about how social and emotional influences alter their course and affect treatment.

In taking a neuroscientific perspective on either abnormal or normal behavioral development, several levels of analysis need to be considered. We organize the discussion of specific psychopathologies into four broad categories—etiology, brain mechanisms, neuropsychology, and the symptom or surface levels (Pennington, 1991)—similar to the four levels proposed by Morton and Frith (1995) in their framework for analyzing developmental psychopathologies.

Before discussing these levels in more detail, it is important to see how they are causally related (Figure 1). Neuroscientists sometimes assume that the causal arrows only run in one direction across these levels of analysis, as depicted in the top part of Figure 1. Etiological factors—namely, gene variants and environmental risk factors—change brain development, which in turn changes neuropsychological development, which leads to changes in behavior. Some of these changes in behavior are the symptoms that define a given disorder. However, the situation is not that simple. A child's behavior changes his or her experience, which in turn changes brain development and the social environment's response to the child, which in turn affects his or her development. Although experience and environment ordinarily do not change genes (i.e., their DNA sequences), such factors can definitely influence gene expression. For example, early stress experiences change the expression of the gene that produces the glucocorticoid receptor (Meaney et al., 1996). Glucocorticoids are hormones important to the stress response. So a more realistic model is provided in the bottom part of Figure 1, where we see that the causal arrows run in *both* directions.

Four Levels of Analysis

Now I discuss these levels of analysis in more detail. The *etiological* level is concerned with genetic and environmental influences that cause the pathology in question. Genetic and environmental influences may act independently, but they may also interact or correlate with each other—the latter situation having some similarities to what developmental psychopathologists call "transactions" (Pennington & Ozonoff,

Unidirectional Causation

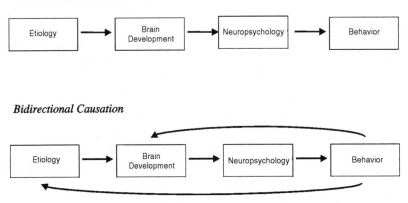

Bidirectional Causation

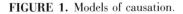

FIGURE 1. Models of causation.

1991). An obvious but frequently overlooked methodological point is that clear answers about environmental etiologies cannot be obtained without controlling for genetic influences. Unfortunately, many existing studies of supposed environmental influences on developmental psychopathology include only non-twin, biological families, in which genetic and environmental influence are inherently confounded. Likewise, until recently, studies of genetic influences on both psychopathology and normal behavior have been indirect, relying on quasi-experiments such as twin and adoption studies, and utilizing fairly simple additive models of genetic and environmental influences. It is now clear that virtually all psychopathologies are caused by a mix of both genetic and environmental factors that likely interact in the process of development to produce a psychopathology, but empirical methods for detecting such interactions have been very limited. Recent advances have made it possible to measure genetic influences on psychopathology directly, as will be discussed later, and to conduct longitudinal studies of individuals with risk alleles to examine gene × environment interactions (Plomin & Rutter, 1998).

The next level of analysis concerns how these etiological influences act on the development of *brain mechanisms*. One of the important recent discoveries in neuroscience is that early experience plays a very important role in sculpting the connectivity of the developing brain; with about 10^{11} neurons and a total of about 10^{15} connections between them, it is logically impossible for 10^5 genes to specify neuronal location and connections in a hardwired fashion (Changeux, 1985). Instead, the developing brain overproduces neurons, dendrites, and synapses, and then lets experience "select" which elements to preserve through a kind of "neural Darwinism" (Edelman, 1987). Later experience also changes brain structure both by adding or subtracting dendrites and synapses, and by modifying existing synapses (Greenough, Black, & Wallace, 1987). So a fundamental account of how experience alters brain structure is emerging within neuroscience; this account is of obvious relevance to psychopathologists who ponder why some experiences are so formative and others are so surprisingly neutral in their long-term effects.

On the genetics side, the substantial heritabilities found for many normal and abnormal individual differences in behavior mean that there are genetically caused variations in brain structure and function within our species. What aspects of brain development are likely targets for genetic influence? Although it has been shown that genetic influences on behavior can "turn on" across the lifespan (Plomin, 1990), it is likely that many genetic influences on brain development, especially those important for developmental psychopathologies, act on early brain developmental processes, such as neuronal proliferation, migration, and differentiation, as well as the formation and distribution of receptors for neurochemicals. There exist numerous animal examples of specific genetic mutations that affect the development of specific brain structures, such as the mouse mutants with specific cerebellar and hippocampal malformations (Changeux, 1985). There is neuropathological evidence of similar early alterations of brain structures in some human pathologies, such as dyslexia and schizophrenia (Nowakowski, 1987). Such mutations not only affect neuronal migration and lamination in a specific brain structure but also alter neural connectivity more widely and presumably alter the computational properties of neural networks. Hence, there is a resolution to the apparent paradox of how a seemingly small, early change in brain development can have major effects despite the sometimes impressive plasticity of the developing brain given a later (and larger) acquired lesion. Other psychopathologies may involve alterations in brain structure on a finer scale, such as changes in the structure or distribution of receptors. Since receptors are proteins coded by genes, variation in their structure is under genetic control.

The next level of analysis, *neuropsychology*, bridges the chasm separating brain and behavior, mind and body, making this level of analysis the most difficult conceptually. Although there are levels of analysis within neuropsychology, by and large, neuropsychology has been focused on a sufficiently molar level of behavioral analysis that the behavioral categories it studies are not completely outside the view of functional psychology. Yet unlike functional psychology, these categories are constrained in neuropsychology by what we know about brain function. Thus, neuropsychology finds spatial cognition an acceptable category but has rejected categories such as a general-purpose short- or long-term memory, and has generally avoided categories such as the self, will, and object relations. (But the fact that both folk and real psychologists use these latter concepts—at times effectively—to predict and to explain behavior is a phenomenon for which neuropsychology must eventually account; see Dennett, 1987.) One can think of neuropsychology as a kind of amalgam of concepts and categories from cognitive psychology, developmental psychology, and neuroscience. Sometimes this amalgam leads to a coherent explanation of the connection between brain and behavior, and sometimes not, as we see when considering specific disorders. Or we could think of neuropsychology as a kind of scaffolding; once we have completed the edifice of neuroscience, neuropsychology in its present form may be nowhere within it. One reason for this eventual outcome is that most of current neuropsychology is not computational. The long-term goal of neuroscience is to provide a computational account of molar functions that explains our current, preliminary notions about the cognitive architecture in terms of the workings of neural systems (Arbib, 1989). To summarize, current neuropsychology is concerned mostly about molar functions that we can recognize, with the constraint that these functions fit what we currently know about how the real brain works; eventually, current neuropsychology will be replaced by a more precise, computational account of how the real brain accomplishes these functions.

For a psychopathologist, it is important that neuropsychology provide an underlying level of behavioral analysis that is closer to and more consistent with brain mechanisms than either the phenomenological account of a syndrome given in the language of symptoms or the purely psychological account couched in terms of Freudian or cognitive-behavioral constructs. In Chapters 3–5, which deal with reviews of specific disorders, we find a great deal of variability in our neuropsychological understanding of psychopathologies. The cognitive neuropsychology of dyslexia is sophisticated and includes neural network models, whereas the neuropsychology of mood and anxiety disorders is much less well developed. In reviewing specific disorders, I label this level of analysis "neuropsychology" and critique both neuropsychological and purely psychological theories. My goal is to highlight the considerable work that is needed to attain a cognitive neuroscientific understanding of psychopathologies.

The *symptom or surface* is the last level of analysis, the one at which most current developmental psychopathologies are defined. A psychopathology is a syndromal cluster of defining symptoms, a putative cluster or "hump" in the continuum of multivariate behavioral space, for which an explanation is sought. The other, lower levels of analysis considered earlier can (1) provide this explanation; (2) organize symptoms according to which of them are primary, secondary, correlated, and artifactual (Pennington, 1991; Rapin, 1987); (3) redefine syndrome boundaries; (4) clarify comorbidities; and (5) explain developmental continuities and discontinuities in the symptoms of a disorder (Pennington & Ozonoff, 1991). In reviewing each of the specific developmental psychopathologies in Chapters 3–5, I consider each of these four levels and also demonstrate how deeper levels of analysis can clarify issues and problems at more superficial levels.

THE MIND–BODY PROBLEM IN PSYCHOPATHOLOGY

The foregoing discussion brings up an issue that is important to consider in greater detail, namely, the mind–body problem in psychopathology. One key point is that work at different levels is interactive and mutually constraining. Genetic and brain studies cannot proceed without a carefully defined behavioral or neuropsychological phenotype, but discoveries at the genetic or brain level can force revisions in phenotypic definitions or boundaries (Pennington, 1997). We see many examples of this key point in the review of research on specific disorders. Such interactions across levels of analysis help to demonstrate the power of a unified approach. I referred earlier to the latent dualism in much of psychology, which means that mental constructs are frequently studied without any consideration for how they are implemented by the brain. A neuroscientific approach to understanding behavior forces us to give up this latent dualism. To draw out this point, let us consider two recent examples of the neural implementation of psychological constructs. Each of these examples may seem initially surprising; I am arguing that this surprise is diagnostic of our latent dualism.

The first example comes from a neuroimaging study of the treatment of obsessive–compulsive disorder (OCD). Both cognitive-behavioral psychotherapy and medications are known to be effective treatments for OCD. In this study, patients' cerebral glucose metabolism was imaged by means of positron emission tomography (PET) scans before and after treatment (Schwartz, Stoessel, Baxter, Martin, & Phelps, 1996). Some patients were treated with psychotherapy and others with medication. Regardless of the type of treatment, patients who responded favorably to treatment showed metabolic changes in the same brain structures. What may seem surprising about this result is that (1) psychotherapy changes brain metabolism, and (2) psychotherapy and medication affect the same neural systems. But unless we are dualists, we know that psychotherapy has to change brain function to change behavior. Because altered activity of certain brain structures (e.g., the basal ganglia) produces the symptoms of OCD, a successful treatment must alter the activity of these critical brain structures. Undoubtedly, the exact means by which psychotherapy and medication produce this similar effect are different. Medication directly alters neurotransmitter levels and hence the activity of certain structures. Psychotherapy teaches strategies for managing obsessive thoughts and compulsive behaviors. But to work, these strategies must somehow affect brain activation.

The second example concerns how a person's personality influences his or her brain's reaction (as measured by functional magnetic resonance imaging [fMRI]) to positive and negative emotional stimuli (Canli et al., 2001). Previous studies have shown that exposure to emotional stimuli activates parts of the brain that process emotions, such as the amygdala, the frontal cortex, and the anterior cingulate gyrus. This study demonstrated that this activation varies as a function of the subject's personality. Two personality dimensions were considered: extraversion (i.e., the tendency to be sociable and optimistic) and neuroticism (i.e., the tendency to be anxious and socially insecure). Subjects with high extraversion had greater brain responses to positive than to negative pictures, unlike subjects with low extraversion. Subjects with high neuroticism had greater brain responses to negative than to positive pictures. What may be surprising about this example is that a psychological construct (personality) mediates brain activity in response to basic emotional stimuli. But, once again, the psychological construct cannot affect behavior unless it affects brain function.

In summary, these examples make it clear that psychological constructs, like expectations or personality, are mediated by the brain, and that altering an individual's psychology (as happens in psychotherapy) changes his or her brain activity. An integrated account of psychopathology must show how both biological and psychological factors influence brain function. The cited examples make it clear that we must take mind–brain relations seriously, and they argue against two possible solutions to the mind–body problem: dualism and reductive materialism. Dualism does not work because it does not provide a way for mind and brain to interact. Reductive materialism does not work because there is not a simple one-to-one relation between psychological states and brain states. But these examples do not tell us which of the remaining solutions to the mind–brain or mind–body problems is correct. Philosophers (e.g., Churchland, 1988) have distinguished several possible solutions besides dualism and reductive materialism, including behaviorism, functionalism, and eliminative materialism. It remains to be seen whether any of these possibilities will work. One interesting point to bear in mind is that none of these solutions to the mind–body problem considers the role of development. Perhaps we cannot solve the mind–body problem without considering how the mind–brain develops. I return to this point later in this chapter, but now discuss issues involved in psychiatric diagnoses.

TO DIAGNOSE OR NOT TO DIAGNOSE?

With few exceptions, the study of developmental psychopathologies begins at the symptom level of analysis. Unlike complex, multifactorial medical disorders such as diabetes or coronary artery disease, whose diagnostic definition depends on pathophysiology, psychopathologies are defined at the symptom level; that is, diagnostic categories for psychopathology are behaviorally defined and purely descriptive. They are based on clinical phenomenology—reports and observations about the behavior and experience of patients. Because understanding of the etiology and pathophysiology of mental illnesses has been so limited, diagnostic reliability could only be achieved at the symptom level. Earlier diagnostic definitions based on presumed underlying psychodynamic mechanisms were found to lack reliability and validity. Hence, moving back to descriptive, behavioral definitions of psychopathologies was, somewhat ironically, a major step *forward* scientifically, one necessitated by the very limited understanding of underlying mechanisms. Obviously, a long-term goal for a scientific psychiatry is to move beyond description to a nosology based on underlying causal processes. One of the main goals of this book is to review our progress toward reaching that goal and to suggest how diagnostic categories will be reformulated as we learn more about their neuroscience.

So psychiatric diagnoses begin when clinicians notice that certain signs and symptoms occur together in certain patients more often than they should by chance, and categorize this cluster of signs and symptoms as a syndrome. This is a dangerous moment for scientific understanding for several reasons.

First, what counts as a sign or a symptom must be defined relative to an empirically based, normative developmental framework (Achenbach, 1991). Some symptoms that at first glance may appear serious can be quite common at certain developmental stages. Kanner (1945, qtd. in Lapouse & Monk, 1958, p. 1136) commented that "a multitude of early breath holders, nail biters, nose pickers and casual masturbators . . . develop into reasonably happy and well-adjusted adults." Lapouse and Monk (1958) found in a random sample of 6- to 12-year-old children that symptoms of anxiety, overactivity, and irritability were quite common, each affecting between 43% and 49% of the sample according to maternal report. With such base rates, a "syndrome" consisting of the presence of all three kinds of symptoms would be found in about 10% of the sample just by chance alone! Such a syndrome would obviously not require a deeper scientific explanation.

Second, even if this first requirement (that signs and symptoms be rare in a random, same-age sample) were met, documentation of greater than chance clustering of symptoms is rarely formally evaluated and tested (initially at least) in population as opposed to clinic samples. Clinicians' memories may be biased toward remembering the striking co-occurrences of symptoms and not the many counterexamples. Referral biases may produce co-occurrences of signs and symptoms in clinic samples that would not be found in population samples. In other words, some co-occurrences may be an artifact of recall or referral biases and not a reflection of the true state of nature.

Third, naming a syndrome can confer a false sense of validity on the diagnostic category, and, worse yet, the impression that there is an explanation for the deviant behavior. (The idea that a name provides an explanation is called the "nominal fallacy," which is discussed later.)

Fourth, nearly all dimensions of behavior are normally distributed, so where we set cutoffs on this continuum for determining the presence of a symptom or diagnosis is somewhat arbitrary. At the same time, both epidemiological research and allocation of treatment resources require that we determine who is and who is not a case. So we need to use diagnoses but must remember that they are provisional. For example, a fundamental issue in research on developmental psychopathology is whether the processes that produce individual behavioral differences lying at the unfavorable, extreme end of the distribution are distinct from the processes that produce individual differences across the rest of the distribution (so-called "normal" variations). We later review methods for addressing this important question. For now, it is important to emphasize that although we use current diagnostic categories in research on developmental psychopathology, we are not prejudging this issue.

A closely related issue is the typological thinking implicit in categorical notions of pathology and normality. One of Darwin's important contributions was to replace typological notions with the concept of variation in a population (Mayr, 2000). Most individual differences in behavior are normally distributed. What we call a "psychopathology" is just an extreme region of a multivariate space, with a somewhat arbitrary threshold for extremity. What we call "normality" is just a central tendency in this multivariate space. So very few "normal" individuals would be close to the mean on all the dimensions on this multivariate space. Moreover, the definitions of categories of psychopathology in the *Diagnostic and Statistical Manual of Mental Disorders* (DSM) are not "monothetic"; they do not consist of a brief set of necessary and sufficient features that all members of the category must share. Instead, they are "polythetic," defined by the presence of a critical number of features in a longer list, few of which are necessary, and none of which are sufficient for the diagnosis (Blashfield & Livelsey, 1999). As a result, members of a given diagnostic category will vary in which features they possess, with some pairs of individuals with the same diagnosis even having nonoverlapping features. For example, the diagnostic category of conduct disorder provides one of the more extreme examples of this situation. There are 15 symptoms of conduct disorder, any three of which are sufficient for the diagnosis. Therefore, five different children could each qualify for this diagnosis without sharing a single symptom. So neither "normal" individuals nor individuals with a given psychopathology are types.

Fifth, what counts as a sign or symptom depends in part on cultural and subcultural values. Culture can undoubtedly affect the perception, manifestation, and treatment of psychopathology. For an epidemiologist, a case is someone in need of intervention (Costello & Angold, 1995), but the determination of who needs intervention occurs in a cultural context, which, unfortunately, includes the level of resources available for interventions. In the context of developmental psychopathology, a case is someone who is not meeting developmental goals. The definition of developmental goals is in turn based on empirical studies of development. While there are undoubtedly some human universals in developmental goals, there will still be cultural variation in these goals and in how much deviation from them is seen as needing intervention.

Another concern about diagnoses has to do with labeling. For some mental health practitioners, diagnoses are aversive because they do not capture the individuality of the patient's problems. Robin Morris (1984) has said, "Every child is like all other children, like some other children, and like no other children"; that is, some characteristics are species-typical, others are typical of groups within the species, and still others are unique to individuals. It is important for diagnosticians and therapists to have a good handle on which characteristics fall into which category. Some patients have symptoms that they feel are unique to them but are in fact virtually species-typical. Other symptoms are fairly specific to a particular diagnosis, and still others are unique to a given patient. Although a good clinician must be aware and make use of a patient's unique attributes, scientific progress in understanding and treating psychopathology depends on there being "middle-level" variation—differentiating characteristics of groups within our species. If not, clinical work is reduced either just to treating the problems in living that everyone faces or to recreating the field for each unique individual. On the one hand, we say there are no psychopathologies because everyone is "in the same boat." On the other hand, we say there are no psychopathologies because everyone is different. A science of psychopathology is not tenable at either extreme. Although there is much confusion and many limitations in the current state of knowledge about psychopathologies in children, this state of affairs hardly means that a science of developmental psychopathology is impossible.

Another potential criticism of this approach to diagnosis is that it is based on the "medical model," which is assumed to posit a single model of physical causality for all behavioral disorders. I have already discussed this issue in the previous section. Moreover, as Meehl (1973) has pointed out, there is no single medical model. Recent medical research on disorders such as heart disease espouses a multifactorial causal model and acknowledges the contribution of genetic, psychological, and cultural factors to etiology. Thus, the medical model that has been castigated by social scientists may increasingly be a straw man. Moreover, our search for the causes of psychopathologies should be just as broad as the search for causes of "medical" disorders and not be hampered by an a priori assumption of what kinds of causes will prove important.

Finally, it is important to remember that the patient has the diagnosis rather than the diagnosis having the patient (Achenbach, 1982); that is, most diagnoses do not provide an explanation for every aspect of the patient's being. A related point is that nosologies classify disorders, not people. Thus, it is important to use "people-friendly" language in talking about diagnoses. Saying "a person with autism" has a distinctly different connotation than saying "an autistic."

In summary, it is very important to remember that behaviorally defined diagnoses are provisional, hypothetical constructs that must be validated. As scientific knowledge accumulates, some currently separate diagnoses will be lumped together, some single diagnoses will be split into two separate diagnoses, and some diagnoses may even disappear altogether. Eventually, the current descriptive, behaviorally defined nosology will be replaced by one that defines psychopathologies in terms of empirically validated causal mechanisms. We next consider how psychiatric diagnoses are validated.

ESTABLISHING THE VALIDITY OF DIAGNOSES

A set of diagnoses, such as those in DSM-IV-TR, constitute a nosology, which is just a classification system or taxonomy for diagnoses. This section considers the issues involved in validating both a nosological scheme and individual syndromes within a nosology. These issues have been well articulated by Fletcher (1985) and Rapin (1987), and I draw on their discussions.

The basic goals of a nosology are to identify clusters of symptoms that reliably co-occur and identify groups of patients that are homogeneous at the level of etiology, pathogenesis, or treatment. These two goals concern internal and external validity, respectively.

Internal validity might also be termed "internal consistency" or reliability. Fletcher (1985) lists five criteria for the internal validity of a nosology: (1) coverage or number of patients classified, (2) homogeneity of the diagnoses, (3) reliability of the classification procedures, (4) replicability across techniques, and (5) replication in other samples. Clearly, a sample- or test-specific diagnosis would necessarily lack reliability. In the last two decades, considerable progress has been made in descriptive psychiatry, and we now have nosologies for child and adult psychopathologies that satisfy these criteria for internal validity.

External validity essentially concerns the explanatory significance of a diagnosis. A subtype may be reliable in terms of the variables used to define it but not have a distinctive relation to any external variables of interest. Fletcher (1985) lists three possible criteria for external validity: (1) differential response to treatment, (2) clinical meaningfulness, and (3) differential relation to processing measures independent of those used to define the diagnosis, such as neuropsychological measures. To this list, we would add (4) differential etiology, (5) differential pathogenesis, and (6) differential prognosis or developmental course.

Fletcher (1985) emphasizes that the search for external validity is essentially a hypothesis-generating and testing affair, much like the search for construct validity (Cronbach & Meehl, 1955). A valid syndrome is a fruitful hypothesis about how to "parse" the domains of both disordered and normal behavior, and the various levels of the underlying causes of behavior. If a syndrome is valid, then it will satisfy tests of both convergent and discriminant validity across levels of analysis: etiology, brain mechanisms, neuropsychology, and symptoms. The ultimate goal of syndrome analysis is to discover a meaningful causal chain across these different levels of analysis. We would like to know which etiologies specifically cause the diagnosis in question, what aspects of brain development they perturb, what deficit in neuropsychological processes this leads to, how this underlying neuropsychological deficit leads to the primary (or core) and secondary symptoms of the disorder, how the symptoms and underlying deficit change with development, and how all of this information helps explain the response to treatment. Thus, a valid syndrome is a construct below the level of observable behaviors or symptoms that provides a meaningful explanation of why certain symptoms co-occur in different patterns across development, and why some treatments are efficacious and others are not.

The concepts of convergent and discriminant validity are closely related to the concept of external validity. We might expect that an ideal nosology would have a complete and unique set of external, converging validators for each of its different syndromes, thereby guaranteeing discriminant validity. However, it has become increasingly clear that complete specificity is not found for psychopathologies. Basically, this lack of specificity is a consequence of the fact that these are complex disorders, as discussed earlier, that lack single causes. So risk and protective factors may be specific to a given disorder, shared by a few disorders, or shared by all disorders (generic). If we cross this distinction with the fact that risk and protective factors are either genetic or environmental, we can see that there are six possible types of risk (and protective) factors (Table 1). On the genetic side, some genetic variations are specific to a single syndrome (e.g., fragile X syndrome), some are shared by a few disorders (e.g., an allele of the serotonin transporter gene appears to be a risk factor for both anxiety and depression), and some turn out to be generic. The same distinctions apply to environmental risk factors: Exposure to a frightening stimulus (e.g., a snake) is an environmental risk event that is specific to a single disorder; stress increases the risk for several disorders; and low socioeconomic status increases the risk for most disorders.

It is more difficult to provide examples of all six kinds of protective factors. Besides the normal alleles of genes that have known risk alleles, we do not know of other specific genes that protect against psychopathology, but it is likely that such genes exist. On the environmental side, we know the most about generic protective factors: good pre- and postnatal care, good nutrition, and good parenting. Again, it is likely that there are more specific protective factors. Identifying both genetic and environmental specific protective factors should have a major impact on the prevention of psychopathology.

A specific psychopathology most likely results from a particular combination of all six kinds of risk factors, not from factors that are all specific to that particular disorder. Similarly, we should expect some overlap in the brain mechanisms underlying different psychopathologies and in their neuropsychology. This state of affairs means that we face the difficult challenge of explaining the overlapping developmental pathways that lead from partly shared risk factors and brain mechanisms to different disorders. The discussion of specific psychopathologies in Chapters 3–5 gives examples of these overlaps at different levels of analysis. This lack of specificity also means that we should expect comorbidity or co-occurrence of developmental psychopathologies, which is indeed the case. I next briefly discuss how to analyze comorbidity.

TESTING THE BASIS OF COMORBIDITY

Explanations for comorbidity have been discussed by Caron and Rutter (1991) and Faraone, Tsuang, and Tsuang (1999b). Essentially, two disorders may co-occur for artifactual reasons or because there is a genuine causal relation between them. Artifactual reasons for comorbidity need to be ruled out before undertaking the usually more arduous process of testing causal hypotheses. Possible artifactual reasons include referral biases, rater biases, and definitional overlap. Comorbidity is more likely to occur in a clinical sample than in a population sample because individuals with more disorders are more likely to seek help (Berkson, 1946). Therefore, some comorbidities observed in clinical samples are simply a product of Berkson's bias. Rater biases may produce artifacts, especially since most psychopathologies are defined by self- or other-report of symptoms. A rater who is very concerned about one set of symptoms may be more likely to endorse other symptoms (a "halo" effect), artifactually producing a comorbidity. Finally, the actual items that define psychopathologies overlap to some extent across disorders. This definitional overlap would also artifactually produce the phenomenon of comorbidity.

Some hypotheses to explain a nonartifactual comorbidity include the following: (1) The two disorders share a risk factor that is consequently not specific to either disorder; (2) one disorder causes at least the symptoms of the second disorder; (3) there is an etiological subtype in which a shared risk factor produces both disorders, but other cases of each disorder do not share risk factors; and (4) there is nonrandom mating such that individuals with transmissible risk factors (either ge-

TABLE 1. Types of Risk Factors

	Genetic	Environmental
Specific	Fragile X mutation	Phobic exposure (e.g., to a snake)
Shared	Allele of serotonin transporter gene	Stress
Generic	?	Low socioeconomic status

netic or environmental) for one disorder are more likely to have children with individuals with transmissible risk factors for the other disorder. In this last case, there would not be a direct causal relation between the two disorders in a comorbid offspring. A more detailed and quantitative treatment of models of comorbidity is contained in Neale and Kendler (1995).

The main methods for testing these four hypotheses include family, twin, and molecular approaches, which are discussed in more detail later. Neuropsychological methods are also helpful, especially for testing the second hypothesis (e.g., Pennington, Grossier, & Welsh, 1993). A family design allows one to evaluate whether there is nonrandom mating and to test whether the two disorders are transmitted independently. To support the nonrandom mating hypothesis, both of these conditions must be satisfied. The presence of a shared familial risk factor, postulated by both hypotheses 1 and 3, will be reflected in nonindependent transmission of the two disorders in families. Specifically, to support hypothesis 1, relatives of probands with only one disorder should have increased rates of *both* that disorder and the other disorder. To support hypothesis 3, in contrast, only relatives of probands with both disorders should be at increased risk for both disorders. Relatives of probands with only one disorder should exhibit increased rates of only that disorder, not the other disorder. However, if the subtype is infrequent, large samples may be needed to test its influence on transmission. Bivariate twin analyses, described later, can determine if the shared familial factor is genetic. If it is, bivariate molecular methods can be used to determine which genes act pleiotropically to produce the two disorders (e.g., Willcutt et al., in press).

In summary, analyzing comorbidity is a crucial task for understanding the development of psychopathology. As we will see, nonartifactual comorbidities appear to be the rule rather than the exception in this field, and evidence is accumulating for genetic risk factors that exert a causal effect on more than one disorder (i.e., pleiotropy). For example, there is evidence for genetic factors that increase the risk for both anxiety and depression, and we have just found that the dyslexia locus on the short arm of chromosome 6 also influences attention-deficit/hyperactivity disorder (ADHD) (Willcutt et al., in press). Such results could lead to a shift in syndrome boundaries and at the very least, influence how we define the phenotype in molecular studies.

WHY A DEVELOPMENTAL APPROACH?

One of the core axioms of this book is that we cannot achieve a complete scientific understanding of psychopathology without knowing how it develops. So the reader may rightly ask, "Why not?" One might imagine that with regard to schizophrenia, if we had total knowledge of the various causal risk factors, as well as total knowledge of the adult brain phenotype, then we would understand the disease. However, the only way to understand how to get from the risk factors to the adult brain and behavioral phenotype is to see how these risk factors change brain *development*. Both brain and behavioral development are very complex interactive processes, so the significance of any risk factor can only be understood by considering its timing and how it interacts with the developmental process.

A developmental approach is necessary at each of the four levels of analysis discussed earlier. At the *etiological* level, the timing of both expression of a risk allele and environmental risk factors will influence their effect on behavioral outcomes. As discussed later in the Neurobiology section of this chapter, the timing of early visual deprivation (an environmental risk factor) critically determines whether it will disrupt the development of an important aspect of visual function, stereopsis (i.e., 3D vision). It is well known that even dominant, single-gene disorders, such as tuberous sclerosis, vary widely across individuals in their phenotypic effects, from a few barely detectable skin lesions to a profound developmental disability such as autism. Why this is the case is poorly understood, but an explanation will very likely depend on a developmental, epigenetic account of how the expression of the tuberous sclerosis gene interacts with the rest of the individual's genome and environmental risk factors.

At the *neurobiological* level, it is well known that the timing of prenatal exposure to teratogens (e.g., alcohol, cocaine, and nicotine) and postnatal exposure to toxins (e.g., lead) determines their effects on brain development. The same appears to be true for social risk factors, such as traumatic stress and deprivation, although the brain effects are not as well worked out. A fairly striking example of this phenomenon (and of how the mind can affect the body) is provided by psychosocial dwarfism, in which young children exposed to chronic severe social stress (e.g., abuse or loss) fail to grow (Vazquez & Lopez, 2001). The underlying mechanism involves the stress hormone, cortisol, which decreases levels of growth hormone. The effect depends on the timing and duration of the social stress. Older children exposed to similar social stress do not exhibit dwarfism. Younger children with psychosocial dwarfism show rapid catch-up growth if removed from the stressful environment but are nonetheless at risk for shortness, cognitive changes, and later depression and anxiety. These long-term effects are more severe if the child remains in the stressful environment past age 5.

At the level of *neuropsychology*, a developmental approach is important for knowing when different neuropsychological functions develop, how they are mediated by brain structures, and how they can be appropriately measured. Localization of brain functions is not innate or static, but changes with both development and the particular environment to which an individual is exposed. For example, in a congenitally deaf individual who has learned a manual sign language, auditory language cortex subserves visual processing of these manual signs (Neville, 1990). In neural network models of cognitive functions, the effects of damage vary considerably depending on whether the damage occurs before or after the network is trained (Thomas & Karmiloff-Smith, 2002). So damage interacts with the developmental process itself.

These examples return us to a claim I raised earlier, namely, that solving the mind–body problem will depend on a developmental approach. If localization of brain functions varies with development, and if the function of artificial neural networks varies with their training and development, then it seems unlikely that we can fully understand brain–behavior relations in the mature human or animal without taking a developmental approach.

Finally, at the level of *symptoms*, a developmental approach is needed because the manifestation of a given psychopathology changes depending on the developmental stage of the individual. The young child with autism who does not engage in pretend play becomes the isolated adult who is obsessed with computers. The overactive toddler with ADHD becomes the adult with poor planning skills.

WHY A SCIENCE OF PSYCHOPATHOLOGY IS DIFFICULT

The preceding sections illustrate some of the conceptual and empirical challenges that a science of psychopathology must meet. In this section, I focus on two main reasons why a science of psychopathology is difficult: (1) Such a science has the extra task of explaining why there are individual differences in a given psychological function, and (2) the study of individual human differences is necessarily quasi-experimental.

Before we can understand individual differences in a given psychological domain (e.g., emotion regulation), we have to have a fairly mature model of normal development in that domain. But understanding individual differences then imposes an extra task, because it requires us to focus on etiology. Our model of normal development would be a neurocomputational model that might also specify the brain systems involved and generally the kinds of environmental inputs needed, but it would not be a detailed model of the *etiology* of normal development in that domain. It would not attempt to specify genes, specific environmental inputs, and epigenetic interactions that lead to a developing brain capable of those kinds of neurocomputations. However, understanding individual differences in a psychological domain requires us to focus on etiology to a much greater extent.

The second source of difficulty is the quasi-experimental nature of the designs that can be used to study human individual differences. The most commonly used method for investigating developmental psychopathologies is the case–control design, in which a group with a given psychopathology is compared to a group lacking that psychopathology on some variable of interest. The important point is that case–control designs are quasi-experimental (Campbell & Stanley, 1966) because the manipulation of group does not involve random assignment. If we could randomly assign diagnoses to individuals, then we could be sure that presence versus absence of the diagnosis is the only factor that distinguishes cases from controls. If we then found that the two groups differed on the variable of interest, then we could be sure of a true causal relation between that variable and diagnosis. (Notice, however, that we would still not know the direction of effects.) Instead, the "manipulation" of group in a case–control design is not experimental, so it is unlikely that cases and controls differ only with respect to diagnosis. To attempt to compensate for this fundamental problem, psychopathology researchers should control for other differences between the groups (i.e., the differences of which they are aware), either by matching other variables or covarying such variables. However, these precautions can never completely compensate for the lack of random assignment. No matter how careful the matching or how extensive the covarying, it is always possible that the finding of a significant group difference on some variable in a case–control design is due to an undetected difference—some other variable that is confounded with group membership. So we can never be sure from the results of a case–control design alone that we have found a true causal relation between diagnosis and some variable.

Sometimes the limitations of case–control designs are forgotten when other, more biological levels of analysis are examined, such as brain structure or function, or alleles of a genetic locus. It is tempting to think that if differences are found at such levels, then they must be primary and part of the causal pathway leading to the disorder. So, if case–control designs find differences at these levels, then we may be tempted to make stronger causal inference than if only cognition or behavior were being examined. But this is a logical error. A brain difference found in a case–control study is, at best, a true correlate of the disorder, one that may only be secondary, since having a developmental disorder alters environmental input to the developing brain. (At worst, the finding is an artifact of some uncontrolled difference between cases and controls.) A difference in allele frequencies at a given genetic locus between cases and controls is unlikely to be secondary to having the disorder (because experience does not change DNA sequences, unless the experience includes exposure to mutagens, such as ionizing radiation), but it could still be due to an uncontrolled difference between cases and controls, such as genetic background. For example, an initial finding that severe alcoholism is associated with a particular allele of the gene for the dopamine 2 (D2) receptor was found to be likely due to an artifact of ethnic stratification differences between case and control groups (Kidd, 1993). I return to this issue in the review of brain and genetic association studies of specific disorders in Chapters 3–5.

So understanding psychopathology is empirically difficult. It is also conceptually difficult, partly because of fallacies and conceptual errors to which we readily succumb when trying to explain abnormal behavior. Some of these fallacies are considered in the next section.

WHAT COUNTS AS AN EXPLANATION

As the foregoing discussion makes clear, the difficult goal of a neuroscientific approach is to provide a comprehensive explanation of psychopathologies. In this section, we consider how a comprehensive neuroscientific explanation relates to other ways psychopathologies have been explained. A crucial issue in such a comprehensive explanation is how to integrate different levels of explanation, including both top-down and bottom-up accounts of psychopathology. A neuroscientific explanation begins with etiological factors that are far removed from the patient's experience and then works forward through the developmental process, and eventually to the symptoms that define the disorders. Traditional psychological approaches work in the opposite direction. They begin with the patient's experience and work backwards, mainly seeking psychological mechanisms that explain the patient's symptoms. Often these mechanisms are beliefs and expectations, perhaps unconscious, that affect the patient's experience and behavior. At first glance, these two ways of explaining psychopathology seem quite different, even incompatible, but since the evidence demonstrates that both bottom-up and top-down factors influence the development of psychopathology, both must be included in a comprehensive account.

Another way of making this same point is to say that we, as humans, are predisposed to explain others' behavior as rational and intentional, given their beliefs and desires. We grant personhood to other people and explain their behavior according to an implicit theory. So we can call such explanations "personal" in this sense. Traditional top-down psychological explanations of abnormal behavior, whether psychoanalytic or cognitive-behavioral, are essentially such personal explanations, but with a wider context. What seems irrational becomes rational given more knowledge of a person's early history, particular learning experiences, or cognitive distortions.

In contrast, a neuroscientific approach to psychopathology makes a more radical claim, namely, that some of the explanation for irrational behavior is "subpersonal." In other words, some of the causes of a given psychopathology lie completely outside of individuals' beliefs and desires, and are completely inaccessible to their phenomenology, no matter how many years of therapy they undertake. Just as the causes of diabetes, heart disease, multiple sclerosis, and Alzheimer's disease are subpersonal, so too are some of the causes of depression, schizophrenia, and ADHD.

A further complication is that scientific explanations of psychopathology, whether of the bottom-up or top-down variety, must contend with potential errors provided by an explanatory framework we all share as humans, namely, folk psychology. Humans inevitably seek explanations of human behavior, and everyday folk psychology provides a stock of ready-made explanations that we use almost unconsciously.

Psychopathology is so puzzling and painful that it is nearly inevitable that patients, relatives, and even clinicians resort to attempts to construct folk psychological explanations. Obviously, psychologists also seek explanations of human behavior, but in doing so, they must first clear their minds of such ready-made explanations. In addition, the public's stigmatizing reaction to psychopathology occurs in part because individuals with psychopathology often violate everyday folk psychology, which holds that a person's behavior is rational in the sense that it is goal-directed and thus understandable in terms of that person's current beliefs and desires. In psychopathology, beliefs and desires may be unusual or even bizarre, and the capacity for planning and executing behavior in accordance with goals may be impaired. One of the important roles for psychologists in the 21st century will be to educate the public about our growing scientific understanding of how psychopathology develops, so as to reduce the stigma currently associated with mental illness.

One potential error to avoid in thinking about the development of psychopathology is the assumption that the beliefs and desires of patients will usually provide a complete explanation of their abnormal behavior. Although belief–desire psychology works very well in everyday social interactions, using it to "explain" psychopathological behavioral borders is often not very informative. For instance, consider the following statements: "Mary tried to kill herself because she believed life was not worth living"; "John tried to kill the President because he desired Jodie Foster's attention." In the first statement, suicidal behavior characteristic of severe depression is explained by a belief. In the second, homicidal behavior in an individual with schizophrenia is explained by a desire. Neither explanation is very satisfactory. What we would really like to know is why these individuals came to have an unusual belief or desire, and why they were willing to act on them. But to answer these questions, we need to move beyond beliefs and desires. So belief–desire psychology has a normative or species-typical aspect; we accept it as a good explanation of what an ordinary person would do in a given situation. Of course, belief–desire psychology does not really provide a scientific explanation of species-typical human behavior. Such an explanation will require evolutionary theory, neuroscience, and cultural anthropology, among other disciplines.

So relying on folk psychology to explain psychopathology commits what I call the "phenomenological fallacy," which is the belief that an explanation for abnormal behavior may be found through close attention to patients' experience of the disorder and their report of symptoms. Part of this report includes patients' usually inaccurate hypotheses about why they are having these symptoms, since people inevitably construct explanations, rationalizations, and attributions for their behavior. Although, in some cases, such erroneous cognitive constructs that arise in *response* to a disorder such as depression or posttraumatic stress disorder serve to perpetuate the disorder, as will be discussed later, in most cases, the actual cause of a psychopathology lies outside the phenomenology of a patient; therefore, it is a fallacy to look for the cause in the patient's phenomenology.

At the same time, partly subpersonal causation for psychopathology raises complex issues for how both practitioners and patients think of the disorder being treated and relate to each other. While parts of folk psychology are undoubtedly misleading about the causes of psychopathology, effective treatment must begin with a patient's and family's understanding of the illness at hand. These issues are captured very movingly in Luhrmann's (2000) *Of Two Minds*, an ethnographic study of the current split between biological and psychodynamic approaches in psychiatric training. Just because some of the causes of psychopathology are subpersonal does not mean that psychiatric treatment should be reduced to dispensing medications. The patient as a person needs to be fully engaged in his or her treatment.

In addition, descriptive psychiatry has undoubtedly made considerable progress by paying close attention to the phenomenology of disorders, and by developing interviews and rating systems to classify disorders reliably. But, as I said in a previous section, this can only be the first step toward a scientific understanding of psychopathology; eventually, our classification of psychopathologies will be based on underlying causal mechanisms, not on surface behaviors. Moreover, what counts as a discrete disorder at the phenomenological level may not be similarly discrete at other levels of analysis. Disorders with different phenomenologies, such as anxiety and depression, appear to derive from common genetic risk factors, and disorders with the same phenomenology may have different etiologies (we say that they are "phenocopies" of each other).

As mentioned earlier, having a reliable descriptive taxonomy for psychopathologies can lead to the illusion that having a name for a disorder provides an explanation. This illusion, called the *nominal fallacy*, is classically illustrated by a character in Molière's *Imaginary Invalid*, who explained that a sleeping potion worked because it had "dormative" powers. As this example makes clear, the nominal fallacy works best if the name that provides the explanation is rather obscure. Although making an accurate diagnosis can be quite helpful in many ways, clinicians should guard against assuming that just naming the disorder provides an explanation for it.

A final fallacy to consider is the fallacy of *reification*, which means inappropriately turning an abstract notion into a concrete thing. Some abstract notions may have no physical basis at all (e.g., deities such as Zeus), while others may be concretized in the wrong fashion. For example, in the Musée des Augustins in Toulouse, there is a statue by Eugene Thivier (1845–1920) titled *La Cauchemar*, which means "the nightmare." The statue portrays a young woman in tormented sleep, with a griffin-like monster perched on her hip. The statue beautifully captures the agony of the nightmares that we all experience, and that are much more common and intense in depression, anxiety, and other psychopathologies. But it is obviously an intended reification, a metaphor in stone, not because it asserts that nightmares have a concrete physical basis, which neuroscientists are discovering in the brain, but because it asserts the wrong physical basis for nightmares (monsters).

The possibilities for reification are more subtle in the case of diagnostic constructs. One error is to forget that the current diagnostic constructs are provisional hypotheses in search of validation and to assume that they too are "carved in stone." The thing that we roughly point to when using a term such as "schizophrenia" undoubtedly exists, but it may not exist in the form currently envisioned by our diagnostic constructs, which in turn select which symptoms count in the definition of schizophrenia. As research progresses, the definition and understanding of schizophrenia will undoubtedly change.

To make this point more clearly, let us consider two historical examples. In the 19th century many inmates of asylums had what was called "general paresis," a mental disorder with a progressive, deteriorating course ending in death. General paresis was a provisional and imprecise label for what was eventually found to be tertiary syphilis. Once this was understood, the key defining characteristic of this disorder became the presence of infection with the spirochete bacteria.

An earlier and more obvious example of the reification of psychopathology is provided by the story of the Gadarene swine in the New Testament. Jesus encounters a man "possessed by demons." After talking with these demons (perhaps the man's thought-disordered verbalizations or his multiple personalities), Jesus cast them out of the man and into an innocent herd of swine, which promptly rushed headlong into a nearby pond and drowned themselves.

In both these cases, the psychopathology is a real thing, but the label used for it is only a metaphor with inaccurate implications. We do not have to search so far back in history to find many examples of similar errors in thinking about developmental psychopathology: "Refrigerator" mothers who fail to deliver their infants from a normal stage of autistic development as an explanation for autism, and seeing things "backward" as an explanation for dyslexia, both come to mind. These reifications are inaccurate and sometimes implicit hypotheses about the nature of a psychopathology. They are harmful in that they may strongly influence diagnosis, treatment, and research. Our descriptive taxonomies for psychopathologies are not theory-neutral; instead, symptoms used to define a disorder depend in part on current conceptions of the disorder. So while our current understanding of psychopathology cannot be theory-neutral, we should always base it very explicitly on a network of hypotheses, some of which have better empirical support than others.

As discussed earlier, another reification error is to assume that diagnoses are discrete, that a sharp boundary exists between psychopathology and normal function. But it could equally well be the case that disorders are just extreme points on a normal distribution, whose variance is determined by a set of risk and protective factors acting on a set of brain systems that mediate both normal and abnormal behavior in that domain. In fact, a comprehensive developmental theory requires a broad-enough set of processes to encompass both normal and abnormal development. If a current theory of development does not explain a given psychopathology, or if a theory of a psychopathology does not explain how it develops, then more work is needed.

A third reification error is to assume that diagnoses are completely separate from each other, with each having totally distinct etiologies, brain mechanisms, and underlying psychological processes. This view of diagnoses would be correct if there were single, specific causes for each diagnosis at each level of analysis. But the field has searched in vain for such single causes of psychopathology. At the genetic level, the OGOD (one gene, one disorder) hypothesis (Skuse, 1997) has been rejected. At the brain level, attempts to explain disorders in terms of single neurotransmitters or single brain regions have failed. At the neuropsychological level, most disorders involve deficits in multiple neuropsychological functions. These various single-cause hypotheses involve reification in that they localize the cause for a complex behavioral phenomenon in a single factor (or level of analysis), instead of acknowledging that the phenomenon is an emergent property of the interactions of factors and levels in development.

As we will see, emerging evidence indicates overlap between disorders, such as anxiety and depression, at all levels of analysis, so what makes two disorders differ may be much more subtle than previously thought. As discussed earlier, disorders are likely regions with fuzzy boundaries in a continuous multivariate space. What will likely distinguish disorders is the weighting of different risk factors, not a distinct set of risk factors, and the different epigenetic and developmental interactions that result from that particular weighting. Small differences in initial conditions may lead to large differences in outcome given the nonlinearity of development.

The goals in this chapter have been to present the basic issues that must be addressed in a scientific understanding of developmental psychopathology and to expose those errors in thinking that almost inevitably occur when we confront the complex and poorly understood phenomenon of psychopathology. Scientific understanding of this phenomenon is difficult because it lies "close to home," affecting either ourselves or those we care about, and because it is so inextricably intertwined with how we think about our own human nature. These issues and errors are elaborated in Chapters 3–5, which discuss specific psychopathologies. I now turn to methods of syndrome analysis, the topic of Chapter 2.

Methods of Syndrome Analysis

Chapter 2 provides an overview of four methods of syndrome analysis—epidemiology, behavioral and molecular genetics, neurobiology, and neuropsychology—each of which is necessary for a scientific understanding of developmental psychopathology. Each method is concerned primarily with a different level of analysis of a developmental psychopathology. To achieve an integrated understanding, these levels must be related to each other. As we will see, much remains to be done to link these levels of analysis.

EPIDEMIOLOGY

Epidemiology, which provides methods for obtaining accurate information about the prevalence, comorbidities, correlates, and courses of different symptoms and syndromes, begins with the symptom level of analysis. We must have such information before we construct theories about disorders and attempt to test their validity. All too often, theories of developmental psychopathology are based on correlations observed in clinical samples but not tested epidemiologically. We do not need a theory to explain the correlation between autism and agility, or between dyslexia and left-handedness, if such correlations simply derive from biased samples.

Costello and Angold (1995) have written about the application of epidemiology to developmental psychopathology; the following summary draws on their account. Epidemiology is a scientific method for understanding the development of diseases. Its aim is to identify key points in the development and transmission of disease, in order to improve prevention and treatment. The key question addressed by epidemiology is "What is wrong with this person and what is it about him or her that has resulted in this illness?" Given this definition, the goal of epidemiology is essentially similar to that of the integrated approach advocated in this book, namely, a comprehensive understanding of the development of psychopathology; as a result, epidemiology is inherently interdisciplinary, but it also provides its own essential methods and concepts for achieving this task, some of which provide the starting point for attempting to understand a developmental psychopathology.

Having used the word "disease" in the definition of epidemiology, I must hasten to define this term in the context of developmental psychopathology. In this case, "disease" is simply the inability to achieve one or more goals of development. Risk factors that cause this inability may be located in the individual, in a dyad, in a family system, or in a social group. Diseases generally differ in their causes and courses. In terms of cause, it is likely that developmental psychopathologies are multifactorial and that feedback loops can exist between risk factors and developing psychopathology (Sameroff & Chandler, 1975). It is also assumed that interactions characterize both normal development and the development of psychopathology. In terms of course, developmental psychopathologies usually have either a chronic or episodic course determined by the interaction between the risk factors and the mechanisms of normal development. Some of the symptoms, which define psychopathologies, may be adaptations given the constraints imposed by other aspects of the disorder. So it is practically a given that the symptoms found in a developmental psychopathology will depend on the developmental stage of the individual. Consequently, the continuities in behavior across time in a given disorder will be heterotypic rather than homotypic; that is, surface behaviors are unlikely to be continuous, but underlying psychological mechanisms may be so. One of the tasks faced by developmental epidemiologists is to provide an explanation for the development of symptoms in a disorder, including, in some cases, recovery from symptoms.

The first goal for an epidemiologist is to provide an accurate picture of the natural history of a developmental psychopathology, so that later experimental attempts to manipulate its course are based on a firm foundation. Consequently, longitudinal studies are needed. Some of the other basic methodological requirements of an epidemiological study are as follows: (1) to obtain a population sample in which to measure the frequency of a disorder, (2) to avoid sampling or ascertainment biases, (3) to disentangle confounding factors from risk factors, when true risk factors have been identified, and (4) to test for the relations among them.

Although the first two requirements seem absolutely fundamental, it is quite striking how much of our information about developmental psychopathologies is based on referred rather than population samples. Although such samples accurately reflect what clinicians actually encounter, they may be very misleading about the true correlates and comorbidities of disorders. This problem, originally pointed out by Berkson (1946), is now termed Berkson's bias by epidemiologists. Berkson was commenting on a common clinical practice in his day, namely, removal of the gallbladder to treat diabetes, a practice derived from the misleading correlation that the rate of gallbladder disease was elevated among patients hospitalized with diabetes. His point was that comorbidities inevitably found in referred populations would not exist in the general population, because patients seeking help were more likely to have multiple maladies than those not seeking help. So Berkson's bias is just a specific case of why correlation does not imply causality. Understanding Berkson's bias is extremely important for developmental psychopathologists whose direct knowledge of disorders and their correlates is almost always based on clinical samples in which biases of ascertainment frequently lead to artifactual associations. The last two requirements highlight the complicated nature of the phenomena studied by developmental psychopathologists. Potential risk factors, for example, poverty and ethnicity, are frequently confounded and usually only quasi-experimental methods are available to disentangle them.

The number of longitudinal epidemiological studies conducted in the field of developmental psychopathology is rather small, so there is much that we still do not know about the epidemiology of these disorders. In Chapters 3–5, I summarize what is known about the epidemiology of specific disorders, including information about prevalence, risk factors, gender ratios, comorbidities, and developmental changes in symptoms.

Here, it is important to summarize the general lessons from large-scale epidemiological studies of developmental psychopathologies. One basic lesson is that in developmental psychopathology, there is considerable but not complete continuity from earlier to later ages. Across seven longitudinal studies summarized in Costello and Angold (1995, Table 2.1, p. 29), the median proportion of subjects with a diagnosis at Time 1 who also received a diagnosis at Time 2 was 51% across a median follow-up interval of 4 years. About half of these subjects exhibit this kind of continuity. The other half of subjects with an earlier diagnosis no longer met diagnostic criteria for any diagnosis, although, as a group, they likely had subclinical elevations of symptoms, an issue not always addressed by these studies. In addition, some children without earlier diagnoses qualified for them at Time 2. Besides this general continuity, there is also evidence for continuity in the kind of disorder, with the degree of specificity correlated with gender. In the Isle of Wight study, 46% of subjects with an emotional disorder in childhood also had one in adolescence; in 75% of subjects with conduct disorder, this diagnosis persisted, as it did in 58% of those with mixed emotional and conduct disorders. This study also illustrates the common finding that developmental continuity is somewhat stronger for conduct disorder than for emotional disorders (i.e., anxiety and depression). The finding that specificity of continuity varies by gender comes from the Dunedin study, which found continuities in boys for both externalizing disorders and an earlier internalizing disorder to a later externalizing disorder. For girls, the only continuity observed was for internalizing disorders. So an earlier internalizing disorder in boys did not significantly increase their risk for a later internalizing disorder; the same lack of continuity was found for girls with respect to externalizing disorders. The causal basis for persistence and desistance in developmental psychopathologies, as well as for gender differences in both prevalence and continuity, is virtually unknown.

BEHAVIORAL AND MOLECULAR GENETICS

Heredity is the last of the Fates and the most terrible.
—OSCAR WILDE

Our increased knowledge of the mechanisms of heredity is perhaps lessening the terror to which Wilde alluded, but much remains to be done. Modern genetics holds the promise of making fundamental improvements in both physical and mental health, partly by abolishing the false dichotomy that separates them. However, in this century, clinicians, scientists, and the general public all need to be *informed* participants in the complex decisions about the ethical use of this genetic information. What follows is an attempt to provide an accessible introduction to genetic methods for clinicians and social scientists. Twin methods for examining extreme traits are presented in greater detail, and some readers may wish to skim or skip that part.

The signs and symptoms that define disorders are the *outputs* of a complicated developmental process. One of the central puzzles of clinical work is that we are usually faced with the end points of a developmental process, about which we usually have only limited understanding. We also know that there are multiple pathways to those particular end points. As researchers, we need to discover how different *inputs* alter this developmental process to produce different outputs. So a scientific explanation of a psychopathology must "begin at the beginning" and recognize that a given output is a joint product of not only genetic and environmental input but also the developmental process itself.

Genetic methods are crucial for understanding the etiology of developmental psychopathologies because there are genetic influences on virtually all developmental psychopathologies, and because we cannot properly study environmental influences without controlling genetic variance. Many studies of social influences on both normal and abnormal development do not use genetically sensitive designs; therefore, finding a correlation between a social influence and a behavior in the developing child does not necessarily demonstrate an environmental influence on development (Scarr, 1992). Suppose we find a correlation between how emotion is regulated in the mother–infant relationship and the child's later emotion regulation in peer relations. It seems straightforward to conclude that the earlier social experience shaped later social behavior. However, if the study sample consisted of biological mothers with their infants, then the design confounds genetic and environmental influences. Besides sharing early social experiences, such mother–infant pairs also share half their segregating genes (genes that vary across individual humans). Consequently, the observed correlation could be partly, or even totally, mediated by genes. So we need genetically sensitive designs to study not only genetic influences but also environmental influences on the development of psychopathology.

This point has influenced contemporary research on parenting (for a review, see Collins, Maccoby, Steinberg, Hetherington, & Bornstein, 2000). Such research has used genetically sensitive and other designs (such as experimental manipulations of human parenting, animal models, and longitudinal studies of the relation between parenting and child adjustment that statistically control for the initial relation) to demonstrate more clearly parenting effects on development. Instead of acting as a shared, main effect across children in a family, parenting effects often emerge in interaction with characteristics of individual children.

In a recent article, Caspi, Taylor, Moffitt, and Plomin (2000) provide a good example of the use of a genetically sensitive design to identify a social-environmental influence on child psychopathology. The authors used a national sample of over 2,000 2-year-old twin pairs for a study in which data on neighborhood conditions and maternally reported child behavior problems were available. As in other studies, about half the variance (55%) in child behavior problems was attributable to genetic factors. Unlike other twin studies, the use of a national sample and direct environmental measures allowed these researchers to identify a clear neighborhood effect that accounted for 5% of the variance in toddler behavior problems. Other, unspecified environmental factors, either shared by family members (15%) or unique to individuals in families (24%), accounted for the remaining variance. Although much previous research has documented a correlation between neighborhood conditions and children's behavior problems, this is the first study to disentangle genetic and environmental contributions to that correlation. Finally, in this study, neighborhood conditions appeared to act as a generic risk factor (Figure 1) for psychopathology, since they affected both internalizing and externalizing behavior problems.

Although there is a long history of controversy about behavioral genetic studies in psychology, the convergence of evidence across studies and methods has provided very convincing evidence of moderate genetic influence on most behavioral dimensions. Some of the controversy derived from misleading claims about the implications of such studies, such as the view that the results of behavioral genetic studies support strict genetic determinism or provide a genetic explanation of group differences in behavior, neither of which is true. As Rende and Plomin (1995, p. 291) point out, it is important to "study nature AND nurture, rather than nature VERSUS nurture." Behavioral development is the emergent product of a complex process of probabilistic epigenesis (Gottlieb, 1991, 1998) to which both genes and environments contribute. Genes do not simply do their work in very early development and then hand the organism over to the environment. Instead, genes are turned on and off across the lifespan, and gene expression is influenced by the environment, including the social environment (Gottlieb, 1998). Neither genes nor environments code for behavior directly; both sides of the nature–nurture debate shared the same erroneous assumption that the instructions for behavior were preexistent in either the genome or the environment and imposed from without on the developing organism (Oyama, 1999). Instead, genetic and environmental influences are inputs to a developmental process, and their impact on behavioral outcome depends on their interactions with all the components of that process. Consequently, it is misleading to speak of the genome as a "blueprint" or to think that genes "code" for a behavior. Genes simply code for protein structure, and variations in the structure of a given protein, in interaction with the developmental process, may push behavioral outcome in one direction or another. So genetic and environmental factors are best conceptualized as acting as risk (or protective) factors in the development of individual differences in behavior; their effects are probabilistic rather than deterministic.

In what follows, I first provide some brief background material on what genes are and how they vary within and across species, then discuss behavioral and molecular genetic methods for studying developmental psychopathology.

Genes and Genomes

A gene is a discrete sequence of base pairs in a deoxyribonucleic acid (DNA) molecule that codes for a protein. The DNA molecule has the structure of a twisted ladder or double helix, the rungs of which consist of pairs of four bases (adenine, guanine, cytosine, and thymidine), whereas the rails of the ladder consist of sugar molecules that do not vary along the sequence. The particular sequence of base pairs carries genetic information, whereas the sugar molecules provide a structural "backbone" for each side of the ladder. Each base uniquely bonds with another base to form a base pair. Consequently, the DNA "ladder" may be split or unzipped down the middle to form two complementary strands (Figure 2).

This unzipping allows the DNA molecule either to copy itself by adding new units of a base attached to a sugar molecule or to be transcribed into messenger ribonucleic acid (mRNA), which participates in the synthesis of proteins. Proteins are strings of amino acids that fold into complex structures (called their tertiary structure) that allow them to perform specific cellular functions, including cell metabolism, gene expression, and intracellular communication. The latter two functions are particularly important in the development of organisms.

Virtually every cell in an organism contains a copy of its entire DNA, called its genome. The DNA in an organism's cells is found in both the nucleus and the mitochondria, which are organelles within the cell that provide energy. In sexually reproducing organisms such as mammals, half of the nuclear DNA comes from each parent, whereas all the mitochondrial DNA comes from the mother. Some neuropsychiatric illnesses involve mutations in mitochondrial DNA, so the transmission of these diseases will be exclusively matrilineal. The nuclear DNA is ar-

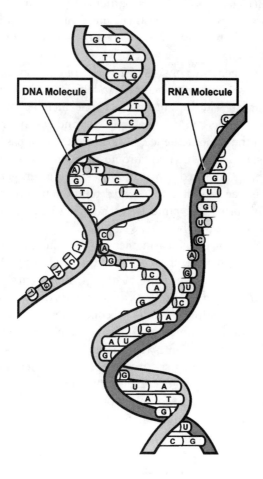

FIGURE 2. DNA and RNA molecules.

ranged on a number of chromosomes, each of which is a single DNA molecule. The number of chromosomes in an organism and the arrangement of genes on them are specific to a species. With the exception of chromosomal additions, deletions, or translocations (pieces of two different chromosomes joined together), individual genetic differences within a species consist of sequence differences in base pairs within genes, whereas the actual genes and their arrangement on chromosomes are common across individuals. So genetic influences on individual differences within a species consist mainly of a small number of sequence differences within a shared genetic architecture. One key goal of genetic studies of behavior is to characterize which sequence differences in which genes influence a particular behavior. Once these genetic variants or "alleles" are known, their influence on development can be elucidated, including their interaction with environmental influences.

The human genome consists of 23 pairs of chromosomes. One pair consists of two sex chromosomes (XX in females and XY in males); the other 22 pairs are called "autosomes." One member of each pair of chromosomes is inherited from each parent, and each pair contains the same genes in the same sequence, but the sequence of base pairs within a gene may vary across the two chromosomes in a pair, since the individual may have inherited different alleles of a given gene from each parent. This is one way in which sexual reproduction increases genetic diversity in offspring; the child is not an exact genetic copy of either parent, but is rather a hybrid.

A second means of increasing genetic diversity in offspring is provided by the mechanism of recombination (Figure 3). An individual may inherit either an exact copy of one of the parent's chromosomes (nonrecombinant) or a hybrid that contains parts of each member of the pair of chromosomes in the parent (recombinant). The bottom of Figure 3 shows two nonrecombinant chromosomes (the outer ones) and two recombinant chromosomes (the inner ones). Recombination occurs in the process of producing sperm and egg cells (called meiosis) and is another way of increasing genetic diversity among offspring in a sexually reproducing species. Recombination quite literally shuffles the genetic deck of cards; parts of a parental pair of chromosomes cross over, break apart, and recombine, producing a chromosome in the sperm or egg that is a hybrid of the parents' two chromosomes. In each meiosis, about 35 crossovers occur across all the chromosomes, or on average about 1.5 crossovers per chromosome. Longer chromosomes will have

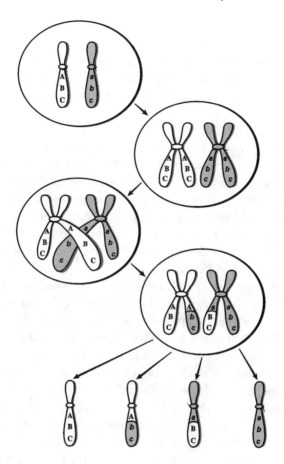

FIGURE 3. Linkage and recombination.

more crossovers than shorter ones. Genes that are close together on a chromosome (the B and C loci in Figure 3) are less likely to get separated in this shuffling process; such genes—those that do not recombine randomly across generations—are said to be "linked." So the probability of a recombination between two genetic loci on a chromosome is roughly proportional to the physical distance between them. If this probability is 50%, then the two loci are recombining randomly (random assortment) and cannot be very close together. As this probability (called the "recombination fraction") gets lower, the physical distance between the two loci is shorter. I say "roughly" proportional because some portions of chromosomes cross over more frequently than others.

Also, an occasional double crossover between two linked loci provides misleading information about the actual distance between them, but there are methods to compensate for this source of error. In summary, if we know the recombination fraction for two loci, we can estimate the physical distance between them. As we see later, this phenomenon of recombination provides the basis of methods for finding genes that influence individual differences.

The amount of DNA in the human genome is roughly 3 billion base pairs. Two convenient measures of genetic distance are a centimorgan (cM), which is 1 million base pairs in length, and a kilobase (kb), which is 1,000 base pairs in length. The centimorgan was named in honor of Thomas Hunt Morgan (1917), who discovered the phenomenon of linkage. With 3 billion base pairs, the human genome thus has 3,000 cM and 3 million kb. This is enough DNA to code for between 2 million and 20 million genes, but, remarkably, the number of human genes is now estimated at roughly only 30,000, although earlier estimates were around 100,000. Although the Human Genome Project has now provided us with a physical map of the entire genome (all the 3 billion base pairs in order), methods of gene identification are still being refined. So determining the exact number and location of all human genes will require further work. Thus, only about 1% of the available DNA codes for genes; the function of the remaining 99% of the DNA in the genome is currently unknown. About 40% of the genes in the human genome are uniquely expressed in the brain, with many of the genes in the remaining 60% also expressed in the brain and other organs, thus making the brain the most genetically complex organ in the body (Hahn, Van Ness, & Maxwell, 1978). This fact, plus the known allelic diversity in many human genes, virtually guarantees some degree of genetic influence on individual differences in behavior.

There is a considerable degree of genetic homology between the genomes of humans and other mammals in terms of the total amount of DNA, the number of chromosomes (24 pairs in the great apes, 23 pairs in humans, and 19 pairs in mice), and the genes and their arrangement on chromosomes. For instance, only about 1–5% of human genes lack a counterpart in mice. In the coding DNA (the DNA that codes for proteins), the base-pair sequence homology between mice and humans ranges between roughly 70% and 90%; between humans and the great apes, the figure is about 98%, being highest between humans and chimpanzees, our closest evolutionary relative. This degree of genetic similarity between humans and other mammals is important for research on developmental psychopathology, because it means animal models can be developed with gene variants similar to those that influence a human disorder. Such animal models allow experimental tests of pathogenic mechanisms, including brain mechanisms, that are not possible in human subjects.

However, one potential limitation of such animal models is that some of the sequence changes that influence psychopathology occur in noncoding regions, such as promoter regions (promoters are DNA sequences adjacent to gene coding regions that influence gene expression). Since noncoding regions exhibit greater cross-species variability than coding regions, animal models of psychopathology may be more difficult to create.

The sequence homology between any two unrelated humans is, of course, even higher, about 99.9%, and that between two full siblings is about 99.95%, so the degree of genetic difference between two full siblings is about half that between two unrelated people.

So a very large part of the genome acts to make all humans alike. Similarly, many of the important environmental influences on development are virtually ubiquitous. The basis of human universals lies in a largely homologous genome and these ubiquitous environmental experiences. As we turn to methods that allow us to detect genetic and environmental influences on individual differences, it is very important to remember that these methods do not measure influences that are shared by all humans. So finding a behavioral trait to be highly heritable does not mean that the environment was unimportant in its development, or that environmental manipulations would be ineffective in changing the mean value of that trait in a population. This point is readily understood if we consider the example of height, which is about 95% heritable. Yet the development of height clearly depends on the environment, and environmental changes in factors such as health care and nutrition have dramatically altered the mean height of human populations in the last century.

Behavioral Genetics

Until fairly recently, the main methods available for evaluating genetic influences on individual differences in human behavior were indirect and did not examine differences in DNA sequences. Instead, the influence of such differences on the development of individual differences in behavior was inferred through careful quantitative analyses of naturally occurring quasi-experiments, mainly twin births and adoptions. It is important to understand that both direct (molecular) and indirect (quantitative or biometric) genetic methods derive their power from a very strong theoretical constraint, namely, that genotypes exert causal influences on phenotypes, but that phenotypes do not change genotypes except in the unusual situation in which the phenotype leads to a mutation, such as through exposure to ionizing radiation. The genome can influence behavior, but behavior cannot influence the genome (although behavior can influence gene expression). Therefore, finding a nonartifactual relation between genotype and behavior means there is some causal pathway leading from that genotype to that behavior, no matter how tortuous or how many other causes also act on the behavior. Thus, genetic studies, unlike other nonexperimental studies of human behavior, detect causal relations, not just correlations.

One may organize the genetic analysis of any trait or phenotype into a series of four questions, one leading to the next, with each answered by a different method:

1. Is the trait familial?
2. If so, is the familiality due in part to genetic influences? In other words, is the trait heritable?
3. If so, what is the mechanism of genetic transmission?
4. What is the actual location of the gene or genes involved?

It is important to point out that some traits having a genetic cause are nonfamilial and therefore nonheritable, so the methods used for these questions would not apply to them. Instead, these conditions are recognized because they produce a characteristic physical and behavioral phenotype, and are proven to be genetic by means of chromosomal analysis, which begins with a karyotype, a photograph of each pair of chromosomes arranged in order of size. These conditions consist of spontaneous changes in either (1) chromosome number (called "aneuploidy") or (2) chromosome size (because of deletions or expansions). Aneuploidy occurs during meiosis in a sperm or egg, such that the embryo has either more or less than the normal number (46) of chromosomes. One of the most common and well-known examples of aneuploidy is trisomy 21, in which there is an extra copy of chromosome 21. Trisomy 21 is the cause of Down syndrome. Chromosome 21 is actually the smallest autosome, with the smallest number of genes, which is likely why fetuses with this aneuploidy survive. Aneuploidies of most other autosomes are not viable, but aneuploidies of the sex chromosomes have a combined prevalence greater than that of Down syndrome. Sex chromosome aneuploidies are viable because the Y chromosome has so few genes and only one copy of the X chromosome, which has a lot of genes, is fully expressed in development. We consider the behavioral phenotypes of some aneuploid conditions in Chapters 3–5, because aneuploidy can cause some of these developmental psychopathologies.

Returning to our four questions, the main methods associated with each, respectively, are (1) family studies, (2) twin and adoption studies, (3) segregation analysis, and (4) linkage and association analysis. Linkage and association analysis are covered in the following section on molecular methods. First, I briefly describe family studies and segregation analysis, then explain twin and adoption studies.

The design of *family studies* is fairly straightforward; the goal is to measure the familiality of a trait, which can be quantified as the correlations among relatives for a continuous trait or as relative risk (the prevalence in relatives divided by the population prevalence) for a categorical trait. These correlations or relative risks are computed separately for different relationships in families and tested for statistical significance. A positive test provides evidence for familiality, which is also expected to decline systematically as the degree of biological relationship decreases. A very useful statistic for genetic studies is the relative risk to full siblings (λ), because the ease of finding genes that influence a trait is proportional to λ. For instance, a λ of 2 means that the relative risk to full siblings is twice the population risk.

It is now established that many psychiatric disorders are familial. For instance, the value of λ is 9 for schizophrenia, 8 for bipolar disorder, and 3 for major depression (Plomin, DeFries, McClearn, & Rutter, 1997). Similar values have been found for childhood psychiatric disorders; the value of λ is around 6 for attention-deficit/hyperactivity disorder (Faraone et al., 1992), about 8 for dyslexia (Gilger, Pennington, & DeFries, 1991), and as high as 100 for autism (Plomin et al., 1997). Although familiality does not prove genetic influence (because familial transmission may be environmentally mediated), data from twin and molecular studies have demonstrated that genetic influences make a large contribution to the familiality of these psychiatric disorders.

As discussed earlier, family studies can also be quite useful for studying the basis of comorbidity. In other words, by studying two (or more) comorbid diagnoses in a family sample, one can test for familial influences on the relation between two disorders. As we see later, evidence of cofamiliality for a number of pairs of disorders indicates that comorbidity in these cases is due at least in part to a shared risk factor.

Familiality for a disorder does not usually depend on the gender of the transmitting parent. That it sometimes does can signal particular mechanisms of transmission, such as mitochondrial inheritance (in which transmission is exclusively matrilineal), or X-linked recessive inheritance, in which males are more liable to express the trait than females and there is never transmission of the trait from fathers to sons (because fathers only transmit a Y chromosome to sons).

Obviously, the validity of a family study depends crucially on the sample studied; a referred sample may have greater or different familiality results than a population sample. A partial correction for referral bias in a referred sample is provided by discarding from the analyses the index case or "proband," the referred individual through whom the family was identified. The difference in results for probands versus nonreferred relatives can be quite striking, as will be demonstrated when we review specific disorders.

Segregation analysis is a particular kind of family study, one that formally tests competing models for the mode of transmission of a trait in families. The data analyzed in a segregation analysis are the correlations among relatives for a particular trait, either categorical or continuous. The fit to the data of a series of nested models is tested; the best supported model is the one with the best fit and the fewest number of parameters (the most parsimonious model). The models tested are (1) vertical transmission versus no vertical transmission (i.e., Is there familiality?), (2) multifactorial transmission versus no multifactorial transmission, (3) major locus transmission versus no major locus transmission, and, if major locus transmission is found, (4) dominant versus additive versus recessive transmission. Obviously, modeling stops if there is no vertical transmission. One of the more complicated models is the mixed model, in which there are both a major locus effect and a multifactorial background. Segregation analysis is computationally intensive and only provides an indirect test of genetic mechanisms. Obviously, if a major locus effect is supported, molecular methods are needed to confirm this result and to identify the location of the major locus in the genome. Some evidence suggests that segregation analysis programs may be biased toward finding major locus effects. For example, segregation analysis of the trait of going to medical school found a major locus effect (McGuffin & Huckle, 1990), even though it seems very implausible that this educational outcome is caused by a single major gene.

Basic Twin and Adoption Methods

The most widely used behavioral genetic methods have been *twin and adoption studies*, which mainly address question 2 concerning heritability. A good introduction to twin and adoption methods is provided by Plomin and colleagues (1997). These methods provide a means of testing models of the etiology of a given behavior, or the relation between multiple behaviors, in a population. Such methods take the population variance in a behavioral trait and test which combination of genetic and environmental components best accounts for it. As in all of science, the meaning of the results naturally depends on the choice and validity of the models tested.

The simplest behavioral genetic model is one in which the population variance in a single trait is modeled as a combination of four components: heritability (h^2), which is the proportion of population variance attributable to genetic influences; common environmentality (c^2), which is the proportion of population variance attributable to environmental influences shared by siblings within a family but differing between families; nonshared environmentality (e^2), which is the proportion of population variance attributable to environmental influences unique to each sibling in a family; and measurement error, which also contributes to the variance of a measure. Since each of those components is a proportion, they can theoretically range between 0 and 1, and they must sum to 1. Of course, the values found for these proportions depend on the particular population that is studied; a population for whom the environment is relatively homogenous will yield smaller estimates of c^2 and e^2. Before saying how it may be tested, it is also important to point out that this model is obviously an oversimplification. It does not distinguish between additive and nonadditive genetic effects (i.e., dominance and epistasis, which are, respectively, the interaction between alleles of a given gene or between different genes), and does not model interactions or correlations between genes and environments. Since such interactions and correlations are very likely important in the etiology of psychopathologies (Rutter, 2001), this limitation needs to be taken seriously. Many of the heritability estimates provided in this book are based on such simple models that incorporate variance attributable to these correlations and interactions in the heritability term. However, the elegance of behavioral genetics consists in part of the fact that, with appropriate designs, more complex models that include such components can be tested against simpler models.

Another limitation of the basic behavioral genetic model is that it tells you very little about developmental mechanisms. Counterintuitively, many life events (e.g., divorce, exposure to combat, and other stressful life events) turn out to be heritable. Obviously, there are not genes for divorce per se, only genetic influences on behavioral and personality traits that increase the risk for divorce.

As another example of this limitation, let us consider how this model treats epigenesis, which is a very important aspect of development. For many behavioral traits, it is common to find moderate heritabilities and more nonshared than shared environmental influences. Some of this nonshared environmental influence may reflect the operation of epigenesis in the developmental process and not environmental factors external to the individual. Hence, it may be very difficult, if not impossible, to identify all the factors that contribute to nonshared environmental variance. Sewall Wright (1920) termed this source of variation "the vagaries of development." Molenaar, Boomsma, and Dolan (1993) have provided examples of this kind of variation in human and animal studies. They argue that "reiterating, chaotic epigenetic processes are capable of creating variability under constant genetic and environmental conditions" (p. 523). Hence, genetically identical animals raised in identical environments will nonetheless vary because of such processes in epigenesis. A rather dramatic example of the role of epigenesis in development is provided by quantitative genetic studies of aging and lifespan. Across species, there is wide variation in lifespan for genetically identical animals reared in highly similar environments. For human twins, the monozygotic (MZ) correlation for lifespan is only .20, while the dizygotic (DZ) correlation is .06 (Finch & Kirkwood, 2000). Although the MZ–DZ difference means lifespan is heritable, 80% of the variance is nonshared. Since a similar degree of variation in lifespan is found in genetically identical animals reared in highly similar environments (Finch & Kirkwood, 2000), it is likely that much of the nonshared variance in human lifespan is due to epigenetic variation and not to environmental factors external to the individual.

Since the brain is the most complex organ in the body, and behavior is the most complex phenotype an animal exhibits, it seems quite likely that some of the variation in brain and behavior reflects similar, chaotic epigenetic processes in development. Hence, some of the variation we observe in psychopathology will likely be epigenetic in origin and not readily explainable. We return now to the basic, quantitative genetic model.

To test this simple four-component model, we need data from a design that allows genetic and environmental influences to be disentangled. The two most commonly utilized designs are twin and adoption studies. Twin studies allow genetic influences to be distinguished from environmental ones, because identical, or MZ, twins share all their genes, since each member of the pair derives from one zygote, a single cell formed when the sperm fertilizes an egg. Fraternal, or DZ ("two zygotes"), twins, like full siblings, share on average half their segregating genes in common, because each member of the pair derives from a different fertilized egg. So, the genetic "manipulation" in this quasi-experiment is the different degree of genetic similarity in MZ versus DZ pairs. The degree of genetic influence on the behavioral trait in question can thus be evaluated by comparing MZ and DZ similarity for that trait. If MZ similarity is significantly greater than DZ similarity, then the hypothesis of genetic influence on the trait in question is supported, and the degree of genetic influence can be estimated. For instance, if the trait in question is measured continuously, then interclass correlations can be calculated separately for MZ and DZ pairs. The proportions of variance contributing to the MZ correlation are both h^2 and c^2, whereas those contributing to the DZ correlation are $\frac{1}{2} h^2$ and c^2. Neither e^2 nor measurement error contributes to twin similarity, so these two components of variance are not part of the MZ or DZ correlation; instead, they are the part of the total variance not accounted for by h^2 and c^2.

It is important that this genetic manipulation not be confounded with environmental differences. Hence, a crucial assumption of the twin method is the "equal environments" assumption: For environmental variables that correlate with the particular behavioral trait being analyzed, MZ pairs are no more similar on average than DZ pairs. Most of us have observed that some environmental variables are frequently more similar in MZ pairs, such as dress, but the critical question is whether such variables relate to the behavioral trait being analyzed. The validity of the equal environments assumption in a twin design can be evaluated by measuring relevant environmental variables, testing whether they are correlated with the behavioral variable of interest, and, if so, then testing whether MZ and DZ similarity for the environmental variable differ. This method evaluates only environmental similarity for the environmental variables that the experimenter chooses to test. Another test of this crucial assumption is to compare results from pairs in which the parents are mistaken about zygosity and from pairs in which parents are not mistaken; this test requires a large sample and only evaluates environmental equality for aspects of the environment that parents control. While neither method provides an exhaustive test of this assumption, existing twin studies that have used these tests have not found violations of the equal environments assumption (Plomin et al., 1997).

The adoption method fairly cleanly unconfounds genetic and environmental influences on development, because the adoptive parents who provide the rearing environment are genetically unrelated to the child. The biological parents provide genes but not the rearing environment, so long as the adoption occurs at birth. (The biological mother does provide the intrauterine environment.) To estimate the four components of variance in the simple model from adoption study data, one computes parent–offspring correlations for both kinds of parents of an adoptive child: biological and adoptive. Twice the biological parent–offspring correlation provides an estimate of h^2, because such pairs share half their genes and nothing else. The adoptive parent–offspring correlation provides an estimate of c^2, because such pairs share c^2 and nothing else. One might expect that these correlations could be attenuated by the fact that parents and offspring are usually being measured at different ages. If the adoptive family also includes biological children, then this possible age attenuation can be avoided by comparing the correlation between adoptive and biological siblings.

The manipulation provided by the adoption design also depends on a crucial assumption, namely, that characteristics of the biological parent or the infant do not influence the choice of adoptive parents. Such an influence on which adoptees are placed with which adopting parents is called "selective placement." If this occurs, then adoptive parent–offspring correlations can be artificially increased, which would then increase the estimate of c^2. Well-designed adoption studies directly test for selective placement. It is very important to note that violations of the crucial assumptions for each design, twin and adoption, have *opposite* effects on estimates of h^2 and c^2. Therefore, if these estimates converge across both kinds of design, we can be more confident that these assumptions have been met.

Using Twin Methods to Analyze Extreme Traits

Of particular relevance for studies of psychopathology is the application of twin and adoption studies to the analysis of extreme variations in behavior rather than the analysis of variance across the whole distribution. Extreme variations may be treated as categories, in which case the appropriate method of analysis is nonparametric and involves comparing the rates of concordance for different degrees of relationship. However, if the trait in question is quantitative (can be measured using an ordinal or interval scale), then treating the trait as categorical does not use all the information contained in the data and is thus less statistically powerful. If we can measure not only whether someone has attention-deficit/hyperactivity disorder or reading disability but also how severely he or she has it, then our data are quantitative rather than qualitative and can be analyzed parametrically. A particularly powerful twin method for analyzing extreme variation in quantitative traits was developed by DeFries and Fulker (1988) and is now called the DF method in their honor. It is based on the phenomenon of differential regression to the mean, first described by Francis Galton (1892).

Let us take, for example, an index case or proband that has been selected because that individual is extreme on some dimension: at the low or high end of the distribution for that trait. Now let us measure the same trait in their relatives. Where do we expect the relative's score to fall on the distribution? If the trait is familial, their relatives' scores will also be toward the same, extreme end of the distribution but on average less extreme than the proband's score. In other words, the relatives' scores move back toward the population mean. This is regression to the mean, which follows from the fact that scores closer to the mean are more probable than scores further from the mean. If the trait were nonfamilial, then the relatives' scores would on average move all the way back to the population mean. So if the trait is familial, two opposing "forces" are acting on the relatives' scores: Regression is "pulling" them toward the mean, and familiality is "pulling" them toward the proband's score. If the familial relation is closer, the familial "pull" should be stronger. Hence, if a trait is familial, the degree of regression to the mean will be inversely proportional to the degree of familial relationship between a proband and a relative. This phenomenon of differential regression to the mean could occur because closer relatives share more of their environments or more of their genes, or some combination of the two.

Using a twin design, we can disentangle genetic and environmental influences on this phenomenon of differential regression to the mean. Co-twins in MZ pairs should regress back to the population mean on average less than the co-twins in similarly selected DZ pairs, if being extreme on that trait is genetically influenced (Figure 4).

The degree of genetic influence on the extreme trait is h^2_g, where the subscript g refers to the extreme group of probands. So h^2_g measures the heritability of the group deficit (or talent), in contrast to h^2, which measures the heritability of variation across the whole distribution. As we will see, the comparison of h^2 and h^2_g provides one test of whether the etiologies of normal and extreme variations differs, which is a fundamental issue in developmental psychopathology. However, before the advent of the DF and molecular methods, empirical methods to address this issue have been mostly lacking. Moreover, the primary earlier method, a test of bimodality, was neither very powerful nor decisive.

To better understand the DF method, it is useful to consider what would happen with different etiological scenarios. For example, what would happen if there were no genetic influence on the extreme trait but significant c^2_g (an effect of shared family environment on the group deficit or talent)? In this case, both the MZ and DZ co-twin means would regress equally back to the population mean (Figure 5), and the DF method would allow us to measure the magnitude of c^2_g. Now consider what would happen if the extreme trait in question were totally nonfamilial (no h^2_g or c^2_g). In this case, both the MZ and DZ co-twin means would regress all the way back to the population mean (Figure 6), and the etiology of the extreme trait would be due to factors unique to individuals with that trait, that is, e^2_g. For instance, the etiology of some forms of severe mental retardation is nonfamilial and reflects either aneuploidy or perinatal accidents; hence, both MZ and DZ co-twins of probands with these forms of mental retardation would, on average, have IQ scores at the population mean.

Obviously, extreme behavioral traits in many cases will be the product of all three factors, h^2_g, c^2_g, and e^2_g, as well as some error of measurement. The advantage of the DF method is that it provides a statistically powerful method of modeling these components of the etiology of the scores of an extreme group. Another advantage is its flexibility; it can readily be extended to (1) the bivariate case, (2) the evaluation of differential etiology (of subgroups, such as males and females, or of extreme and normal variations), (3) tests for linkage, which are discussed later, or (4) the examination of interactions in etiology.

Multivariate Behavioral Genetic Methods

Both twin and adoption methods may be generalized to the multivariate case in order to examine genetic and environmental relations among

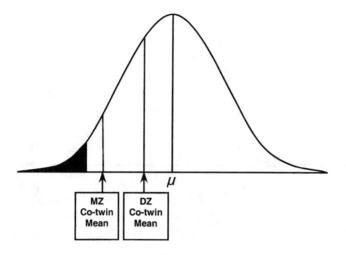

FIGURE 4. Co-twin means if extreme scores are due to genetic influences.

correlated traits. Say, for example, we would like to know why there is a phenotypic correlation between Wechsler Verbal and Performance IQ, or among Wechsler subtests. Multivariate behavioral genetic methods allow us to estimate the degree to which such phenotypic correlations are due to shared genetic and environmental influences. However, since in the case of psychopathology we would like to answer this question with respect to extreme rather than normal variations, we need multivariate methods specific to this situation. Such multivariate models are needed to answer a key question in developmental psychopathology: What is the causal basis of the comorbidities so commonly found among developmental psychopathologies? Different methods are used depending on whether the trait is measured categorically or continuously. If the trait is measured categorically, the bivariate extension involves the comparison of cross-concordances. For instance, let us say that we want to test the etiology of the comorbidity between the categorical diagnoses of anxiety and depression. We could select a sample of MZ and DZ pairs in which at least one twin had one of these two diagnoses, say anxiety, and then test for the diagnosis of depression in the co-twins, computing rates of cross-concordances between anxiety and depression for MZ and DZ pairs. Significantly higher cross-concordance in MZ than in DZ pairs would support genetic influence on the relation between anxiety and depression. If the extreme traits were measured

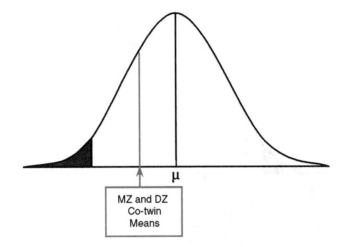

FIGURE 5. Co-twin means if extreme scores are due to shared and nonshared environmental influences.

continuously, then the bivariate extension of the DF method could be utilized to calculate bivariate h^2_g, c^2_g, and e^2_g, which provide information about the degree to which the relation between the two extreme traits is due to shared genes, shared common family environments, or shared nonfamilial environmental influences (shared by the two traits but not by siblings within a family), respectively.

I discuss specific findings from these bivariate methods when considering specific disorders in Chapters 3–5. For instance, these methods have found considerable genetic overlap between anxiety and depression. These bivariate results can be used to calculate two related statistics that answer somewhat different questions about the etiological relation between two correlated phenotypes.

One question we would like to answer is what proportion of the phenotypic overlap is due to shared genes or environments? The proportion due to shared genes (termed PG) can be calculated as follows:

$$PG = \frac{\text{bivariate } h^2}{\text{phenotypic correlation } (r_p)}$$

The proportions due to shared common family environments (PC) or to shared nonfamilial environments (PE) can be calculated similarly.

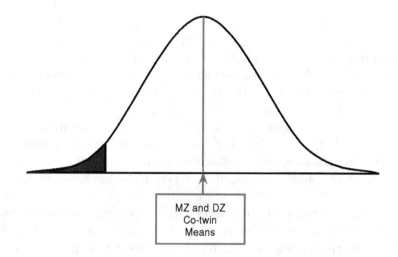

FIGURE 6. Co-twin means if extreme scores are due to nonshared environmental influences.

A second question is what proportion of all the genes or environments acting on either phenotype are shared by *both* phenotypes? The genetic proportion in this case is called the genetic correlation (r_g) and can be calculated as follows:

$$r_g = \frac{\text{bivariate } h^2}{h_x \cdot h_y}$$

The terms h_x and h_y are the square roots of the heritabilities of each of the two correlated phenotypes. The proportions due to shared common family environments (r_c) and to shared nonfamilial environments (r_e) can be calculated similarly.

Although each of these proportions, PG and r_g, are related because each is a function of bivariate h^2, in some cases they can differ considerably. Obviously, if bivariate h^2 is 0, then both PG and r_g must be 0 as well. Similarly, if bivariate h^2 is 1, then r_g and PG must be 1 as well. (Demonstrating this requires the knowledge that the maximum possible values for PG, r_g, r_p, and $h_x \cdot h_y$ are 1 and then substituting a value of 1 for bivariate h^2 in the first and second equations.) However, for intermediate values of bivariate h^2, say, .5, PG and r_g can differ considerably because the phenotypic correlation (r_p) and the individual heritabilities

(h^2_x and h^2_y) are free to vary. For instance, if bivariate $h^2 = .5$, $r_p = .5$, and both h^2_x and $h^2_y = 1.0$, then $PG = 1.0$, but r_g equals only $.5$. These values mean that *all* of the phenotypic correlation is due to shared genes, but that those shared genes are only half of all the genetic influences acting on either phenotype. In a different case with bivariate $h^2 = .5$, but $r_p = .8$ and h^2_x and $h^2_y = .50$, then PG is lower, $.63$, and r_g is at a maximum of 1.0. These values mean that 63% of the phenotypic correlation would be due to shared genes (and the other 37% would be due to environmental influences shared by the two phenotypes). However, those shared genes would constitute *all* the genetic influences acting on either phenotype.

As a transition to the next section, it is important to point out that a given DZ twin or sibling pair could share more or less than half of their segregating genes. Since each member of such a pair gets a random half of each parental genome as a result of the mechanisms of meiosis and recombination discussed earlier, some of these sibling pairs will actually be genetically more like identical twins, whereas others will be more like two unrelated individuals. Obviously, for a given stretch of DNA (a genetic locus), the likelihood of within-pair variation in the degree of genetic similarity is much greater. At a given genetic locus, a given sibling pair may share both transmitted alleles, one from each parent (hence, their "identity by descent," or ibd, is 1.0), only one transmitted allele (an ibd of .5), or no alleles (an ibd of 0). As we will see, molecular genetic methods exploit this within-pair genetic variance at particular loci to identify genes that influence phenotypic traits. If degree of phenotypic similarity in sibling pairs is correlated with their ibd status at a locus, then it is likely that a gene influencing that trait is nearby.

Molecular Methods

In contrast to the methods discussed earlier, molecular methods can provide direct evidence of genetic influence on a trait or on the relation among traits. All of these methods test for a relation between phenotypic and DNA sequence variations, so they require precise measures in both domains and theoretically sound, quantitative methods of relating genetic and phenotypic variation. As discussed earlier, it is important to understand that the relation being tested is not simply a correlation; rather, it is the hypothesis that sequence variation in a particular part of the genome causes, at least in part, the phenotypic variation.

We can divide molecular methods into tests of *linkage* and of *association* (Table 2). Generally, we use linkage methods to screen broadly for loci influencing a trait, whereas tests of association are usually used once we know at least the approximate location of candidate loci.

Linkage Methods

The initial goal of linkage methods is to find the approximate locations of genes influencing a trait. As explained earlier, the phenomenon of linkage depends on the fact that, as it were, the croupier in the genetic casino does not shuffle perfectly. The phenomenon of recombination shuffles genes (cards in this metaphor) in the process of forming gametes, but genes (cards) that are close together are less likely to be separated in a shuffle because they are physically close together—linked. So, linkage represents a deviation from Mendel's second law of the independent assortment of genes (see Figure 3). For example, say we are searching the deck for a gene or genes whose location is unknown, such as a gene influencing a particular behavioral trait, such as dyslexia. As explained earlier, the deck in question, the genome, is vast,

TABLE 2. Molecular Methods

Method	Use	Issues
Linkage		
Parametric	Find approximate location of a major locus influencing a phenotype	Transmission parameters of complex behavioral phenotypes are often unknown
Nonparametric	Find approximate location of genes influencing a phenotype	Less powerful
Association		
Case–control	Identify an allele that influences a phenotype	Ethnic stratification; multiple mutations of the same gene
Family-based		
Transmission disequilibrium test (TDT)	Same	Multiple mutations
Haplotype relative risk (HRR)	Same	Multiple mutations

since it contains approximately 30,000 genes in its coding regions and a much larger amount of noncoding DNA. Our job is to find a sequence variation (a particular card) in this huge deck that influences the trait we are studying. Moreover, in this deck are many, many other sequence variations influencing other traits and many more sequence variations in noncoding regions. A very few of these other sequence variations will happen to lie close enough to the sequence variations we are searching for, so as to be linked to them. If we have a map of sequence variations or "markers" across the genome that are roughly evenly spaced and close enough together to detect linkage to most or all of the adjacent genes, then we can use these markers to search for the location of sequence variations that influence the trait in which we are interested.

A somewhat more formal hypothesis is that there are sequence variations in genes (risk alleles) that influence the trait in question. Presumably, this hypothesis is based on studies of the trait with the indirect behavioral genetic methods discussed earlier, so that we already know that the trait is familial, heritable, and perhaps even subject to major gene influence. If our hypothesis is correct, then individuals with more of this trait on average will have more of these risk alleles than individuals with less of the trait. In other words, our hypothesis implies that these particular risk alleles are cotransmitted with levels of the trait across generations (in the case of a single gene and a categorical trait, we would say that they cosegregate). So levels of the trait are a proxy for the unknown causative alleles, if our hypothesis is correct. Because of the phenomenon of linkage, nearby sequence variations, some of which are markers in our genomic map, are also cotransmitted along with levels of the trait and the unknown risk alleles. Hence, two out of the three cotransmitted items are known to us: levels of the trait and sequence variations in markers. Knowledge of these two items allows us to know the approximate locations of the third unknown item, the risk alleles. Thus, if we find linkage between particular markers and levels of the trait, we infer that there is a nearby gene, an allele of which influences the trait we are studying. In summary, cotransmission of genetic markers and a behavioral trait helps us to map the approximate location of genes whose alleles influence that trait.

A student of statistics and experimental design will quickly notice that our hypothesis (somewhere out there are some genes that influence this behavioral trait) is not very constrained and will almost inevitably lead to multiple statistical tests, one for each marker considered. A genomic map with markers spaced 10 cM apart requires 300 markers to cover the genome, so with an alpha level of .05, 15 linkages would be found by chance alone in a whole genome search. So it is necessary that the quantitative methods used in linkage studies protect against spurious significance. One strategy for conducting a whole genome search is a two-step process. The initial screening step has liberal significance levels (e.g., an alpha of .01, which would lead to three spurious positive results on average, or even an alpha of .05). It is followed by a rigorous confirmation step employing multiple markers in the regions identified in the screening step. Because the degree of deviation from random assortment is inversely proportional to actual genetic distance, markers in the region of an allele influencing the trait will exhibit gradations of linkage proportional to their distance from the unknown gene and from each other. This systematic pattern of linkage across markers in a chromosomal region, increasing and then falling off, can be detected with multipoint methods that consider the data from multiple markers in a region simultaneously. Such methods produce probability maps of the region, indicating the most likely location of the unknown gene. Obviously, the probability of obtaining spurious positive results for a series of markers in a region is much less than the probability of obtaining a spurious result in the initial screening step. This probability is proportional to the number of markers utilized and their degree of polymorphism (how many alleles in the marker and how frequently the different alleles occur in the population).

One multipoint method that is useful for mapping genes that influence extreme, quantitative traits is called "interval mapping," which is an extension of the DF method discussed earlier; it was developed by David Fulker and colleagues at the Institute for Behavioral Genetics in Boulder, Colorado (Fulker, Cherny, & Cardon, 1995). Interval mapping is particularly useful in studies of psychopathology because (1) it is appropriate for extreme traits that are measured quantitatively; (2) it is quite powerful statistically; (3) it readily tests whether the same chromosomal region is linked to different levels of the trait, even levels from either end of the distribution; and (4) it is quite flexible and can be readily extended to consider dominance, bivariate linkage (which is needed to find genes responsible for comorbidities), or interactions with other factors, such as gender. I illustrate some of these applications of interval mapping in Chapter 5, in the discussion of dyslexia.

Linkage methods are broadly divided into those that require specification of the mode of transmission and degree of penetrance (essentially, how close to 1:1 is the mapping between a hypothesized allele of a single gene and the behavioral trait in question, so that with a pene-trance of 0.80 there is 80% probability that someone with the allele will have the trait) and those that do not. The former, which require specifi-cation of these parameters of transmission, are called "parametric," and the latter are called "nonparametric." Parametric linkage methods were developed first, partly because of geneticists' historical emphasis on Mendelian traits. For a student of behavior, it is quickly apparent that parametric linkage analysis is testing a very strong hypothesis indeed, namely, that a single Mendelian gene has a major causal influence on the trait in question. If penetrance is modeled at a high value, then the finding of only a very few subjects in a family who have the relevant marker but not the trait (or the reverse) disconfirms this hypothesis. For most behavioral traits, transmission is unlikely to be Mendelian, be-cause multiple genes and environmental risk factors will influence the trait, so the parameters of transmission will be unknown. Hence, to use parametric linkage methods, we have to make assumptions (specify pa-rameters) that are likely to be incorrect. Parametric linkage methods do have the advantage of statistical power (because they are testing such a strong hypothesis, namely, consistent cotransmission in an extended family between a marker and a trait) and can be useful in analyzing data from very large extended families, especially if these are considered one at a time. Since genetic heterogeneity may occur across such families, combining their data may be misleading.

Nonparametric methods require fewer assumptions and are gener-ally preferable in linkage studies of behavioral traits. They also do not require large extended families and often utilize sibling pairs from nu-clear families. As discussed earlier, there is variability in degree of with-in-pair genetic similarity for a given genetic marker across a sample of sibling pairs. Each sibling has two alleles for a given marker, one inher-ited from each parent. If the parental alleles are known and distinguish-able (multiple markers help here, as well as genotype data from grand-parents), then we can determine for each member of a sibling pair which of their two alleles came from the mother and father, respectively. As discussed earlier, a sibling pair might share no parental alleles, just one parental allele, or both parental alleles of that marker. Thus, for that marker, the pair can be genetically unrelated (their ibd is 0), can have one of the two parental alleles in common (an ibd of .5), or have both of the parental alleles in common (an ibd of 1.0). All sibling-pair linkage methods relate genetic similarity at a locus (the ibd value) to phenotypic similarity. Finding a significant relation supports the hypothesis that a gene influencing the trait is located near the marker in question.

In summary, to conduct a nonparametric, sibling-pair linkage study of an extreme behavioral trait (e.g., a developmental psychopathology), we need a fairly large sample of sibling pairs (say, around 150) in which at least one member of each pair has the trait in question; genetic marker data from these pairs, their parents, and, preferably, their grandparents; and appropriate statistical methods for analyzing the relation between genotypic and phenotypic similarity within pairs.

Association Methods

We now consider association analysis, which tests for a correlation between a particular allele of a candidate gene and a phenotype. To appreciate the difference between linkage and association analysis (Hodge, 1993), it is important to understand the difference between linkage and linkage disequilibrium. In the case of linkage, the particular allele of a given locus that is linked to a behavioral trait will vary across families, because recombination will have sorted different alleles of the marker with the particular risk allele of the linked gene that influences the trait. Say that we found linkage between dyslexia and the gene for the ABO blood type. In some families, most or all of the dyslexics would have type A blood, and the nondyslexics would have types B or O. In other families, the dyslexics would have type B blood, and in still others, they would have type O blood. So linkage between dyslexia and the ABO gene does *not* mean that all dyslexics have a particular blood type. In this case, the gene that influences dyslexia and the ABO gene are close enough together that recombination (shuffling) is reduced but not eliminated. In the thousands of years since the mutation in the dyslexia gene, recombination has shuffled that gene with different alleles of the ABO gene across families. But what if the dyslexia gene and the ABO gene are so close together that little or no reshuffling has occurred over those thousands of years? In this case, we would say the two genes are in linkage disequilibrium and, as a result, virtually all dyslexics across families would have a particular ABO blood type, say Type A. In this case, there is both linkage between dyslexia and the ABO gene, *and* there is association between dyslexia and the A allele of that gene. However, the ABO gene would not in this case play a causal role in the development of dyslexia.

In summary, if there is allele sharing for a marker gene among individuals with a given trait (e.g., dyslexia) that is found within but not across families, we say there is linkage. If there is allele sharing both within and across families, we say there is association. Hence, there are three possible reasons for a finding of association: (1) As just discussed, there is linkage disequilibrium between the candidate allele and a nearby risk allele; (2) the candidate allele is the risk allele (in which case, there would be no recombination); or (3) an artifact produces association but not linkage.

One prominent artifact that has been identified in case–control association studies is ethnic stratification. Allele frequencies vary considerably in human populations, even within groups labeled as "Caucasian," "Hispanic," or "African American" (see, e.g., Seaman, Fisher, Chang, & Kidd, 1999). Therefore, an ethnically matched case–control association study may nonetheless confound allele frequencies with group, thus producing a spurious association. To avoid this confound, within-family association methods are used, such as the transmission disequilibrium test (Spielman, McGinnis, & Ewens, 1996) and the haplotype relative risk method (Falk & Rubenstein, 1987; Terwilliger & Ott, 1992). Both these methods test whether the candidate allele is more frequently transmitted to affected than to nonaffected family members. These methods are now being generalized for use with continuous traits and covariates.

Nonetheless, even within-family association methods will fail to detect a causative gene in which different mutations across families each produce the disorder. In this case, there would be linkage to markers close to this gene but not association to a particular allele of the gene.

As stated previously, association analysis is usually appropriate only if there is a candidate location, either from a linkage study, or based on a hypothesis about which particular gene is influencing a trait. That hypothesis could come from knowledge of the neurobiology of the trait (e.g., the trait involves dopamine transmission; therefore, genes for dopamine receptors may be involved in its cause) or from previous linkage studies (a gene in this region influences the trait, and one of the known genes in this region has a function that makes it a possible candidate gene). However, a new association method has been proposed for whole genome searches. It involves pooling DNA samples from family members and then conducting a genomewide association search (Risch & Merikangas, 1996).

Linkage and association methods have complementary strengths and weaknesses. Linkage can be detected over a much broader genetic distance, but linkage methods are less statistically powerful than association methods (Risch & Merikangas, 1996). If searching for a risk allele for a complex phenotype, such as a psychopathology, we may not find risk alleles with low effect sizes using linkage methods. New methods are being developed to overcome these shortcomings. One method uses linkage methods with evenly spaced markers to conduct a whole-genome search to identify promising regions. Such regions can then be searched more intensively using association methods.

The ultimate goals of both linkage and association methods are to identify the mutations in the genes that causally influence the trait in question and to characterize how these mutations alter the function of these genes in the development of brain and behavior. So identifying genes that influence psychopathologies is only the first step. The real promise of genetic methods is the information they will provide about pathophysiological brain mechanisms. What if we could only work "backward" from behavior to underlying brain mechanisms, say by using neuroimaging techniques? Then we would have much less power to identify the brain mechanisms underlying a psychopathology. In Chapters 3–5 of this book, which review specific disorders, I discuss the initial progress made toward this important but difficult goal of working "forward" from genes to identify pathophysiological brain mechanisms.

NEUROBIOLOGY

Behind every crooked thought there is a crooked molecule.
—ANONYMOUS

If neuroimaging is the answer, what is the question?
—ANONYMOUS

This section is concerned with the next level of analysis necessary for understanding the development of psychopathology, namely, that of brain mechanisms. The two quotations highlight some of the conceptual issues we face in mapping behavior onto the brain. At this point, the reader should recognize *both* the truth and error in the first quotation. Thoughts are reducible to the physical substrate of the brain (monism or reductionism), but a given thought, whether crooked or straight, is not reducible to a single cause. To be explained, it must be reconstructed (from the interactions of multiple causes and their impact on neurocomputation). The second quotation reminds us that the value of any technology for the understanding of behavior depends on the questions posed.

As discussed earlier, virtually all etiological influences on developmental psychopathologies, both genetic and environmental, act by changing the trajectory of brain development. However, we are only beginning to understand the alterations in brain development that underlie developmental psychopathologies. There are several reasons for this lack of knowledge: (1) Some of the necessary methods have only recently become available; (2) the brain level of analysis has not always been viewed as relevant by psychologists studying abnormal development; and (3) brain studies of psychopathology have been more focused on identifying potentially causal brain variables than on explaining how changes in such variables produce the symptoms that define the disorder. I consider the two latter reasons in more detail.

Accounts of psychological development too often take brain development for granted or assume that it operates separately from psychological development, which is part of the latent dualism in psychology, discussed earlier. One implicit assumption is that the basic structure of the human brain is genetically programmed, and that genes act mainly during prenatal development to set up this basic structure, and then the environment takes over to shape postnatal development. This resolution to the nature–nurture problem might be called the partition solution: A civil war is uneasily settled by dividing the country in two! The problems with this assumption are that (1) both genes and environments act together throughout lifespan development, (2) basic brain structure does not appear to be genetically hardwired, and, most importantly, (3) the scope of developmental theory is unduly restricted. Development is a central problem for both modern biology and modern psychology; it would be very odd indeed if the theories of development in each field had nothing to do with each other. Complex systems theory is beginning to be applied to understanding development in both fields, which at least points to one way in which an integrated developmental theory might be achieved.

A complementary problem is found in much biological research on psychopathology. More than 10 years ago, in an *Annual Review of Psychology* article, DePue and Iacono (1989, p. 458) pointed out that there "is a serious limitation to much of the neurobiologic research and modeling in psychopathology" due to its focus on "the integrity of functioning of a biological variable *per se*," rather than "the larger neuro-behavioral framework within which the variable operates." In other words, biological research on psychopathology is often overly focused on the physical reduction side of the neuroscience paradigm, and too little focused on the reconstruction side. A complete explanation of a psychopathology will require that we know not only its biological causes but also how those causes act to change psychological functions. As discussed earlier, this second task ultimately requires neurocomputational models. In what follows, I first provide examples of some of the ways genes and environment can alter brain development, then discuss the larger neurobehavioral framework in which such brain changes operate; finally, I turn to methods for studying brain mechanisms.

What have we already learned about different ways genes and environments alter brain and behavioral development? There are three broad classes of known genetic effects on brain development: (1) on brain size, by altering the number of neurons or synapses; (2) on neuronal migration, sometimes in a regionally specific fashion; and (3) on neurotransmission, by changing either levels of neurotransmitter, or the binding properties of receptor proteins. The best understood environmental example involves deprivation of sensory experience during a critical period. I briefly discuss examples of each of these four kinds of influences on early brain development to illustrate how they can explain changes in behavioral development.

For example, with regard to the first effect, it is well known that brain size is affected in many genetic syndromes. Thus, there is microcephaly in Down syndrome and other mental retardation syndromes. In contrast, macrocephaly occurs in about one-fourth of individuals with autism and in fragile X syndrome. The mechanism underlying macrocephaly in fragile X syndrome appears to be failure to transcribe a gene that regulates synaptic pruning; this failure of transcription is caused by the accumulation of repetitive DNA sequences that characterize the disorder. Neurocomputational models support the straightforward intuition that having too few or too many connections in brain networks would affect cognitive development in different ways. For instance, a network with too many connections recalls specific inputs well but generalizes across them poorly, a pattern reminiscent of some of the symptoms of autism and fragile X syndrome.

With regard to the second effect, there are well-studied genetic mutations in both mice and fruit flies that affect neuronal migration (Changeux, 1985), and evidence for migrational anomalies in several human syndromes. Nonhuman cases have sometimes demonstrated that the migrational anomalies cause particular behavioral deficits.

One example of the third kind of effect, on neurotransmission, has been demonstrated in phenylketonuria, in which an enzyme defect prevents the conversion of phenylalanine into tyrosine, which is the rate-limiting precursor for the synthesis of dopamine. So even the mild elevations of phenylalanine found in treated phenylketonuria can produce dopamine depletion in prefrontal cortex, which in turn causes somewhat selective executive function deficits (Diamond, Prevor, Callender, & Druin, 1997; Welsh, Pennington, Ozonoff, Rouse, & McCabe, 1990).

Another way neurotransmission can be affected is through alterations in the binding properties of receptors for neurotransmitters. These receptors are proteins coded for by genes. Their binding properties depend on their tertiary structure, which is determined by the way they fold up. Base-pair differences in the gene for a receptor can cause differences in its tertiary structure and, hence, in its binding properties. These changes can in turn make a particular neurotransmitter more or less available at the synapse. As will be discussed later, attention-deficit/hyperactivity disorder has been found to be associated with an allele of the DRD4 gene. There is initial evidence of allelic differences in other receptor genes in other psychiatric illnesses, so this kind of effect could contribute to many psychiatric disorders, since most of them involve neurotransmitter imbalances.

The classic example of an early environmental effect on brain development involves the formation of ocular dominance columns in primary visual cortex that segregate the input from each eye. This segregation in turn is necessary for stereoscopic vision. Extensive experimentation established that binocular visual experience during a critical period is necessary for these ocular dominance columns to form (see Greenough, Black, & Wallace, 1987, for a review). In fact, the formation of ocular dominance columns is a good example of how global form emerges from local interactions, in this case, between adjacent neurons in visual cortex, which initially receive projections from both eyes. Competitive interactions between adjacent neurons strengthen some synapses and weaken others, such that neurons receiving input from a single eye come to be grouped together. There are also successful neural network models of both the development of ocular dominance columns (Miller, Keller, & Stryker, 1989) and of stereoscopic vision itself (Churchland, 1995). All of this research taken together provides an integrative neuroscientific explanation of a pathology of visual behavior: the lack of stereoscopic vision in individuals with early binocular deprivation (e.g., because of infantile cataracts). In this example, we know the environmental cause, we know how it changes brain development (lack of ocular dominance columns), and we know how that structural change alters neural network function to prevent the development of a specific behavior, stereopsis.

These examples, especially the last, are meant to give the reader a feel for what an integrated neuroscientific explanation of a psychopathology will look like. The relevant risk factors will be specified, their effect on the development of brain structure will be understood, the effect of that structural change on neurocomputation will be worked out, which in turn will explain how psychological development is altered. So this kind of explanation involves both a physical reduction (a change in brain structure) and a reconstruction (an alteration in neurocomputation that changes behavior).

Such an integrated explanation begins to solve the mind–body problem, at least for one aspect of mind. One aspect of conscious visual experience, stereopsis, is explained by an anatomical feature of the brain (ocular dominance columns) and the computations it permits. (A philosopher would object, of course, that this explanation does not tell us why or how a stereoscopic representation of the visual world enters consciousness. How consciousness arises and why we have it are the really hard parts of the mind–body problem, ones that I certainly do not claim to solve.) As we see later, we do not have as complete an explanation of any psychopathology as we have for either the failure of stereopsis given binocular deprivation, or the executive deficits found in early-treated phenylketonuria. But these examples can help us evaluate how close we are to adequate explanations. Indeed, just as in the stereopsis example, there are also critical or sensitive periods in infant development for input from the social environment. Although we do not know exactly which neural networks are involved, we do know that early environmental input is necessary for the development of emotion regulation and empathy, which are crucial for mental health.

There are undoubtedly many other genetic and environmental mechanisms underlying brain development. For instance, work is under way to identify other candidate genes that affect brain development (Vicente et al., 1997) and to test whether these genes influence behavioral disorders. I next consider methods for studying brain mechanisms in psychopathology.

As mentioned earlier, many potential brain mechanisms explain alterations in behavioral development, some concerning the large-scale structure of the brain and others the structure at the level of individual neurons and synapses. The overall conceptual point to bear in mind is that it is currently very much an open question as to which level of brain structure and function is most relevant for understanding many psychopathologies. With the advent of these modern techniques, many brain variables can be studied, but there are many fewer theoretical constraints on which variables are relevant for the development of psychopathology than exist at the cognitive or even genetic levels of analysis. Moreover, unlike genes, all of these brain variables may be changed by the individual's environment. So, if a group with a psychopathology differs from controls on some brain variable, all we know is that we have potentially identified a brain correlate of the disorder. This correlate may be a by-product of a difference in some other brain variable that is causal in the disorder, or it may be produced by the different experiences encountered by individuals with this particular disorder, rather than being directly involved in pathogenesis. Thus, while modern neuroimaging techniques represent unprecedented advances in our ability to study the brain noninvasively, important conceptual and technical limitations remain.

The methods that are used to study brain mechanisms in psychopathology can be broadly divided into those that focus on lesions, neurochemistry, and neuroimaging. All three methods may be utilized in human or animal models. In humans, a case–control design is employed, so that, as discussed earlier, the manipulation of having a naturally acquired lesion or psychopathology is only quasi-experimental. In animal models, the lesion or the modeled cause of the psychopathology is experimentally manipulated, thus permitting stronger inferences about brain–behavior relations. I briefly describe lesion and neurochemical studies, then devote more time to neuroimaging studies.

Lesion Studies

A lesion study examines changes in behavior after a particular part of brain is damaged or removed; these changes are typically observed after recovery from the acute effects of the lesion. A simple but misleading assumption, often implicit in the interpretation of lesion studies, is the subtraction assumption, namely, that the functioning of the brain after damage is equal to its functioning before damage *minus* the functions of the damaged part. In other words, the subtraction assumption holds that brain functions are localized and additive. If brain functions are neither localized nor additive, then the subtraction assumption is wrong, and the interpretation of lesion studies becomes more complicated. If the brain is a highly interactive dynamic system, then damage to one part will alter the interactions of all the other parts, making it much more difficult to infer the normal function of the part that was damaged. Problems with the subtraction assumption in psychological experiments were pointed out by Donders more than 100 years ago, yet these problems remain important issues in modern neuroscience, affecting the interpretation of both lesion and neuroimaging studies. Converging evidence from these two kinds of studies provides strong support for the conclusion that a particular part of the brain is necessary for a given function, but it does not demonstrate that it is sufficient for that function.

There are further problems with studies of naturally occurring lesions in humans, including the typical lack of detailed measures of behavior before the lesion and the difficulty inherent in determining exactly what parts of brain were damaged by an accidental lesion. Despite these important caveats, lesion studies by neuropsychologists have convincingly demonstrated that there is some specialization of function in the brain and have provided us with a rough map of structure–function relations. Moreover, some of the symptoms observed after lesions resemble those found in psychopathology; I review lesion data relevant to specific psychopathologies in Chapters 3–5.

Neurochemical Studies

Neurochemical studies either measure or manipulate levels of a given neurochemical to test its relation to behavior. I first briefly explain the relevant neurochemicals and then discuss methods for testing their influence on behavior.

For the nervous system to function, there must be communication between cells, both within the nervous system (between neurons) and between the nervous system and the rest of the body (e.g., between a peripheral nerve and a muscle fiber). This communication is accomplished by chemical messengers (neurotransmitters and neuromodulators) that are released by one cell and bind to receptors on another, like a key in a lock.

Figure 7 depicts a synapse with receptors and neurotransmitters, and illustrates several of the ways that the amount of neurotransmitter available at the synapse can be manipulated by medications. A medication can inhibit (or accelerate) the degradation of neurotransmitter by enzymes in the presynaptic neuron (Panel A, Figure 7). For instance, the earliest antidepressants inhibited the action of monoamine oxidase and were thus called monoamine oxidase inhibitors (MAOIs). A medication can also inhibit or facilitate the binding of a neurotransmitter to a receptor on the postsynaptic neuron (Panel B, Figure 7). To understand the third way a medication can manipulate neurotransmitter levels, it is important to notice that there are also receptors on the presynaptic neuron that play a role in regulating neurotransmission. Some of these presynaptic receptors are involved in the process of reuptake of neurotransmitters (Panel C, Figure 7). Inhibiting reuptake is one way to increase the amount of neurotransmitter available at a synapse. So Prozac is a selective serotonin reuptake inhibitor (SSRI). Finally, the binding of a neurotransmitter to some postsynaptic receptors releases a G protein that sets off a cascade of "second messenger"

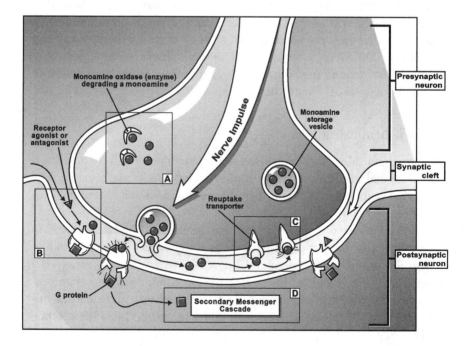

FIGURE 7. Neurotransmission at the synapse.

reactions (Panel D, Figure 7). Manipulating these second messenger re-actions is yet another way to alter neurotransmission with medications.

Once binding between a neurotransmitter and a receptor occurs, changes in the physical shape of the receptor lead to chemical changes in the cell of which the receptor is a part. Anything that can bind to a receptor is called a *ligand*. Ligands include not only neurotransmitters and neuromodulators (of course) but also similar but not identical molecules that can modify intracellular communication by binding (sometimes partially) to receptors. For instance, such a ligand can block a receptor without causing a complete change in shape, just as a "bad" key can fit into a lock without turning it. In this case, we call the ligand an "antagonist" because it interferes with the normal function of the receptor. Many natural toxins (e.g., curare and snake venom) work in just this way; they are potent antagonists that block neurotransmission in circuits involved in vital functions, such as breathing. Ligands can also bind to parts of receptors in a way that facilitates neurotransmission, in which case we call them agonists. For example, the benzodiazepines (e.g., Valium) used to treat anxiety disorders are agonists of GABA (gamma-aminobutyric acid) neurotransmission; they bind to GABA receptors in a way that facilitates neurotransmission. Since GABA is one of the main inhibitory neurotransmitters in the brain, these particular agonists increase inhibition of neuronal firing and thus produce a calming effect.

So what is the difference between a neurotransmitter, such as GABA, and a neuromodulator, such as cortisol, or an endogenous opiate (such as an endorphin)? First of all, there is not a sharp boundary between these concepts, because some neurotransmitters have modulatory effects (e.g., dopamine). Typically, a neurotransmitter is a smaller molecule, either an amino acid (e.g., GABA or glutamate) or something derived from a single amino acid (hence "monoamine," such as dopamine). Neurotransmitters generally act quickly at a synapse to change cellular functions (e.g., help cause a neuron to fire or a muscle fiber to contract). Neuromodulators may act at the synapse, or elsewhere, and be carried in the bloodstream; they act more slowly than neurotransmitters to regulate the state of a system. The next distinction, between intrinsic and extrinsic neurotransmitters, will, I hope, clarify the boundary between neurotransmitters and neuromodulators.

The rapid and precise neurotransmission required by neural networks to process information is accomplished by excitatory (mainly glutamate, but also aspartate) and inhibitory (mainly GABA, but also

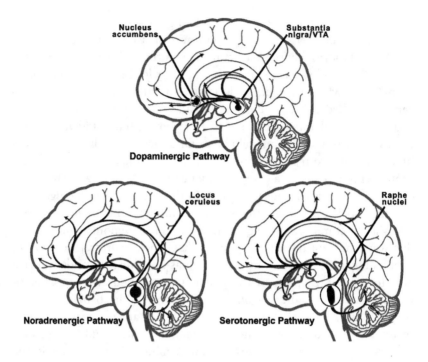

FIGURE 8. Extrinsic neurotransmitter pathways.

glycine) neurotransmitters. Each of these neurotransmitters is an amino acid. These intrinsic neurotransmitters bind to ligand-gated receptors, causing a pore or channel in the receptor itself to open, thus letting in positive or negative ions, thereby quickly changing the electrical potential of the postsynaptic neuron.

A slower modulation of the function of whole networks is accomplished by extrinsic neurotransmitters that are released by groups or neurons (nuclei) that mainly have their cell bodies in the brainstem, but whose axons project up into the neocortex, limbic system, and basal ganglia (Figure 8). So both motivation and action selection, as well as perception, can be modulated by these extrinsic neurotransmitters. Most of these extrinsic neurotransmitters are derived from single amino acids (they are monoamines) supplied by food. The catecholamines (they all share a catechol nucleus in their chemical structure) all derive from the amino acid tyrosine. There are three catecholamines: dopamine, norepinephrine (also called noradrenaline), and epinephrine (also called adrenaline). Dopamine is released by two sets of brainstem nuclei, the substantia nigra and the ventral tegmental area. Very roughly speaking, dopamine modulates reward detection and approach behavior. Norepinephrine is released by the locus ceruleus; again, roughly speaking, it coordinates behavioral arousal in response to stress. Serotonin is formed from the amino acid tryptophan and is released by the raphe nuclei. Very broadly speaking, it has a stabilizing effect on neurotransmission. A final important extrinsic neurotransmitter is acetylcholine, which is derived from choline and released by nuclei in the basal forebrain.

But it is a reification either to ascribe a single function to these extrinsic neurotransmitters or to localize the cause of a given disorder to a putative excess or deficiency of one of them, because there are multiple tracts and receptor types for these extrinsic neurotransmitters, and extrinsic neurotransmitter systems interact with each other. The same extrinsic neurotransmitter may thus act in an inhibitory fashion in one location and in an excitatory fashion in another.

Because of large diurnal and episodic fluctuations in the levels of neurochemicals, and because many neurochemicals are produced both in the brain and in the rest of the body, measuring levels of neurochemicals in groups with different psychopathologies has been difficult. Invasive procedures, such as a spinal tap, have been required to sample central as opposed to peripheral neurochemicals but can only be ethically justified in certain situations. Even with such invasive procedures, the presence of other, large sources of variation has often made it difficult to detect variation related to the psychopathology in question. These ethical and methodological problems are more pronounced in the study of children with psychopathology, where development adds yet another source of variation. Manipulation of the level of a given neurochemical by administration of a drug (e.g., Ritalin [methylphenidate], which is a dopamine agonist) gets around some of these problems and can be a powerful test of a hypothesized relation between a brain variable and a behavior, especially if the manipulation is parametric and dose–response relation is found. I review relevant neurochemical studies in Chapters 3–5 on specific psychopathologies but next turn to neuroimaging methods.

Neuroimaging may be broadly divided into methods that measure brain structure and brain function. Except for electroencephalography and evoked potential measures, neuroimaging methods are relatively new and have dramatically increased our ability to study relations between brain and behavior.

Structural Neuroimaging

The main, current method of structural neuroimaging is magnetic resonance imaging (MRI). An MRI scanner consists essentially of a tube inside a very strong electromagnet, along with some sophisticated recording equipment. The electromagnet produces transient pulses of a strong magnetic field, which induces magnetic resonance in the hydrogen atoms in the subject's brain (or other tissues). As these hydrogen atoms relax from this state of resonance, they release energy that is detected by the recording equipment. Amazingly, the shape of the underlying brain structure can be reconstructed from these energy values. Because different tissues in the brain or the rest of the body differ in their water (H_2O) content, they also differ in their density of hydrogen atoms, and thus in the amount of energy they release as their hydrogen atoms relax from resonance. At every point in the circumference of a circle around a subject's body, the energy released will differ somewhat as a function of the density of tissues lying on a diameter line below that point. The set of energy values for all the points in the circumference uniquely specifies the shape of the structure in that slice. Hounsfield (1979) ingeniously devised a mathematical algorithm for reconstructing the underlying structure from the circumferential energy values, for which he won the Nobel Prize. Once the shape of structures is specified, semiautomated methods outline particular structures and compute their area or volume. One problem with such methods is the considerable degree of variability across subjects' brain anatomy, so that we cannot always be confident that a given anatomic definition is identifying the same structure across subjects. Moreover, even with a similar structural anatomy, the areas activated by a given task may vary across subjects. Although this variability does not invalidate the method, it undoubtedly adds noise to group studies and contributes to some of the differences in results across studies. Despite this problem, there is some degree of convergence for some disorders on which brain structures are most involved. Notice that if brain structure is only a weak correlate of the underlying brain pathogenesis, then we would expect less agreement across structural studies. This could be a reason why brain structure results are less consistent for some disorders than for others.

Functional Neuroimaging

Functional neuroimaging measures brain activity during performance of a task by either recording the brain's electrical activity (by means of electroencephalography, or EEG), the magnetic fields generated by that activity (by means of magnetoencephalography or MEG), or measuring the changes in the flow of blood, glucose, or oxygen that are closely correlated with neuronal activity in a particular brain region. Examples of the latter type of measures include positron emission tomography (PET) and functional magnetic resonance imaging (fMRI). Both PET and fMRI use the mathematical algorithms described earlier to reconstruct the location of metabolic changes associated with task performance throughout the whole brain.

All of these techniques have different strengths and weaknesses in terms of spatial and temporal resolution. EEG or MEG studies of activity changes evoked by stimuli and tasks have excellent temporal resolution, on the order of milliseconds. But neither method is good for localizing activity changes below the cortical surface, and only MEG accurately localizes activity from the cortical surface. The temporal resolution of PET is roughly a minute and that of fMRI, a few seconds. The spatial resolution of each is measured in millimeters, with fMRI providing better spatial resolution than PET.

A good overview of both the technical and theoretical aspects of fMRI can be found in Cohen, Noll, and Schneider (1993). Sarter, Bernston, and Cacioppo (1996) provide a broad discussion of some of the important conceptual issues involved in interpreting functional neuroimaging studies, including the subtraction assumption discussed earlier (see also Van Orden & Paap, 1997) and the possibility that the mapping between brain structure and function may be very complex, limiting the ability to localize functions. Thus, while we may find functional neuroimaging differences between cases with a given psychopathology and controls, what those differences mean in terms of the functions of neural circuits is much less clear.

Despite these technical and theoretical limitations, modern functional neuroimaging studies (using mainly PET or fMRI) have provided a wealth of exciting new information about brain systems important for psychopathologies. Indeed, a book such as this would hardly be possible without this new information. For each psychopathology reviewed later, I consider what we have learned from structural and functional neuroimaging studies, and discuss how these findings contribute to our understanding of the disorder.

NEUROPSYCHOLOGY

This next level of analysis is concerned with identifying underlying functional deficits that explain the symptoms that define psychopathologies, and eventually explaining those functional deficits in terms of both etiological and brain mechanisms. Underlying functions may be cognitive processes, such as action selection or attention or memory, but may also include processes not usually thought of as cognitive, such as mood regulation or empathy. So the domain of neuropsychology is hardly fixed; rather, it continues to expand as we learn more about the brain bases of species-typical human functions. All of these functions are neuropsychological because they are mediated by the brain, perhaps by specialized circuits. It is important to emphasize that this level of analysis is different from that of observable behaviors (Morton & Frith, 1995), even though we must use behavioral tests to make inferences about the intactness of underlying functions. Since there are multiple determinants of a given behavior, converging evidence across different designs is needed to make an inference about the causal role of an underlying neuropsychological function in producing that behavioral symptom, as I discuss shortly.

The value of this level of analysis lies in its theoretical strength and parsimony. Due to the efforts of cognitive and developmental psychologists, our theories about underlying functions are much stronger than theories about brain mechanisms. With a small number of underlying functions, we can construct testable explanations for a broad range of behaviors. So one chief goal of neuropsychological research on developmental psychopathologies is to identify an underlying functional deficit or set of deficits that explain the behavioral symptoms that define the disorder. It is important to bear in mind that it may not be just a single functional deficit. It may take the interaction of two or three functional deficits to produce the full syndrome picture, or there may be subtypes of the same behaviorally defined disorder, each with different underlying functional deficits. Most importantly, a single neurobiological cause (e.g., a neurotransmitter deficiency) will likely affect several neuropsychological functions. Before proceeding to discuss neuropsychological systems involved in psychopathology, it is important to discuss briefly how neural network models may help us to bridge the psychological and brain levels of analysis.

As noted in the previous section, one important gap in our integrated account of psychopathologies is the lack of a strong theory for relating brain structure and function to these underlying psychological functions. This gap, of course, is due to the formidable mind–body problem. Basically, we need an intermediate level of analysis between brain structure and physiology on the one hand and psychological functions on the other. Computational neuroscientists are beginning to provide this level of analysis with research on artificial neural networks. Through the interaction of idealized neurons, these networks learn and perform the input-to-output mappings that implement psychological functions. Moreover, these functioning networks can be "lesioned," and the performance of the lesioned network can be compared with that of patients with deficits acquired as a result of brain damage. More relevant for understanding the development of psychopathology are manipulations of the network architecture before learning takes place (see Oliver, Johnson, Karmiloff-Smith, & Pennington, 2000). Such neural network models of a few developmental psychopathologies have been implemented; I review these in Chapters 3–5 on specific disorders. These models must build on a fairly mature understanding of the neuropsychology of a disorder, which must be developed through studies of patients and their relatives. Later in this section, I discuss the designs used to gain that mature understanding. Such a computational model provides a rigorous, specific implementation of a theory and often leads to novel predictions about actual behavior. In the future, as these artificial networks become more realistic, it may be possible to relate their functions to those of actual neural networks, and thus build stronger theories of how the changes in brain development produce changes in psychological development that underlie the symptoms of a disorder. In what follows, I next consider which neuropsychological systems are most relevant for understanding psychopathology.

Very broadly, one may follow Luria (1966) and divide the human central nervous system into three functional systems: (1) the arousal/motivation system, which has cortical, limbic, and brainstem components; (2) the perception/memory system, consisting chiefly of the posterior neocortex and the hippocampal formation; and (3) the action selection system, consisting chiefly of the frontal neocortex, the basal ganglia, and parts of the thalamus. Figure 9 is a schematic of these three functional systems. If one imagines this figure superimposed on a side view of the human brain, then there is a rough anatomical correspondence between each system in the figure and the parts of the brain that belong to it. Interactions between systems subserve psychological functions; some illustrative examples are used to label the arrows connecting systems. For instance, representations generated in posterior cortex are "transmitted" to prefrontal cortex, where they are maintained in active working memory. These same representations, when transmitted to the motivation system, permit emotional conditioning.

Obviously, this model is a simplification because of the high degree of interactivity of the human brain and organism; for example, the arousal/motivation system reaches outside of the central nervous system to the endocrine and peripheral nervous systems. The three systems interact with each other, so a neat line cannot be drawn between them. But this simplistic model does provide a useful starting point for understanding the brain bases of psychopathology.

Of these three systems, the two most important for the development of psychopathology are the arousal/motivation system and the action selection system. Psychopathology is traditionally defined as disturbances of mood, behavior, and thought. As we will see, action selection and thought selection are intimately related; thus, our two brain systems cover the three traditional domains of psychopathology. Chapters 3–5, which discuss specific developmental psychopathologies, are organized around these brain systems. The point of this organization is to suggest how our classification of psychopathologies would look if it were based on pathophysiology rather than on symptoms. So disorders of arousal/motivation include depression and dysthymia, bipolar illness, anxiety disorders, and posttraumatic stress disorder. Disorders of action selection include attention-deficit/hyperactivity disorder, conduct disorder, Tourette syndrome, obsessive–compulsive disorder, schizophrenia, and possibly autism. However, I must admit that neither autism nor schizophrenia fits neatly into this classification system, because each includes disturbances in all three areas of function: motivation, action selection, and perception/memory.

Disorders of perception and memory include mental retardation syndromes and developmental language disorders, including dyslexia, which are not always thought of as psychopathologies but undoubtedly influence the development of mood, behavior, and thought.

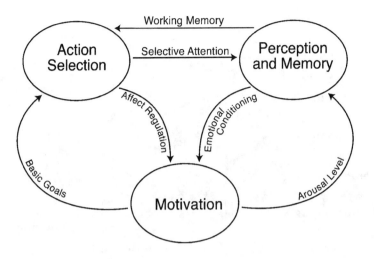

FIGURE 9. Neuropsychological systems.

Figure 10, a medial view of the human brain, shows the location of the main cortical and subcortical structures important for psychopathology (i.e., those in the motivation and action selection systems). The orbitofrontal cortex, amygdala, hypothalamus, and pituitary gland are all important structures in the motivation system. The entire prefrontal cortex (dorsolateral, medial, and orbital), the basal ganglia (which include the caudate nucleus, the putamen, and the globus pallidus [not shown in the figure]), and the thalamus are important structures in the action selection system. Structures that mediate between the motivation and action selection systems include the orbitofrontal cortex, which is part of both systems, and the anterior cingulate gyrus, which plays a role in both emotional arousal and attention. In the following two sections, I discuss the functions of these and other structures involved in motivation and action selection.

Motivation System

The motivation system accomplishes one of the key adaptive tasks for any behaving organism, which is to allow goals and values to influence both perception and action selection rapidly and to adjust motivational state to fit changing environmental circumstances. In other words, the motivation system must interact with the action selection system to per-

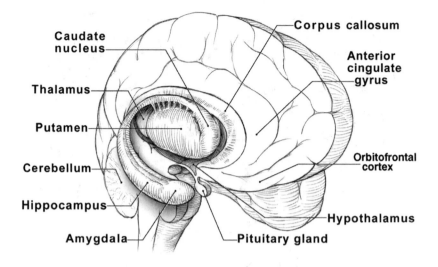

FIGURE 10. Brain structures involved in psychopathology.

mit rapid selection of adaptive actions *and* flexible responses to ever-changing contexts. These two goals are partly in conflict. Rapidity could be maximized by a hardwired system, with an invariant link between motivational states and specific actions, a situation found in simpler organisms and part of the evolutionary core of our own brains. Flexibility might be maximized by a completely open system, which would, however, face a combinational explosion, with every possible action a candidate for every possible context. So some kind of compromise is needed. Because evolution is conservative, this compromise has likely been accomplished by adding new brain structures to modify the functions of older ones rather than radically redesigning the whole brain.

So we can think of the motivation system in the primate brain as consisting of levels or layers, somewhat like an onion. Rolls (1999) and Panksepp (1998), among others, have reviewed research on the function of different levels of the motivation system. Here, we briefly consider three levels: brainstem, limbic, and cortical (Figure 11). Figure 11 identifies some of the relevant brain structures and the main function of each level. At the lowest level, nuclei send diffuse projections up to higher levels and release modulatory, extrinsic neurotransmitters, as discussed earlier in the neurochemical section. Thus, the locus ceruleus (LC) releases norepinephrine, the ventral tegmental area (VTA) and the substantia nigra (SN) release dopamine, and the raphe nuclei (RN) release serotonin (see also Figure 8). These extrinsic neurotransmitters adjust arousal in the rest of the brain to match current goals. Also, circuits in the midbrain and brainstem mediate automatic behavioral responses to primary reinforcers, such as a sweet or bitter taste. Such responses come close to being innate. At the two higher levels, structures modify these automatic motivational responses. For instance, at the limbic level, the amygdala allows the rapid extraction of valence from environmental input and the learning of associations between primary and secondary reinforcers, but it is slow to unlearn these associations (LaBar & LeDoux, 1997). At the highest level, the orbitofrontal cortex (OFC) is specialized for rapidly reversing the link between reinforcers and actions as the context changes (Rolls, 1999). In summary, there are virtually innate motivational states mediated by the lowest level of the system in the brainstem. This motivational core is amplified by emotional learning, mediated in part by the amygdala. The motivational learning of the amygdala is rapid, which can be important for survival, but not flexible, which can be disadvantageous (as we will see when we consider mood and anxiety disorders). Finally, the OFC provides a way to inhibit or reverse motivated behaviors mediated by the lower structures.

Thus, as will be further elaborated, affective neuroscience has made

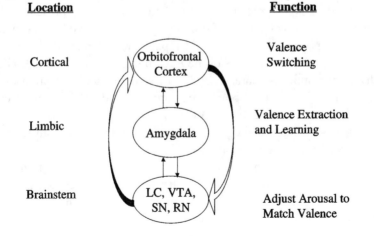

FIGURE 11. Three levels of the motivation system. LC, locus ceruleus; VTA, ventral tegmental area; SN, substantia nigra; RN, raphe nucleus.

considerable recent progress in delineating more completely the brain structures involved in motivation. It is also worth emphasizing that the term "motivation," as used here, is broader than the terms "emotion" or "affect." So hunger, thirst, and pain are all examples of motivational states as are the emotions of joy and fear. "Emotion," in turn, as used here, is broader than the term "affect." Affect, arousal with a positive or negative valence, is a component of emotion, which has the additional components of subjective experience and facial expression. These distinct facial expressions serve in part as social signals (they may also serve less social functions, such as preparation for actions such as looking or biting). Nonetheless, what is striking at the brain level is the *commonalities* among circuits for both emotions and other motivational states. For instance, work on the negative emotion, disgust, suggests that the neuropsychology of taste may have much in common with the neuropsychology of moral aversion (Rozin, Haidt, & McCauley, 2000). Let us now consider the structures in the three levels of the motivation system in more detail.

Brainstem and Midbrain Level

At this level, midbrain circuits in the periaqueductal gray (PAG) matter and the parabrachial nucleus of the pons mediate core affective responses. Brainstem nuclei control arousal level in the brain by releasing extrinsic neurotransmitters. (I discussed extrinsic neurotransmitters in the preceding Neurobiology section.) Panksepp (1998) presented data supporting the involvement of different parts of the PAG in seven core affective responses: seeking, rage, fear, panic, lust, care, and play. Stimulation of these different parts of the PAG in experimental animals elicits behavioral responses characteristic of these core affective responses. Of course, these low-level responses are regulated and amplified by circuits in the limbic and cortical levels of the motivation system. Nonetheless, as is discussed later, some of these midbrain circuits are sufficient to produce a basic affective response.

Turning now to the brainstem nuclei, the three monoamine (i.e., derived from one amino acid) neurotransmitters—norepinephrine, serotonin, and dopamine—are of particular importance for disorders of affect regulation. As discussed earlier, each of these extrinsic neurotransmitters is released by the axons of different brainstem nuclei (LC, VTA, SN, and RN in Figure 11); these axons project widely throughout the brain. Of great relevance for understanding disorders of affect regulation is the fact that both norepinephrine and serotonin-producing neurons synapse on the amygdala and the hypothalamus, among other structures. Therefore, manipulating norepinephrine and serotonin levels (e.g., by means of drugs or diet) can change the function of these two structures that play a central role in regulating emotions.

Limbic Level

There are three structures at the limbic level: the amygdala, the hypothalamus, and the nucleus accumbens. The *amygdala*, just one synapse away from the thalamus, through which most sensory inputs pass, can therefore mobilize a rapid response to some sensory inputs, without waiting for slower cortical processing of the input. The amygdala is well positioned to coordinate emotional responses, because it regulates the autonomic nervous system, partly through connections to the hypothalamus, and because it sends projections to all areas of the cortex, providing an emotional influence on cortical processing (Bownds, 1999). The amygdala's role in negative emotion has been most extensively studied and is clearly documented as necessary for the classical conditioning of a fear response (including an autonomic response) to a previously neutral stimulus. Such fear conditioning can occur rapidly (hence, it is called one-trial learning) and has obvious relevance to the development of anxiety symptoms, such as those seen in specific phobias and posttraumatic stress disorder. The conditioned fear response may be extinguished (which has obvious relevance for the treatment of phobias). Animals or humans without an amygdala cannot acquire a new conditioned fear response (LaBar & LeDoux, 1997), although they can still generate an autonomic fear response to aversive events. Extinction of a conditioned fear response depends on cortical inhibition (e.g., by the orbitofrontal cortex), rather than weakening of synaptic connections within the amygdala itself. Therefore, lessening cortical inhibition could cause reemergence of conditioned fear responses, a mechanism that might help explain some aspects of anxiety disorders (Bownds, 1999).

The *hypothalamus* helps coordinate rapid behavioral expression of emotional and motivational states, and provides a key link between brain and body. Electrical stimulation of the lateral hypothalamus elicits different appetitive behaviors related to sex, thirst, hunger, and temperature regulation. The hypothalamus accomplishes its regulation of the sympathetic nervous system through the hypothalamic–pituitary–

adrenal (HPA) and the sympatho–adreno–medullary (SAM) axes, which are crucial to the stress response system (Chrousos & Gold, 1992; Gold, Goodwin, & Chrousos, 1988a, 1988b), and important for understanding the symptoms of mood and anxiety disorders (Figure 12). The hypothalamus activates the SAM axis by means of the vagus nerve in the spinal cord; the SAM is able to act within seconds to generate a short-term stress response. The vagus nerve also connects to a separate, ancient nervous system in the gut, the enteric nervous system, which has receptors for the major extrinsic neurotransmitters (norepinephrine, dopamine, and serotonin) discussed earlier. The anxiety symptom of "butterflies in your stomach" can be explained in part by this vagal connection to the enteric nervous system. The HPA axis takes minutes to activate and mediates a longer term stress response, lasting hours and days. It regulates the release of cortisol, whereas the SAM axis regulates the release of epinephrine and norepinephrine, each from different parts of the adrenal glands. These axes consist of bidirectional connections that, under normal circumstances, act as a negative feedback loop to stop the release of these messengers that activate the autonomic and central nervous systems, and thereby terminate the stress response. However, if these axes become dysregulated, the stress response is not terminated, and the individual is subject to the persistent state of negative arousal that in somewhat different ways characterizes both anxiety and depression. Dysregulation of yet a third hypothalamic axis, the hypothalamic–thyroid–adrenal (HTA) axis, is also important for understanding aspects of depression.

Whereas the amygdala mainly mediates negative affect, the *nucleus accumbens* (NA), the third limbic structure, is involved in positive affect and approach behavior. It lies just below the prefrontal cortex (see Figure 8) and is sometimes considered part of the ventral striatum (Depue & Iacono, 1989), that is, the limbic portion of the basal ganglia. This limbic portion of the seeking/expectancy affective circuit identified by Panksepp (1998) receives dopaminergic input from the VTA and also has close connections with the prefrontal cortex. It has turned out to be an important structure in the neurobiology of addiction and could well play a role in other psychopathologies that involve too much reward seeking (e.g., mania and attention-deficit/hyperactivity disorder).

Cortical Level

The amygdala and other parts of the limbic system interact closely with the *orbitofrontal cortex* (OFC), which is one part of prefrontal cortex.

Various parts of prefrontal cortex maintain different kinds of information in active or working memory to guide action selection; the kind of information depends on reciprocal connections to other parts of the cortex and limbic system (Goldman-Rakic, 1987b). Thus, dorsolateral prefrontal cortex maintains spatial information in working memory through its extensive reciprocal connections with the parietal cortex. The OFC, through its extensive reciprocal connections with the limbic system, can be thought of as maintaining motivational information in working memory. So this structure likely plays a key role in the conscious or subjective experience of emotion. Crucially, unlike the amygdala, the OFC can rapidly switch motivational contingencies, permitting flexibility in motivated behavior (see Rolls, 1999). More specifically, as reviewed in Goldman-Rakic (1987b), the connectivity of the OFC supports a role in both the motivation and the action selection systems. The OFC receives inputs from distinct thalamic nuclei, the olfactory system, the amygdala, and the temporal pole and entorhinal temporal cortex, which mediate the processing of high-level object representations. Thus, the OFC has connections that permit it to assign and switch motivational valence to highly processed representations of

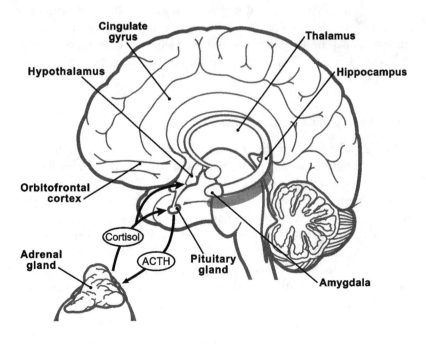

FIGURE 12. Hypothalamic–pituitary–adrenal axis.

input (Rolls, 1999). Its descending projection to a cholinergic nucleus in the basal forebrain permits the OFC to regulate its own arousal level and that of other parts of the brain. It also connects with distinct parts of the caudate nucleus, providing a role in action and thought selection (this orbital–caudate circuit plays a role in obsessions and compulsions, as I discuss later). Finally, through its connections with the autonomic nervous system, stimulation of the OFC can cause changes in cardiac and respiratory function.

Damasio (1994) has developed a theory of "somatic markers" to explain the function of the OFC. In this theory, the OFC is important because it quickly attaches an emotional "tag" to each ever-changing context, which is an important input into selecting a response to that context. These tags are called "somatic markers." Lack of a system that provides a fast, "gut-level" sense of what to do next, and what to avoid, results in harmful errors, and action selection can become too slow and deliberate. Human patients with orbital lesions have trouble making very simple, everyday decisions, such as selecting a restaurant, and they also make disastrous errors in judgment. When tested physiologically in a gambling paradigm, unlike controls, they neither avoid high-risk conditions nor do they generate an autonomic response to these conditions.

We now consider several key issues regarding the motivation system, all of which are important for understanding its role in the development of psychopathology, including (1) how this system develops, (2) its relation to consciousness, and (3) how it "solves" the mind–body problem.

Development of the Motivation System

With regard to development, the lowest level of the motivation system may be thought of as mediating basic, virtually innate mammalian behaviors, whereas higher levels mediate motivational learning and flexibility in motivated behavior. What evidence supports innate motivational behaviors? Experiments have identified key, low-level circuits necessary for core motivational responses, such as a facial reaction to a taste. These circuits include the PAG matter (Panksepp, 1998) and the parabrachial nucleus (PBN) of the pons (Berridge & Winkielman, in press). Stimulation of these structures by electrode or neurotransmitter microinjection is sufficient to trigger affective behavioral responses. If only these brainstem circuits are present, as occurs in an anencephalic infant or a decerebrate rat, a given taste can nonetheless produce a characteristic behavioral response (Berridge & Winkielman, in press). Moreover, across primate and mammalian species, similar facial reactions to sweet (i.e., tongue protrusions) and bitter (i.e., gaping and head shaking) tastes are observed. These facial reactions can also be observed in human infants, indicating that they develop very early.

Despite this evidence for innateness, the motivation system as a whole is an open and developing system that can be modified by both genetic and environmental influences. It is susceptible to environmental influences because its regulatory feedback loops extend into the social domain, such that relationships with others play a very important role in the regulation of mood and arousal. Research shows that early experiences of intense, unmodulated arousal have lasting effects on the nervous system, making it more vulnerable to mood dysregulation (Sanchez, Ladd, & Plotsky, 2001). It is clearly a developing system, because the young child's capacity for mood regulation changes dramatically over the first years of life and coping with stress is a lifelong developmental task. Individual differences in reactivity to stress and novelty are partly genetically influenced (Sanchez et al., 2001). One possible pathway through which these genetic influences might act is through structural differences in the protein receptors for the four extrinsic neurotransmitters mentioned earlier. DNA sequence differences in the genes that code for these receptor proteins could change the tertiary structure of the protein and thus affect how efficiently it binds to a neurotransmitter. In summary, in the case of the motivation system, individual differences in both genes and environments act on the *same* developing neural system to produce individual differences in a key psychological process for mental health, mood or affect regulation, particularly in response to stress.

Relation of the Motivation System to Consciousness

We now consider the relation of motivation to consciousness. Although psychology has traditionally required that the definition of an emotion include its being consciously experienced, recent evidence indicates that some unconscious motivational states may nonetheless affect both perception and action. Subliminal inductions of affective state (e.g., by a briefly presented emotional face) changed subjects' consumption of a flavored drink, *without* any changes in subjective reports of mood (Berridge & Winkielman, in press). In other words, the lower levels of the motivation system, such as the brainstem circuits and the amygdala, may operate to influence behavior *without* conscious awareness. Psychopathologists, beginning with Freud, have long recognized that unconscious motives can play an important role in abnormal behavior, but they lacked empirical methods for measuring this hypothetical construct. It is exciting that social neuroscience is beginning to provide these methods, so that we can soon objectively evaluate how much of a role unconscious affect plays in the development of psychopathology.

How Motivations Bridge Mind and Body

We now consider how the motivation system "solves" the mind–body problem. Part of this problem is artificial and derives from the latent dualism discussed earlier. From a monist or materialist perspective, mind is never separate from body, so no special mechanisms have to be invoked to account for the interactions between events we regard as "mental" and "physical" or bodily. Nonetheless, it is worth discussing the mechanisms that serve these interactions, which are perhaps most evident in the case of disorders of affect regulation, because symptoms of these disorders are both mental (changes in moods and cognitions) and physical (changes in appetite, sleep, heart rate, and immune functions). In addition, the risk factors are both genetic and environmental, and effective treatments are both psychological and pharmacological. Clearly, an adequate explanation of these disorders must be based on a system that permits intimate, bidirectional communication between phenomena that we typically (and wrongly) divide into the mental and physical categories.

The mind–body problem, as it applies to mood regulation, can be readily appreciated if we consider how quickly we blush or get sweaty palms in response to a thought about an imagined or recalled situation. How is it that a thought can change our heart rate, respiration, and so on? The mystery goes in the other direction as well. Alterations in parts of the endocrine system, for example, changes in thyroid function due to an autoimmune illness, can produce a negative mood and depressed thoughts.

To allow "mind" to talk to "body," and to allow "body" to talk to "mind," the different parts of the motivation system must be integrated in a bidirectional fashion. The different parts of the motivation system are a distributed network. The interactions among the components of this network regulate arousal level or mood, which is a coordinated response of *all* the systems involved. A mood is not just in one's mind or body; it is in both. To avoid substance dualism (and to solve Descartes' mediation problem), the parts of this system must have a shared, physical method of information exchange. Essentially, this means that there must be a mechanism of communication among cells in the brain, in the autonomic nervous system, and in the rest of the body. This mechanism is provided by a common set of (1) chemical messengers that either circulate in the bloodstream or are released by the synapses of neurons, and (2) receptors for the messengers in the membranes of these different kinds of cells. These messengers include neurotransmitters (e.g., norepinephrine and serotonin) and neuromodulators (e.g., hormones such as estrogen or cortisol, and neuropeptides such as endorphins). Some of these substances (e.g., norepinephrine) can serve in both roles, as neurotransmitters when released at the synapse, and as hormones when carried in the bloodstream. Receptors for these messengers are in both the brain and the body, such that behavior arises from brain–body interaction (Pert, 1997). So not only is it inaccurate to separate mind and body but it is also misleading to consider the central and autonomic nervous systems as acting separately of either each other or other systems (e.g., the immune system). The fact of bidirectional interaction among these systems has led to a new interdisciplinary field of study called "psychoneuroimmunology" (Booth & Pennebaker, 2000).

Given the multiple components of this system, a problem in the regulation of arousal and motivation could be due to dysfunction at a number of different levels. Cognitive factors could influence processing and appraisal. Neurotransmitter imbalances, perhaps due to genetically mediated changes in receptor properties, could dysregulate the system. Changes in orbital or amygdala functioning, perhaps due to early trauma, could have an impact. Or changes in endocrine function due to an autoimmune disease could change the function of the HPA or HTA axes. Despite these widely varying etiologies, the phenomenological experiences of the patients with each etiology would have some commonalities, because the same interdependent systems are disrupted.

Action Selection System

In addition to appraising the adaptive significance of the ever-changing environmental context and generating an appropriate motivational state, the organism must plan and execute actions to deal with that context. Especially in humans, these actions may be directed at a simulated, future context and may be in competition with motivations and actions evoked by the immediate context, thus giving rise to the distinctively human virtues of foresight, resistance to temptation, and courage.

How is action selection mediated by the brain? As mentioned earlier, at a computational level, one of the very difficult problems faced by an action selection system is the so-called "frame" problem. Since the range of possible actions is infinite, a computational device obviously cannot sort through all of them in real time. How can it narrow the range very quickly to a small, relevant list of alternatives? Humans effortlessly use a representation of the current reference frame or context to do this, but programming computers to solve this frame problem turns out to be very difficult. As Damasio (1994) and Rolls (1999) have argued, one important input to the human action selection system comes from the motivation system; the motivational state evoked by the current context quickly narrows the field of possible actions. Selection from that much narrower list becomes a tractable, computational problem. Anatomically, this must mean that there are extensive reciprocal connections between the two systems, some of which I have already described. Moreover, there is structural overlap, since the OFC is part of both systems.

Another important constraint on the action selection system is that while we can think of many possibilities rather quickly, we can generally only do one thing at a time, and to do it properly, some degree of monitoring is required. Launching competing actions at the same time or during the execution of another action will not do. Thus, while the brain is massively parallel, action is relentlessly serial. Step-by-step, we make our way through our lives, mostly doing one thing at a time. This second constraint means that action deselection must work closely with action selection; in other words, inhibition of irrelevant inputs and actions must be an important part of the action selection system. As we will see, there are important inhibitory connections within and between the structures that make up this system.

A final consideration is that the mechanisms involved in thought selection are quite similar to those involved in action selection. Many thoughts are candidate actions, plans to resolve real or imagined problems. So the circuits to be described next also play a role in pathologies of thought selection, such as those observed in depressive ruminations, the obsessions that characterize obsessive–compulsive disorder, and the delusions and hallucinations found in schizophrenia.

As mentioned earlier, three main brain structures interact in the action selection system: the frontal cortex, the basal ganglia, and the thalamus. The basal ganglia consists of the caudate nucleus and putamen (together called the striatum) and the globus pallidus.

As shown in simplified fashion in Figure 13, there are three broadly different action selection circuits or loops, each with feedforward connections from distinct parts of frontal cortex to distinct parts of the basal ganglia (i.e., different dorsal portions for the motor and cognitive loops, and ventral portions for the emotional loop). These in turn make feedforward connections to distinct parts of the thalamus (ventral lateral thalamus in the motor loop, ventral anterior thalamus in the cognitive loop, and the medial dorsal thalamus in the emotional loop). That part of the thalamus sends a feedback connection back to the particular part of prefrontal cortex (see Alexander, 1995; Casey, Durston, & Fosella, 2001; Mahurin, 1998, for more detailed discussions).

Each level of this system performs a somewhat different function. The prefrontal cortex mediates the highest level of planning in the brain, including long-range planning. It receives inputs from all the rest of the brain and is thus well-positioned anatomically to integrate current constraints on action selection so as to help select the action that best fits the current context. It exerts top-down control over primary and secondary frontal cortex and the basal ganglia and cerebellum, all of which are more directly tied to motor output. It also appears that memories of motor sequences are stored in these other structures, and under certain conditions, these automated sequences may be implemented as actions without prefrontal input. Different portions of the frontal cortex maintain different kinds of information about the current context in active or working memory and broadly plan actions appropriate to that context. In the cognitive loop, the relevant portion of prefrontal cortex is the dorsolateral prefrontal cortex (DLPFC). In the motor loop, it is the premotor cortex (PMC) and supplementary motor area (SMA). In the emotional loop, it is the OFC (especially its medial portion) and the anterior cingulate gyrus (ACG).

While integration and maintenance of evidence relevant to candidate actions are functions of the frontal cortex, selection or deselection of such actions depends on the next two levels of the system. The basal ganglia appear to be a high-threshold detection system for initiating actions (O'Reilly & Munakata, 2000). This is necessarily a conservative, high-threshold system, because actions are energetically expensive, and mistaken actions can have very negative adaptive consequences. When sufficient evidence accumulates that a given action is warranted, this threshold is met and circuits within the basal ganglia fire, leading to re-

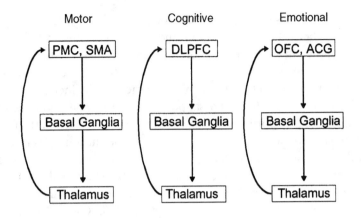

FIGURE 13. Three circuits in the action selection system.

duced thalamic inhibition of the given areas of prefrontal cortex. There are actually two opponent pathways within the basal ganglia. The first, just described, is called the "direct pathway" and facilitates action initiation. The second, called the "indirect pathway," has an opposite effect and inhibits candidate actions. In some disorders, this balance between initiation and inhibition is disturbed, and inappropriate actions are initiated.

Both the basal ganglia and frontal cortex receive dopaminergic input from the substantia nigra (SN) and ventral tegmental areas (VTA), with each loop receiving somewhat different inputs that serve to modulate the activity of particular action selection circuits. Alterations of these dopaminergic inputs, whether pathologically or therapeutically, will alter the action selection process. A dopamine deficit in the SN pathway leads to a paucity of action initiation in Parkinson's disease. Excess dopamine in the VTA input to the limbic loop is postulated to produce the delusions and hallucinations observed in schizophrenia.

From the foregoing discussion, it should be clear that pathologies of thought and action selection can involve either too little or too much inhibition, and can arise at various levels of the system. So failure of inhibitory control over automated action sequences is one mechanism for psychopathology and can be observed in hyperactivity, tics, compulsive actions, and impulsive antisocial behaviors.

However, to explain these disorders a simple inhibition deficit conceals an important problem. Such an explanation implies that all individuals are similar in their impulses, and that what distinguishes individuals is how successfully they inhibit inappropriate impulses. It seems unlikely that individuals have equivalent impulses to be overactive, to make motor tics, to wash their hands over and over, or to violate the rights of others! Moreover, it is difficult to verify empirically the existence of impulses not manifested in behavior. Instead of a simple inhibition explanation, it seems more likely that disinhibitory disorder results from a *combination* of stronger or different impulses *and* deficits in inhibition. Work is proceeding to map particular inhibitory pathologies onto deficits at different levels in different loops (see, e.g., Casey et al., 2001).

The action selection system, like the motivation system, is an open and developing system that can be modified by both genetic and environmental influences. It is open to the environment because actions are nearly always embedded in a social context that is either immediately present or simulated, so relationships help to regulate action selection, either quite directly in young children, or more indirectly in older children and adults. Moreover, one of the important functions of a protracted human childhood is to allow for the parental and cultural transmission of patterns of action. Obviously, action selection develops: from the infant, with little motor control except for eye movements; to the toddler, whose attempts at consolidating autonomous action control are evident in the "terrible twos"; to the domination of action selection by peer culture in middle childhood and early adolescence; and, we would hope, on to the more flexible and long-term patterns of action selection characteristic of adulthood. As we will see, there are genetically influenced individual differences in the action selection system. Again, one mechanism through which genes exert their influence is differences in receptors, especially dopamine receptors, which are more dense in the prefrontal cortex and basal ganglia. In summary, just as in the motivation system, both genes and environments act on the *same* developing neural system to produce individual differences in a key psychological process for mental health—action selection.

This concludes the description of the two neuropsychological systems most important for understanding psychopathology. I next turn to methods for studying neuropsychological functions.

Designs for Neuropsychological Studies

A neuropsychological understanding of a developmental psychopathology depends on a close, reciprocal interaction between research on normal neuropsychological development and work on disorders. The former provides models and paradigms for probing the basis of psychopathology; the results from studies of abnormality can, in turn, force revisions in our basic scientific understanding of normal function.

As useful as neuropsychology is for understanding developmental psychopathology, some important limitations in traditional neuropsychology need to be addressed. The first limitation was discussed earlier. Traditional neuropsychology has focused on the parts of the brain that are least relevant for understanding psychopathology. The neuropsychology of visual perception and long-term memory is much better developed than the neuropsychology of action selection or emotion regulation.

The second limitation is that traditional neuropsychology has not focused on development and has generally been too fixated on localization of function. But strong modularity theories (e.g., Fodor, 1983) that posit innate localized functions in the brain do not fit with what we know about brain development (see Elman et al., 1996, and Oliver et al., 2000). In addition, the main method for inferring localized functions (the double dissociation method) has serious logical problems (see Van Orden, Pennington, & Stone, 2001). It relies on contrasting patterns of deficits across "pure" cases. But there is not a theory-neutral way of defining pure cases, and the inference from a double dissociation to two independent modular functions presupposes that modules exist. Since such double dissociations can arise in a nonmodular cognitive system (e.g., a connectionist model), a finding of double dissociation does not prove modularity. I now turn to neuropsychological methods.

Neuropsychological research on a developmental psychopathology proceeds by addressing the following series of questions, with different designs appropriate for different questions:

1. What is the neuropsychological phenotype of adults with the disorder (case–control studies of adults)?
2. Which aspects of that phenotype are specific to the disorder (mental-age-level designs and designs contrasting disorders)?
3. How does the phenotype change with development, and which aspects of that phenotype are a consequence of the disorder (cross-sectional and longitudinal designs, and studies of compensated individuals or those with subclinical variants)?
4. If the disorder is familial, which aspects of the phenotype are familial (family studies)?
5. If the disorder is genetically influenced, which aspects of the

familial phenotype are genetically influenced (twin, adoption, and molecular studies)?

6. Does a specific neuropsychological deficit cause the symptoms of the disorder (treatment studies and animal models)?

Case–Control Studies

The initial phase of a neuropsychological investigation of a developmental psychopathology is necessarily exploratory and descriptive. Partly because measures have been more available for adults, this initial phase often compares adult cases with the disorder and control subjects without it on a broad range of neuropsychological measures. Cases and controls should be otherwise comparable on demographic variables such as age, gender, ethnicity, and parental social class. If we matched cases and controls according to their own social class, we might create an artifact, since having a developmental psychopathology often lowers individuals' educational and occupational attainment. The main goal of this design is to limit the field of candidate deficits. If we find that cases and controls do not differ on some neuropsychological domains, then those domains are unlikely to be related to the development of the disorder, as long as the measures utilized are psychometrically appropriate (in terms of reliability and sensitivity) for the groups studied. (Such unaffected domains could nonetheless represent areas of compensation or enhanced development in the disorder and thus provide clues for understanding the development of the disorder.) However, this design does not tell us why the two groups differ in the domains for which we find positive results. These aspects of the neuropsychological phenotype could be consequences or correlates of having this disorder, or a developmental disorder in general, or they could be the cause of the disorder. To address these possibilities, other designs are needed.

Besides missing potential confounds, matching and covarying each have other problems that merit mention. Matching can lead to a regression artifact that may produce spurious positive results. Say, for example, we are comparing a group with autism to a group without autism, both randomly selected from the population, to test the hypothesis that a verbal memory deficit is associated with autism. The group with autism will have a lower mean IQ than the group without autism, because about 75% of children with autism have mental retardation. If we match a subset of each group on IQ, then the subset with autism will of necessity have a higher mean IQ than the remaining sample with autism, and the IQ-matched subset without autism will necessarily have a lower mean IQ than the remaining sample without autism. Verbal memory measures are correlated with IQ (in fact, virtually any cognitive or neuropsychological measure is correlated with IQ). Because of this correlation, the mean of each subset on the verbal memory measure will regress back toward the mean of the sample from which it was drawn; thus, the subset with autism will obtain a mean verbal memory score that is lower than its mean IQ, and the subset without autism will obtain a mean score that is higher. Hence, the regression artifact will produce the predicted group difference on the dependent variable!

Covarying avoids the regression artifact but makes certain assumptions about the relation between the dependent variable and the covariate, namely, that the relation is linear and similar in both groups. If these assumptions are not met, then covarying may not remove the effects of the covariate. A further problem with covarying a potentially confounding variable is that a possibly erroneous and usually implicit assumption can be made about the relations among the independent variable (diagnosis), the dependent variable, and the covariate. On the one hand, if both IQ and diagnosis have separate relations to verbal memory in individuals with autism, then we would like to control for IQ. On the other hand, the relations may not be separate. If, for example, a verbal memory deficit is a true correlate of autism, which in turn *leads* to a lower IQ, then covarying IQ might eliminate a true verbal memory difference. In this case, covarying would be unduly conservative.

Most case–control studies of developmental psychopathologies use school-age children or adolescents, so that a number of years have elapsed since the "onset" of the disorder. Obviously, growing up with a disorder can have many effects on development across most levels of analysis—from brain structure and function to neuropsychological functions, to observable signs and symptoms. Many of the differences observed with case–control designs may be secondary either to this particular disorder or to just growing up with a developmental disorder, rather than primary and specific to the disorder in question. One method for addressing this problem is a longitudinal study that begins before the disorder can be diagnosed. However, especially for rare disorders, such studies can be difficult and expensive to undertake. A partial solution is provided by two kinds of control groups, either younger, typically developing children matched to the group with the disorder on a relevant variable, such as mental or reading age, or a group of children similar in age, with a different developmental psychopathology that has some of the same effects on development as the disorder being studied. For instance, say that an investigator is studying Down syndrome. To control for the general effects of mental retardation, he or she could select a group with another retardation syndrome, such as fragile X, that is otherwise similar (in age, IQ, gender, and parental socioeconomic status) to the group with Down syndrome.

The first kind of control adjusts for the delay in at least some aspects of development that is inevitably found in developmental psychopathologies and detects weaknesses (and strengths) that cannot be accounted for just by developmental delay. For instance, children with Down syndrome lag behind their age-mates in performance on Piagetian tests of cognitive development; the important question is whether this lag is greater (or less) than would be predicted given their mental age. To give a second example, children with reading disability almost always perform worse than age-mates on reading pseudowords (a measure of phonological coding); the important question is whether their level of performance is worse (or better) than would be predicted by their level of reading development.

While mental-age or reading-age controls adjust for level of development, they obviously do not control for other effects of growing up with a developmental disability. That is provided by a control group composed of individuals with a different disability, one that can also contribute to detecting whether performance in a given area is better or worse than developmental level would predict. A relative strength or weakness that is found using both kinds of controls is more likely to be specific to the disorder in question, but other designs (either a longitudinal study or a treatment experiment) are needed to test whether the specific feature is primary. In some cases, available animal models of the disorder permit experimental tests of the causal relation that would be impossible or unethical in humans.

In summary, many developmental disorders have an effect on overall level of cognitive function, albeit for different reasons. Because most cognitive abilities are positively correlated, a finding of an apparently specific cognitive deficit in a given developmental psychopathology might just be secondary to a lower IQ. Three commonly used methods test this possibility: (1) using a mental-age-matched control group (younger, typically developing subjects matched on mental age to the group with the disorder); (2) covarying IQ; and (3) using a group with another developmental disorder matched on both chronological age and mental age to the group of interest. Converging positive results across two or three of these methods provide fairly convincing evidence that a candidate-specific cognitive deficit cannot be explained by an overall level of cognitive function. Null results are, as usual, more ambiguous, since a specific cognitive deficit in the disorder in question could lower overall cognitive function.

Cross-Sectional, Longitudinal, and Subclinical Designs

Using the designs just described, we may find a cognitive deficit that is specific to a disorder, but it obviously could still be a consequence or correlate rather than a cause of the disorder. If a consequence, then it should be less apparent at earlier ages and not present before the onset of the disorder. This possibility can be tested by cross-sectional and longitudinal designs. The ideal design is a longitudinal study that begins before the onset of the disorder itself. A primary neuropsychological deficit that causes the symptoms of the disorder should be present either before or at least at the same time as the onset of the disorder; if the deficit appears after the onset of the disorder, it cannot logically be primary. This ideal design is more feasible for disorders with later onsets and higher prevalences (e.g., dyslexia) than for disorders with earlier onsets and lower prevalences (e.g., autism), although a few prospective studies of autism have recently been undertaken.

Two other designs that test whether a deficit is a consequence of the disorder per se involve studies of individuals who have compensated for the disorder, or of subclinical cases (those who never had the disorder but have elevated symptoms of the disorder). If the same specific cognitive deficit is found in both groups, then it is unlikely to be a consequence of having the disorder, but one could always argue that it is a consequence of having some of the symptoms of the disorder. So these designs by themselves are not conclusive.

Family Designs

A more powerful version of the subclinical design is provided by designs that study relatives of the affected person. If the disorder is familial, then its neuropsychological cause should be familial as well. If the disorder is also dimensional rather than categorical, then relatives without the disorder should show some evidence of the neuropsychological deficit. Likewise, relatives of probands selected for the neuropsychological deficit without the disorder should nonetheless have higher rates of the disorder. Such results would indicate that the disorder and the deficit are cotransmitted in families. To test whether such cotransmission is due in part to genes, the bivariate genetic methods described in the earlier section on Behavioral and Molecular Genetics can be utilized. Positive results from such tests still do not absolutely prove cause. A deficit could appear in development before the onset of a disorder and be coheritable with it, yet still be a correlate of the disorder instead of the neuropsychological cause of it. To test cause, the presumed causal variable needs to be manipulated, which is what is done in treatment designs.

Treatment Designs

If a neuropsychological deficit partly causes the behavioral symptoms of a disorder, then amelioration (or, in some cases, exacerbation) of that deficit should produce some change in these symptoms. Such a treatment may not necessarily cure the disorder, either because the disorder may have more than one neuropsychological cause or because all the developmental consequences of having had the disorder would not be expected to disappear immediately, if at all. But a treatment study provides another test of a presumed causal mechanism. The treatment might be behavioral, such as training phonological skills in children with (or at risk for) dyslexia, or it could be pharmacological, such as giving Ritalin to children with attention-deficit/hyperactivity disorder. In either case, the treatment should modify both the neuropsychological deficit and symptoms in a proportional manner; that is, there should be a dose–response relation between the intensity of the treatment and the degree of improvement in both the neuropsychological deficit and the behavioral symptoms of the disorder.

However, even a positive result from such a treatment study does not prove the hypothesized causal mechanism. There may be a third, unidentified variable that mediates the observed changes in the symptoms. Another possibility is that the original etiology of the symptoms is independent of the hypothesized causal factor, but this factor and the symptoms share a bidirectional causal relation. For example, say the symptom is increased perceptions of stress originally caused by socialization. These perceptions increase neurotransmitter (i.e., norepinephrine) levels related to anxiety, which in turn heighten perceptions of stress. A treatment that reduces norepinephrine could therefore lessen perceptions of stress, but this positive result would not warrant the conclusion that the original cause of the symptom was an excess of norepinephrine. This example illustrates the bidirectional relation between mind and brain emphasized throughout this book.

Animal Models

In some cases, the candidate neuropsychological function is also present in another species (obviously, this is not true for most language skills and may not be true for some aspects of social cognition). If we have some understanding of the genetics or neurobiology of the disorder in question, we can manipulate those factors in an animal model and test how that manipulation affects both the candidate neuropsychological function and behavioral symptoms. An example of an animal model (of the effects of phenylalanine on prefrontal dopamine levels; Diamond et al., 1997) was discussed briefly in the preceding section on brain mechanisms.

Flint (1999) and Skuse (2000) have reviewed the use of genetic manipulations in animal models to explore the role of specific genes in the development of learning, memory, and some aspects of social behavior (i.e., maternal behavior). Such models have great promise for helping us to trace pathways from specific genes to brain development to behavior, but realizing that promise will require more integration between systems and molecular neuroscience (Flint, 1999).

If, in an animal model, the genetic or neurobiological manipulation impairs the candidate neuropsycholgical function selectively and worsens symptoms, this result is consistent with that function playing a causal role in the disorder. However, it is still possible that some other, unmeasured neurospychological function is the real culprit.

In summary, no single design conclusively establishes a causal relation between a candidate neuropsychological deficit and the symptoms of a disorder. Converging evidence across the designs considered here would be very strong evidence for a causal relation, but it could still be possible that our neuropsychological theory was inadequate. This inadequacy could result in our misnaming or omitting the relevant causal function.

Having concluded the discussion of methods for analyzing developmental psychopathologies, I now examine how these methods have been applied to specific disorders and review treatments and possible preventive interventions. Three broad classes of disorders are covered: (1) disorders of motivation (Chapter 3), (2) disorders of action selection (Chapter 4), and (3) disorders of language and cognitive development (Chapter 5). After a brief historical introduction, the review of each disorder follows a common format: (1) definition, (2) epidemiology, (3) etiology, (4) brain mechanisms, (5) neuropsychology, and (6) treatment.

Disorders of Motivation

Four disorders are included in this chapter: (1) depression and dysthymia, (2) anxiety disorders, (3) posttraumatic stress disorder, and (4) bipolar illness. As discussed earlier, all four disorders represent disruptions in the development of the arousal/motivation system, which includes portions of both the central and peripheral nervous systems.

DEPRESSION AND DYSTHYMIA

> How weary, stale, flat, and unprofitable
> seem to me all the uses of this world.
> —HAMLET, Act 1, Scene 2

> There is a certain slant of light,
> On winter afternoons,
> That oppresses, like the weight
> Of cathedral tunes.

> Heavenly hurt it gives us;
> We can find no scar,
> But internal difference,
> Where the meanings are.
> —EMILY DICKINSON

Shakespeare's Hamlet is suicidally depressed because of a traumatic loss, the murder of his father by his uncle. Emily Dickinson reminds us that milder changes of mood are associated with seasonal change. The mood disorders that we call depression and dysthymia have been recognized since classical times and frequently have been depicted in literature. Hippocrates (ca. 460–377 B.C.), who proposed a humoral theory of mood problems, is credited with the first physiological explanation of mental disorders. In his theory, mood depended on the proper balance among four bodily fluids or humors: blood, phlegm, yellow bile, and black bile. An imbalance involving an excess of black bile (in Greek, *melan choler*) was seen as the cause of depression, hence our term "melancholy." In the Renaissance, Burton (1621/1948) described the phenomenology of depression in *The Anatomy of Melancholy*. More recently, author William Styron (1990) provided a compelling account of his own major depression in *Darkness Visible*.

Despite this long history, a neuroscientific explanation of depression has emerged only in the last few decades, due to advances in both the pharmacological treatment of depression and the psychobiological understanding of the effects of stress, including psychosocial stress. I review these advances in the section on Brain Mechanisms.

Depression and dysthymia illustrate several key issues in developmental psychopathology, including continuity versus discontinuity, lumping versus splitting of diagnostic categories, and how the interaction between a constitutional vulnerability (a diathesis) and environmental stressors leads to a distinct developmental course of a disorder. In terms of the first issue, it was long believed that depression exhibited a marked developmental discontinuity, such that depression was not possible in children because they lacked the necessary intrapsychic structures postulated by Freudian theory for the emergence of depression. It is now clear that depression occurs across the lifespan, even in infants, although the symptoms naturally vary somewhat as a function of the developmental level of the patient. In terms of the second issue, syndrome boundaries, evidence from twin studies finds shared genetic influences on both anxiety and depression; so for some purposes, it makes sense to lump these two diagnostic categories together. In terms of the third issue, depression has an episodic course in which a progressively smaller environmental stress appears sufficient to trigger an episode. This distinctive course would qualify as a transaction (Sameroff & Chandler, 1975), in which the repeated interaction between risk in a developing individual and risk in the environment produces a positive feedback loop. In depression, this transaction has a physiological basis that has been explained by a kindling model, to which I return later.

Definition

DSM-IV-TR (American Psychiatric Association, 2000) defines a major depressive episode as a significant decline in mood or pleasure/interest (including sexual interest) persisting for at least 2 weeks and accompanied by significant changes in at least four out of seven other possible symptoms. So the key symptom in depression is loss of pleasure, or "anhedonia." The other symptoms can be roughly grouped into (1) three cognitive symptoms: feelings of worthlessness or guilt; diminished ability to think, concentrate, or decide; and recurrent thoughts of death, or suicidal ideation or action; and (2) four somatic symptoms: significant changes in weight or appetite, reduced or increased sleep, psychomotor agitation or retardation, and extreme fatigue. In children, a change toward an irritable rather than a depressed mood also meets the first requirement. As in other DSM-IV-TR definitions, the symptoms must cause clinically significant distress or functional impairment and not be better accounted for by exclusionary conditions (in this case, a mixed episode, bereavement, or direct effects of a substance).

Dysthymia is defined as a milder and more persistent depressed mood (at least 2 years in adults and 1 year in children) accompanied by at least two other cognitive or somatic symptoms (psychomotor agitation or retardation is not included in the list of symptoms for dysthymia, and the suicide cluster is replaced by feelings of hopelessness).

Although everyone experiences negative mood changes in response to disappointment or stress, a diagnosable depressive disorder differs from normal mood fluctuations in (1) the extent to which it disrupts normal functioning, (2) its persistence, and (3) the cognitive and somatic symptoms that co-occur with the depressed mood. So major depression and dysthymia are not just changes in mood, but rather are disabling syndromes characterized by a puzzling co-occurrence of changes in mood, cognition, and somatic functioning. Nonetheless, as is the case for most disorders considered in this book, the definition of major depression provided by DSM-IV-TR likely imposes a categorical distinction on an underlying continuum. For instance, a recent twin study found that subsyndromal symptoms of depression in index twins predicted both their own future depressive episodes and those of their co-twin in a linear fashion (Kendler & Gardner, 1998).

Epidemiology

Major depression and dysthymia are common disorders and major public health concerns that are not fully recognized. About two-thirds of persons with major depression are not treated, even though the disorder carries about a 15% risk for suicide, as well as an increased risk for other medical illnesses, including heart attack and stroke. In addition, in the Global Burden of Disease Study, Murray and Lopez (1997) documented that major depression was the fourth leading cause of disability across the world, behind respiratory infections, diarrheal diseases, and perinatal disorders, but ahead of ischemic heart disease, cerebrovascular disease, and other medical conditions. Moreover, they forecast that by the year 2020, major depression will rise to second place, due mainly to the declining impact of infectious diseases. They concluded that the substantial burden of depression and other neuropsychiatric conditions is underrecognized in terms of global public health policy.

The prevalence of depression and dysthymia is greater (1) in adults and adolescents than in children, (2) in females than in males after puberty, and (3) in younger cohorts than in older ones. At any one time, 5–9% of adult women and 2–3% of adult men have major depression (point prevalence), whereas the lifetime prevalence is 10–25% in females and 5–12% in males (DSM-IV-TR). The adult point prevalence of dysthymia (with or without major depression) is roughly 3%, with a lifetime prevalence of roughly 6%; dysthymia is about two to three times more common in adult females than in males (DSM-IV-TR).

Children and Adolescents

The point prevalence of major depression is about 1% in preschoolers, 2–3% in children ages 6 to 11, and 6–8% in adolescents (Hammen & Rudolph, 1996), with the gender ratio being essentially equal before adolescence, then mirroring the adult pattern of female predominance in adolescence. Rates of dysthymia are lower, roughly about 1%. However, rates of elevated depressive symptoms short of diagnostic cutoffs are considerably higher in adolescents than adults, reaching about 50% in one study (Hammen & Rudolph, 1996). So in terms of both major depression and depressive symptoms, adolescents are at greater risk than adults.

Cohort Differences

This high prevalence in adolescents may partly reflect cohort as well as developmental differences. It is now well documented that the prevalence of depression is greater and the age of onset is younger in more recent age cohorts across a number of developed countries (Hagnell, Lanke, Rorsman, & Ojesjo, 1982; Klerman & Weissman, 1989; Lewinsohn, Rohde, Seeley, & Fischer, 1993). These cohort differences are not just due to increased detection. Because these increases in prevalence are too rapid to be genetically mediated (unless the genetic mechanism involves "anticipation," which is discussed later in the section on fragile X syndrome in Chapter 5), they are likely due to some environmental difference between cohorts, such as the decreases in family and community support that have occurred across this century.

Gender Differences

Something about gender interacts with development to produce different gender ratios for depression across the lifespan, and it is unlikely that these gender effects are entirely biological. Before adolescence and after age 30 (Satcher, 1999), the gender ratios are equal. For instance, the change in gender ratios for depression at adolescence is an important but unexplained developmental phenomenon. It is not simply explained by the hormonal changes that accompany menarche, since the rate of depression was not found to be related to pubertal status in females once age was controlled (Angold & Rutter, 1992). Moreover, the gender ratio for depression is equal in some cultures, raising the possibility that sociocultural factors contribute to gender differences in depression. For example, among the Amish, the overall rate of depression is four times lower than the rate in the rest of the United States, and the gender ratio is equal (Egeland, Hostetter, & Eshleman, 1983). At the same time, some influence of biological factors is suggested by the impact of hormonal fluctuations on mood, as seen in premenstrual syndrome and postpartum depression. In addition, one study has found a higher heritability for depression in females than males (Bierut et al., 1999). In summary, the explanation for gender differences in depression appears to be due to an interaction between biological and psychosocial factors that is not fully understood.

Developmental Continuity

Evidence from longitudinal studies indicates a fairly specific continuity in depression from childhood to adolescence, and on to adulthood. Kovacs, Akiskal, Gatsonis, and Parrone (1994) found that children with dysthymia have an 81% rate of later major depression. In a follow-up of a large sample of individuals who came to clinical attention for persistent depressed mood in childhood or adolescence, 60% were found to have suffered at least one episode of major depression as adults (Harrington, Fudge, Rutter, Pickles, & Hill, 1990). This rate was four times that found in the follow-up of individuals who had been seen for psychiatric problems other than depression in the same clinical setting (Harrington, 1992). The specific continuity of depressive disorders is stronger in children who do not have comorbid conduct disorder (Harrington, Fudge, Rutter, Pickles, & Hill, 1991).

Sociocultural Differences

The National Comorbidity Study (Kessler et al., 1994) found that the rate of mood disorder in blacks was two-thirds that found in whites and Hispanics, but that there were few differences as a function of social class or poverty. In contrast, an earlier report found no ethnic group differences once socioeconomic status was controlled (Smith & Weissman, 1992).

Comorbidities

Finally, there is a high risk of comorbid disorders among adults, adolescents, and children with major depression or dysthymia, including anxiety disorders at all ages, substance abuse and personality disorders in adults, and disruptive behavior disorders in children and adolescents (Cicchetti, & Toth, 1995; Hammen & Rudolph, 1996).

Etiology

There is now convincing evidence of both genetic and environmental influences on the development of depression. I first examine evidence for familiality, heritability, mode of transmission, and gene locations, then consider evidence for environmental risk factors.

Familiality

Depression is clearly familial. Among adults, first-degree relatives of probands with major depression have a relative risk that is two to three times the population risk for this disorder (Barondes, 1993; Nurnberger & Gershon, 1992). They also have a similar elevation in risk for bipolar illness (Barondes, 1993). Interestingly, this cofamiliality between unipolar and bipolar illness goes in both directions. First-degree relatives of bipolar probands, besides having about an eightfold increase in risk for bipolar illness, have about a twofold increase in risk for unipolar depression (Barondes, 1993). This finding of bidirectional familiality suggests that there are partially overlapping risk factors, either genetic or environmental, for these two mood disorders. The familiality of major depression is higher in children than in adults. Children of depressed parents have about a sixfold increase in risk for depression (Downey & Coyne, 1990). One interpretation of this greater familial risk in children is that having a depressed caregiver poses an additional environmental risk beyond the familial risk shared by first-degree relatives in general. In other words, children of depressed parents may get a "double whammy." They are more likely to inherit risk alleles for depression, and they suffer the environmental stressor of a less responsive primary attachment figure (Cicchetti & Toth, 1995).

Heritability

A recent, large-scale twin study (Kendler, Neale, Kessler, Heath, & Eaves, 1992b) found a heritability of 33–45% for major depression, with most of the remaining variance due to nonshared rather than shared environmental influences. These results would fit with a diathesis–stress model of the etiology of depression, in which genetic risk interacts with stressful life events particular to individuals in a family to produce depression. A follow-up study of this same population found that the heritability of major depression increased to 66% for lifetime history diagnoses, reliable over a 5-year period. Moreover, the comorbidity of anxiety disorders was more prevalent in those with these reliable diagnoses (Foley, Neale, & Kendler, 1998).

Fewer studies have examined the familiality or heritability of depression and dysthymia in children and adolescents, but the results are broadly similar to those found in adults. Several studies have found that the recurrence rate in relatives is greater for child than for adult probands (Knowles, Kaufmann, & Rieder, 1999; Todd, Neumann, Geller, Fox, & Hickok, 1993), which is consistent with the hypothesis that a higher number of familial risk factors lowers the age of onset. Rende, Plomin, Reiss, and Hetherington (1993) found a moderate heritability of .34 for symptoms of depression in an adolescent twin sample. In a somewhat older, adolescent twin sample, Thapar and McGuffin (1997) found a heritability of .70 for symptoms of depression. In a sample of child and adolescent school-age twins, we found a heritability of .39 for symptoms of depression (Willcutt & Pennington, 1997). These studies address the heritability of depressive symptoms rather than that of a depressive disorder. Other studies have failed to find a significant difference between the heritabilities of depressive symptoms and disorders, which is consistent with the hypothesis that the same genetic risk factors act on both normal and extreme (i.e., diagnosable) individual differences in depressive symptomatology. However, more research is needed to test whether there is continuity in the genetic risk factors for depression across both age and degree of severity at a given age.

Mode of Transmission

The mode of transmission of major depression does not appear to be Mendelian (Faraone, Kremen, & Tsuang, 1990), consistent with results for other developmental psychopathologies. It is likely that multiple genes and environmental risk factors are involved, consistent with a multifactorial model.

Gene Locations

Efforts to identify actual genes involved in the etiology of depression so far have not been definitive. An association study found that an allele of a serotonin transporter promoter region (i.e., regulating transcription of the serotonin transporter gene, which codes for a receptor involved in reuptake of serotonin) was more frequent in individuals with both unipolar and bipolar depression (Collier, Arranz, Sham, & Battersby, 1996). Another study (Lesch et al., 1996) had found an association between this allele and the personality trait of neuroticism (which is defined by symptoms of anxiety and depression). However, two subsequent studies (Ball et al., 1997; Ebstein et al., 1997) failed to find this association with neuroticism.

Once risk alleles for depression are identified, much clearer tests of several important issues can be conducted, including (1) better identification of environmental risk factors, (2) determination of whether there are shared genetic risk factors for unipolar and bipolar illness, and (3) whether there is a shared etiology for both normal and extreme variations in depressive symptomatology.

Environmental Risk Factors

The fact that the heritabilities for depression are considerably less than 1.0 means that its etiology cannot be entirely genetic. There must be environmental risk factors as well. Although many environmental and psychological correlates of depression have been identified, firmly establishing which correlates play a causal role is difficult, because we cannot ethically manipulate most of these in humans and perform a true experiment. Very few of these correlates have been studied using a genetically sensitive design. So some of them may be partly a *result* of depression rather than a cause. In what follows, I discuss environmental and psychological correlates of depression and indicate which of these have been supported as playing a causal role in the development of depression and which have not. Some of the evidence for a causal role comes from animal models in which the environmental risk factor was experimentally manipulated. This evidence is discussed in the following section on Brain Mechanisms.

It is well documented that adult depression is correlated with *loss* and lack of social support, such as early parent loss, later loss of a close relationship, or lack of a confidant (Brown & Harris, 1978). Moreover, the onset and relapse of depression is more likely following a major loss of either a close relationship or a source of self-worth, such as a job (Monroe & Depue, 1991). Other stressful life events increase the rate of depression. Particularly convincing examples are provided by unpredictable stressors that affect a whole group. Unlike some stressful life events, there is no way these events could be secondary to depression in the individuals affected. So long as the comparison group is carefully chosen, these natural experiments come close to providing causal information. For instance, after a bank failure, there was a 29% rate of depression among depositors compared with a 2% rate among controls

(Ganzini, McFarland, & Cutler, 1990). Months after the Three Mile Island nuclear power plant disaster, residents living close to the plant experienced a higher rate of depressive symptoms and a lower rate of coping behaviors compared to residents of a similar neighborhood not close to the plant (Baum, Gatchel, & Schaeffer, 1983).

However, not all depressions are preceded by a stress or a loss, and not all individuals exposed to a stress or a loss develop depression. For these reasons, a diathesis–stress model of the development of depression is widely accepted. However, directly testing this model awaits a clearer specification of the genetic diathesis.

If social stressors such as loss and lack of social support are risk factors for adults, it seems plausible that these factors might pose an even greater risk for children, who generally have less ability to escape social stress in their families, and whose development depends crucially on social input. There are higher rates of depression in children who have been abused or neglected by their parents (Cicchetti & Toth, 1995), although such children are also at increased risk for a variety of other psychiatric problems, such as conduct disorder. There has also been considerable research on the social effects of having a depressed caregiver, much of it based on attachment theory (see Cicchetti & Toth, 1995; Hammen & Rudolph, 1996). There is indeed considerable evidence that parent–child interactions are compromised when a parent is depressed. For instance, in families with a depressed parent, there is more parental discord and parental hostility directed toward children (Rutter & Quinton, 1984). In interaction with their infants, depressed mothers exhibit less positive affect, and are more critical and less attuned than are nondepressed mothers (Cohn, Campbell, Matias, & Hopkins, 1990). Attachment theory posits that both self-concept and models for interpersonal interactions are based on early interactions with a primary caregiver. Thus, both of these factors are hypothesized to be altered in a permanent way when children interact with a depressed caregiver, thereby increasing the risk for depression. However, as plausible as this pathway to depression may be, there is not yet direct causal evidence for it. Children of depressed parents are undoubtedly at greater risk for depression, but some of that increased risk is mediated genetically. We need genetically sensitive designs, such as adoption studies, to measure depressed parents' social transmission of depression. Moreover, the environmental risk posed by a depressed parent may operate in ways other than changing the attachment relation, such as by increasing stress, as is discussed later.

While stressful life events are a likely environmental risk factor for depression, it is important to realize that these events are not necessarily randomly assigned. Individual differences in personality could plausibly be correlated with rates of stressful life events. To the extent that such personality differences are heritable, we would expect to find evidence for genetic influences on the occurrence of stressful life events. Two large twin studies have found just that (Kendler, Neale, Kessler, Heath, & Eaves, 1993a; Plomin, Lichenstein, Pedersen, McClearn, & Nesselroade, 1990). In these studies, the MZ concordance was higher than the DZ concordance for accidents, injuries, financial problems, and crime victimization. Interestingly, there were not MZ versus DZ concordance differences for life events less likely to be correlated with an individual's personality, such as the death of friends and relatives. A later, follow-up twin study did find evidence for a causal role of stressful life events in the etiology of major depression (Kendler, Karkowski, & Prescott, 1999). Hence, twin studies have clarified the relation between stressful life events and depression, some of which is due to shared genes (Thapar, Harold, & McGuffin, 1998) and some due to such events acting as environmental risk factors for later depression.

In summary, aspects of the environment such as stress and loss increase the risk for depression, but exactly how they exert their effect is difficult to determine in studies of humans. As we see in the next section, a better understanding of the mechanisms by which stress and loss increase the risk for depression is provided by animal models.

Brain Mechanisms

Sachar (1981) provides a summary of the early discoveries that led to the first effective pharmacological treatment for depression. In 1950, it was discovered that treatment of hypertension with the drug reserpine produced a severe depression in about 15% of persons treated. The mechanism underlying this unexpected effect turned out to be the depletion of two monoamine neurotransmitters, norepinephrine and serotonin. Around the same time, it was found that treatment of tuberculosis with the drug iproniazid produced a period of mania in some patients. Iproniazid effectively increases levels of monoamines by inhibiting the enzyme monoamine oxidase (MAO), which breaks down monoamines. Moreover, in experimental animals, reserpine produced a depressive syndrome that was reversed by treatment with iproniazid. Subsequently, it was found that MAO inhibitors such as iproniazid were effective antidepressants in human patients. Hence, it appeared that a reduction of monoamines led to depression, whereas an increase led to mania, at least in some individuals.

Norepinephrine

These and other observations led Schildkraut (1965) to formulate the biogenic amine hypothesis of mood disorders, which focuses on the role of norepinephrine. Stated simply, depression results from a deficiency of norepinephrine (NE), and mania results from an excess of it. Nemeroff (1998) reviewed the support for this hypothesis; I summarize his main points. Many studies have documented lower NE metabolites in the urine and cerebrospinal fluid (CSF) of depressed individuals. In post-mortem studies of depressed suicide victims, there are *increased* densities of NE receptors in the cortex. One mechanism for regulating neurotransmission is for postsynaptic neurons to increase or decrease the number of receptors depending on neurotransmitter levels. If those levels are low, receptor number would be increased, although this increase still might not compensate for very low levels of neurotransmitter. Further support for this hypothesis is provided by the efficacy of recently developed drugs—selective norepinephrine reuptake inhibitors, or SNRIs—that selectively block the reuptake of NE by presynaptic neurons.

Serotonin

Although there is ample evidence implicating NE in depression and mania, other neurotransmitters are involved, particularly serotonin. Prange, Wilson, Lynn, Alltop, and Stikeleather (1974) formulated the "permissive" hypothesis to account for the role of serotonin in mood disorders. This hypothesis holds that a fall in serotonin levels "permits" a decrease in NE levels. This is plausible, because the brainstem neurons in the raphe nucleus that release serotonin project onto neurons that release NE. A role for serotonin in mood disorder is supported by (1) lower peripheral serotonin metabolites in depressed individuals, (2) increases in serotonin receptors in brains of depressed suicide victims, and (3) the remarkable effectiveness of selective serotonin reuptake inhibitors (SSRIs), such as Prozac, Paxil, Zoloft, and Luvox, in treating depression (Nemeroff, 1998).

These simple hypotheses relating levels of monoamines to mood have required elaboration because, even though antidepressant medications immediately change monoamine levels, the normalization of mood takes several weeks. Moreover, not only the amount but also the stability of monoamine levels are important for normal mood. Nonetheless, most current drug treatments of depression act by manipulating levels of monoamines, especially levels of NE and serotonin.

Thus, at this point, levels of NE and serotonin are regarded as a final common pathway in mood disorders, but, as discussed earlier, this does not mean that altered levels of these neurotransmitters necessarily cause mood disorders in the first place. Moreover, it is important to remember that neurotransmitters can only affect function by acting on neural networks. Depression is an emergent property of the whole system. So reducing mood disorders to neurotransmitter levels is an error, much in the same way as reducing behavior to a gene. As I have already stated, it is because there are receptors for NE and serotonin at various points in the arousal/motivation system, including the amygdala and the amygdala's connections to the hypothalamus, that manipulating neurotransmitter levels can change the function of the system.

Hypothalamic–Pituitary–Adrenal Axis

To understand the symptoms of depression, we must also understand what happens when the hypothalamic–pituitary–adrenal (HPA) axis is dysregulated, perhaps because of neurotransmitter imbalances. As discussed earlier, the HPA axis mediates the longer term stress response by means of neuromodulators that act more slowly than neurotransmitters. These neuromodulators include peptides (short strings of amino acids) and hormones (proteins or longer strings of amino acids). The neuroendocrine system, which is regulated by the hypothalamus, and of which the HPA axis is a part, uses neuromodulators, mainly released into the bloodstream, to communicate. To control the longer term stress response, the hypothalamus releases a peptide, corticotropin-releasing factor (CRF), which in turn stimulates the pituitary gland to release adrenocorticotropic hormone (ACTH). ACTH stimulates the adrenal glands to release glucocorticoid hormones, such as cortisol, which in turn mobilize the stress response in various organ systems (see Figure 12).

Cortisol is carried by the bloodstream back to the hypothalamus and ordinarily provides a negative feedback signal to inhibit further release of CRF, thus terminating the stress response. However, the HPA axis may become chronically activated because of either persistent environmental stress, or genetically mediated differences in its physiology, or a combination of the two (a diathesis–stress interaction). In such cases, we would expect a number of changes in HPA axis function, including (1) increased cortisol levels in blood and CSF; (2) increased levels of CRF and ACTH; and (3) size increases in the pituitary and adrenal glands, because CRF and ACTH, respectively, also have a trophic effect on these two glands. Indeed, changes in these detectable markers of chronic hyperactivity of the HPA axis have been repeatedly demonstrated in animal models of stress (Sapolsky, 1994). As we will see, these markers of HPA axis overactivity are also found in both human depression and animal models of depression.

Chronic cortisol release has a number of harmful effects, including immune suppression, atherosclerosis, digestive disorders, and accelerated aging and death of hippocampal neurons (Bownds, 1999; Sapolsky, 1994), that help account for the increased risk of heart attack and stroke in people with major depression, as well as some of the memory impairments in people with depression and anxiety disorders (since the hippocampus is crucial for long-term memory function).

I next turn to evidence that the HPA axis is overactive in depression, which comes from neuroendocrine measurement in both human patients with depression and experimental animals. The very impressive converging evidence of HPA-axis hyperactivity in human depression (Nemeroff, 1998) includes (1) increased cortisol levels in the urine, blood, and CSF of unmedicated patients with depression; (2) elevated levels of CRF, which are reduced by successful medication treatment of the depression; (3) enlargements of the adrenal and pituitary glands; (4) increased numbers of CRF-producing neurons and increased expression of the CRF gene in the hypothalamus in postmortem studies; and (5) other neuroendocrine alterations in the pituitary (i.e., blunted release of growth hormone) and thyroid (alterations in response to exogenous thyroid-stimulating hormone) glands. Moreover, direct delivery of CRF to the brains of lab animals produces symptoms of depression: insomnia, decreased appetite and libido, and increased anxiety.

Animal models of the effects of stress and loss have demonstrated that these environmental risk factors change levels of NE and serotonin, and alter the function of the HPA axis. For example, Stone (1975) reviewed evidence that a variety of stressors, both physical (electric shock, heat, and noise) and social (separation and fighting) lead to reduced levels of NE and serotonin in a dose-dependent fashion. Other studies have documented that such stressors also lead to changes in the

HPA axis, including increased cortisol release and enlarged adrenal glands (Mineka, Gunnar, & Champoux, 1986; Sapolsky, 1994). The animals in these studies also exhibit behavioral symptoms of depression, such as passivity and social isolation. Monkeys switched from high to low social rank by changing their social group had decreased serotonin levels and increased cortisol (Raleigh, McGuire, Brammer, & Yuwiler, 1984). So low social status is a stressor in monkeys, and very likely in humans as well.

Animal models utilizing infant animals have illuminated the role of early loss and stress in the development of depression. Nemeroff (1998) found that neonatal rats subjected to repeated early separations from their mothers and then reared in a standard rat colony had HPA alterations as adults. Specifically, they had elevations of cortisol, ACTH, and CRF. Some of these effects were normalized by treatment with an SSRI (Paxil), but the HPA abnormalities returned when this treatment was stopped. Hence, early social separation, such as occurs in neglect or loss, creates a lasting vulnerability in the HPA axis that is partly reversed by medication treatment. In another animal model, Nemeroff (1998) induced anxiety in bonnet macaque mothers by making the availability of food unpredictable. The anxious mothers then ignored their infants, who exhibited symptoms of anxiety and depression; they froze in novel situations, were less active, and withdrew from social interactions. As adults, they had elevated CRF levels. Suomi (1991) found that about 20% of rhesus monkeys subjected as infants to a separation from their mothers had lasting changes in their cortisol levels and greater emotional sensitivity as adults. Other studies (Caldji et al., 1998; Liu et al., 1997) have found that maternal care during infancy influences the development of the HPA-mediated stress response (i.e., appropriate maternal care lessens vulnerability to later stress).

In summary, both physical and social stress cause alterations in neurotransmitter levels and overactivity in the HPA axis. Early social stress causes a permanent vulnerability in the HPA axis, such that it will be more reactive to later stresses. In contrast, early positive attachment experiences buffer the HPA axis and make it less vulnerable to stress.

So, in humans, the risk factors of early loss, neglect, or a depressed parent may act *directly* on both the stress response system and the development of interpersonal cognitions. Both the vulnerable HPA axis and the altered interpersonal cognitions may then persist as risk factors for the development of depression after a later stress.

These animal models also begin to explain the distinct developmental course of mood disorders. In many patients, episodes of mood disorder recur more frequently with successive episodes and the apparent environmental stressor needed to trigger an episode becomes less and less severe. Eventually, episodes can occur with no environmental stressor. This course implies a positive feedback loop in the arousal/motivation system, such that the threshold for HPA overactivity is lowered with each successive episode. To account for this phenomenon, Post (1992) and colleagues (Post, Rubinow, & Ballenger, 1986) proposed two well-studied models of similar, positive feedback loops: behavioral sensitization and electrophysiological kindling. In the latter, a model of seizure disorders in which electrical stimulation is applied to the amygdala, with each successive stimulation episode, the amount of current needed to induce a seizure decreases, until seizures become spontaneous. The kindling hypothesis of mood disorders in effect describes the episodes as a kind of limbic, HPA-axis "seizure," with each episode lowering the threshold for a future episode. Both the infant animal models and the kindling hypothesis stress the importance of continued medication treatment in mood disorders to prevent relapses.

Neuroimaging Studies

In several recent reviews of neuroimaging findings in major depression (Byrum, Ahearn, & Krishnan, 1999; Davidson, Abercrombie, Nitschke, & Putnam, 1999; Dubovsky & Buzan, 1999), the main structural findings are enlarged lateral ventricles, especially in late-onset major depression, and decreased volume of the frontal lobes and parts of the basal ganglia (caudate nucleus and putamen). The main functional findings include (1) *decreased* blood flow in prefrontal cortex and cingulate gyrus, with the decrease often being greater in the left hemisphere, and (2) *increased* blood flow in the amygdala. Supporting a relation between brain metabolism and depressive symptoms, Davidson and colleagues (1999) found a correlation of .56 between metabolic rate in the right amygdala and negative affect. Another neuroimaging study of depression (Bench, Frackowiak, & Dolan, 1995) found that successful drug treatment of the symptoms of depression also normalized blood flow in the left frontal lobe. We can speculatively interpret these findings as suggesting an imbalance between top-down (prefrontal) and bottom-up (amygdala) components of the affect regulation system.

Neuropsychology

In this section, I first review major psychological theories of depression and then consider the difficult problem of how to integrate biological and psychological theories. Before considering specific psychological theories, it is useful to recapitulate what an adequate theory of depression must do. First, it must be supported by rigorous evidence that the mechanism it proposes actually *causes* depression. Second, it must explain why there are individual differences in the susceptibility to depression. Both human and animal studies provide ample evidence that after exposure to the same environmental risk event, some individuals develop depression and others do not. Third, it must explain *all* the symptoms of depression—in the areas of mood, cognition, behavior, and somatic functioning. Fourth, it must be comprehensive and provide a way to integrate findings about depression from all the levels of analyses considered here. As we will see, no existing psychological theories of depression meet these four criteria.

Freud's Theory

Freud postulated (1917/1963) that depression is related to loss and that the resulting anger toward the lost person, because it is unacceptable to the superego, is turned against the self. His insight about the role of loss was seminal, but other aspects of the theory are problematic. Because children in his theory do not have a fully developed superego, they cannot undergo this intrapsychic transformation of anger and therefore cannot have depression. The existence of depression in children (and experimental animals) clearly argues against Freud's theory, not to mention the difficulty of testing psychoanalytic theories empirically.

Later psychological theories developed by learning and cognitive-behavioral theorists included Lewinsohn's (1974) reinforcement model, Seligman's (1975) learned helplessness model, and Beck's (1987) cognitive theory.

Reinforcement Model

According to the reinforcement model, depression results from receiving fewer rewards and more punishments. It is not too surprising that individuals with depression actually receive fewer social rewards and that they perceive their lives as less rewarding and more punishing. Holmes (1997) reviewed studies that have found these correlates of depression but concluded that such findings could be a result rather than a cause of depression. If this is the case, depression could set in motion interpersonal transactions whereby depressed behavior leads to fewer rewards, which exacerbates depression. In other words, the reinforcement theory may help explain factors that maintain depression and may even suggest some helpful interventions, without being an adequate theory of the etiology of depression. Another reason the reinforcement theory is an inadequate etiological theory of depression is that it does not adequately address the key issue of individual differences in the susceptibility to depression. The only answer a simple reinforcement theory provides to this question is essentially chance differences in experience. Because of bad luck, some people get fewer rewards and more punishments. But how does a learning theory then explain the fact that not everyone exposed to the same punishment develops depression? As soon as we try to modify the reinforcement theory to explain such individual differences in a nonchance way, we have to introduce constructs from other theoretical paradigms. The reinforcement theory does not explain all the symptoms of depression, unless it posits that reduced rewards and increased punishments cause stress. But then it becomes very similar to a stress theory. Finally, reinforcement theory is not comprehensive. In summary, reinforcement theory does not meet the four criteria for an adequate theory of depression. It nonetheless makes a contribution to our understanding of depression by identifying a positive feedback loop (a transaction) that may contribute to the development and maintenance of depression.

Learned Helplessness

Seligman's (1975) learned helplessness theory, which, interestingly, grew out of research on animals' responses to uncontrollable stressors, holds that uncontrollable, stressful life events lead to a sense of helplessness, which leads to depression. The phenomenon of learned helplessness was discovered accidentally. Dogs that were previously subjected to inescapable shocks, unlike dogs previously exposed to either escapable shocks or no shocks, made no effort to escape in a later testing session when exposed to escapable shocks. In other words, they had learned to be helpless in the face of shock, even though they could have escaped the shocks in the later testing session. A similar effect was then demonstrated in humans, leading to the development of the learned helplessness theory of depression.

The key construct in this theory is a belief about lack of control, thus making it a cognitive theory of depression. Two kinds of evidence question whether the construct of beliefs about control is central either to depression or to the learned helplessness phenomenon (reviewed in Holmes, 1997). The first kind of evidence is the lack of predictive value of beliefs about control for later depression. The second is the failure to find a belief in lack of control in human subjects who exhibited experimentally induced learned helplessness. So what about the dogs who looked depressed? They may have indeed been depressed, not because of cognitive belief about control, but because of a physiological response to inescapable stress.

Later versions of the learned helplessness theory have focused on the negative attributional style shown by people at risk for depression (Abramson, Seligman, & Teasdale, 1978). This style attributes negative outcomes to enduring characteristics of the self and positive outcomes to factors outside the individual's control. Given that any person experiences both positive and negative outcomes over time, persons with a negative attributional style would accumulate a lot of evidence that they cannot control their lives. As in the earlier learned helplessness theory, this belief in lack of control decreases self-esteem, mood, and motivation, and eventually leads to depression. As in the reinforcement theory, a feedback loop is proposed, but this time the feedback strengthens a maladaptive cognitive style rather than a behavioral style.

Although this revised theory might help explain the maintenance of depression and point to a treatment, it fails as a causal theory because it does not explain where the negative attributional style came from in the first place. Notice that the learned helplessness theory started as a theory about the cause of depression—uncontrollable external events— but then became a theory about individual differences in the susceptibility to depression. But it does not explain the etiology of those individual differences. It is possible that individual differences in attributional style could be caused by socialization differences, including cultural differences. But such differences could also arise from genetically influenced differences in personality or a combination of socialization and genetic differences. The important overall point is that the learned helplessness theory is not a totally adequate theory because it does not explain individual differences in susceptibility.

Beck's Theory

Beck's (1987) cognitive theory is based on information-processing concepts such as associative networks, selective attention, and selective recall. The basic idea in this theory is that activation of negative self-schema by stress biases information processing such that the person makes systematic errors in thinking about events. Attention and recall are biased in a negative direction by the presence of a negative self-schema in the person's associative networks, leading to a focus on negative thoughts that then cause depression. The theory is developmental in that the negative self-schemas arise from the child's early interactions with the environment, such as interactions with a caregiver. The systematic errors in thinking include overgeneralization, magnification, minimization, and personalization. Again, a feedback loop is postulated to reinforce this cognitive style, leading eventually to Beck's cognitive triad of automatic, repetitive, and negative thoughts about the self, the world, and the future.

What have empirical studies found about the validity of Beck's cognitive theory of depression (see review in Holmes, 1997)? Past research has documented that as a group, people with depression have more negative thoughts, although these are most pronounced in a subgroup of patients with depression. Given that DSM-IV-TR includes negative thoughts among the defining symptoms of depression, a current study of this question would inevitably and tautologically find this result. There is also evidence that individuals with depression selectively attend to and recall negative information. In summary, negative thoughts and biases in information processing have been found to correlate with depression.

But the key questions follow: Do negative thoughts precede the onset of depression, and can inducing negative thoughts produce depression? Lewinsohn, Steinmetz, Larson, and Franklin (1981) conducted a 1-year prospective study of 1,000 subjects to answer the first question and found that earlier negative thoughts did *not* predict later depression. Although mild depressive feelings can be induced by having subjects read negative statements (and thus have negative thoughts), this only shows that cognition can affect mood, not that negative thoughts cause depression. A review of research on whether negative thoughts cause depression (Haaga, Dyck, & Ernst, 1991) concludes that cause has not been documented empirically. Instead, it is more likely that depression causes negative thoughts that contribute to the maintenance of depression. As I discuss later, cognitive therapy based on Beck's model is effective in treating depression.

Given the bidirectional nature of the connections between parts of the motivation system, it should be the case that mood or arousal level affects cognition *and* that cognition can affect mood. Obviously, learning bad news, even from a neutrally worded telegram, quickly affects both mood and physiological arousal in the peripheral nervous system. At the same time, the experience of a marked change in physiological arousal, such as occurs in major depression, affects cognition in a variety of ways. One process is likely to be confabulation (Bownds, 1999), the construction of "explanations" to justify the altered mood and physiological arousal ("I must be a very bad person to feel so bad" or "The only solution to these terrible feelings is for me to die"). The cognitive system seeks explanations for behavior and mood, and will construct an explanation even when the real basis of the mood or behavior is not accessible to it. Such confabulation has been dramatically documented in hypnosis and in patients with some neurological conditions, such as split-brain patients or those with anosognosia (denial of illness). Another process by which mood affects cognition is the input from the amygdala and brainstem nuclei to the cortex.

Review of Theories of Depression

We have considered four psychological theories of depression, none of which meets our four criteria for an adequate theory. In particular, none has proven cause or is comprehensive. Each theory has contributed to our understanding of the maintenance of depression and to therapies for depression.

The physiological theories of depression reviewed earlier, such as the biogenic amine theory, the permissive theory, or the neuroendocrine theory, have different weaknesses. Although they identify relevant biological variables, they, too, have neither proven cause nor are they comprehensive. So what is needed is a theory of the normal and abnormal development of affect regulation that is both comprehensive and incorporates what we have already learned.

We can see the outline of such a theory in the material that has been reviewed. Genetic studies provide a basis for understanding individual differences in susceptibility to depression. Stress and loss can cause depression, and early stress and loss can create a lasting vulnerability, as well as exacerbate vulnerability in individuals at genetic risk.

Affect regulation, a key, early developmental as well as lifelong task, depends crucially on socialization. Self-cognitions and attributional style make important contributions to affect regulation, as do social support, exercise, sleep, nutrition, and certain illnesses. Perhaps because of the evolutionary advantage provided by being able to mobilize a stress response quickly, the amygdala and the HPA axis have a built-in Achilles' heel: They are easily overactivated. The immune system provides an interesting parallel; disorders involving an exaggerated immune response are quite common. Natural selection quickly weeds out genes for weak immune responses or slow fear conditioning, but there is probably little selection pressure against extremes in the opposite direction. A comprehensive theory will need to integrate what we know about depression and affect regulation, and to interpret them in terms of the neural systems I described earlier. In other words, we need a developmental neuropsychology of emotion regulation that accounts both for human (and mammalian) universals in emotional development and the extreme individual differences seen in mood and anxiety disorders.

Treatment

The efficacy of various treatments for depression has been much better studied in adults than in children and adolescents. Two broad conclusions emerge from this work. First, pharmacological and psychosocial treatments are about equally effective in the treatment of depression in adults, and a combination of the two types of treatment is somewhat more effective. However, for severe depression, biological therapies (i.e., drugs or electroconvulsive therapy) appear to be more effective than psychosocial ones. Second, there are differences between adults and younger individuals in terms of which drug treatments work and how long they take to work.

There are numerous, well-designed studies of either behavioral or drug treatments for adult depression, as well as a few large-scale studies comparing their efficacy (see review in Holmes, 1997). Three different kinds of psychosocial therapy—interpersonal psychotherapy, learning therapy, and cognitive therapy (based on Beck's theory)—have all been found to be about equally effective in treating mild to moderate depression. This suggests that something common to the three approaches, such as social support, may underlie their effectiveness, rather than the specific process the particular therapy was designed to manipulate. A similar rate of effectiveness is found for each of the three broad classes of antidepressant medications: MAOIs, such as phenelzine (Nordil); tricyclics, such as impramine (Tofranil) and amitriptyline (Elavil); and SSRIs, such as fluoxetine (Prozac) and paroxetine (Paxil).

About 20% of patients with depression respond neither to drugs nor to behavioral therapy. In these patients, and in other patients with severe depression, electroconvulsive therapy (ECT) has been shown conclusively to be an effective treatment. ECT produces improvement faster than drugs or behavior therapies, which may be a life-saving difference in suicidal patients, and it has few side effects. So despite the stigma that still attaches to ECT, it is important to understand that modern ECT is a safe and effective treatment for severe depression and has undoubtedly saved many lives.

Psychosocial therapies (i.e., cognitive-behavioral therapy and interpersonal therapy) also appear to be effective in the treatment of depression in children and adolescents, although there is much less research on this topic. In contrast, tricyclics and MAO inhibitors have not shown treatment efficacy in this age group and are not recommended, particularly given some of their potential side effects (Kutcher, 1998). Consequently, current drug treatments for depression in children and adolescents mainly involve SSRIs. As in adults, evidence from current treatment studies with SSRIs supports a response rate of about 65–75% (Kutcher, 1998). Another important difference between adults and younger patients in response to antidepressant medication is the length of treatment needed before a therapeutic response is evident. In adults, this is typically 3 to 4 weeks. In children and adolescents, it is more than twice as long, about 8–12 weeks. Although it has not been systematically studied, there are likely benefits to combining behavioral and drug treatments in children and adolescents, just as there are in adults.

The final topic to be covered in this section concerns prevention. There are exciting recent developments in the prevention of depression in children, adolescents, and young adults. As reviewed by Seligman, Walker, and Rosenhan (2001), several prevention trials using the techniques of cognitive therapy in an educational fashion have demonstrated reduced rates of later depression in the treatment group compared to the control group. In each study, individuals at risk were randomly assigned to treatment or no-treatment and then followed up for a year or more. The definition of "at risk" varied across studies: a pessimistic explanatory style in studies of college and high school students, and either parental conflict or mild symptoms of depression in studies of children. Because there were substantial treatment effects in each study, widespread preventive education of this sort could be quite promising as a way to reduce the epidemic of depression among young people.

Given the information reviewed earlier, we can also identify other risk factors that could be targeted by preventive interventions, including abuse, neglect, and other sources of stress in the lives of children. Continued education of the public and primary care providers about depression is obviously important given the large majority of cases of untreated depression.

ANXIETY DISORDERS

Research on anxiety disorders raises important questions about syndrome boundaries, both among different anxiety disorders and between anxiety disorders and depression. A case can be made for lumping some, but not all, anxiety disorders, and for merging some, but not all, of them with depressive disorders. Thus, anxiety disorders provide an interesting test case of how the various methods of syndrome analysis address the issues of construct and discriminant validity of diagnoses, and also illustrate how different tests of external validity can give different answers to the question of whether two diagnoses are distinct. Thus, as more research evidence accumulates, it is likely that our taxonomy of anxiety disorders will change. I suggest one possible direction for change by considering obsessive–compulsive disorder separately in Chapter 4. I also discuss posttraumatic stress disorder, the one anxiety disorder that is defined etiologically, in its own section. Thus, I now cover phobic disorders (agoraphobia, social phobia, and specific phobia) and two of the anxiety states (generalized anxiety disorder and panic disorder), as well as the two anxiety disorders specific to childhood (separation anxiety disorder and overanxious disorder; the latter is included in DSM-IV-TR under generalized anxiety disorder).

As was the case for depressive disorders, a neuroscientific understanding of anxiety disorders has begun to emerge only in the last few decades due, again, to serendipitous pharmacological discoveries and to psychobiological research on the stress response system. As we will see, the brain mechanisms underlying both depressive and anxiety disorders partially overlap.

Definition

Whereas the key symptom in depressive disorders is anhedonia, or loss of pleasure, in anxiety disorders it is unrealistic fear that interferes with adaptive functioning. As is true for depressive disorders, anxiety disorders are characterized by alterations in mood (anxiety, tension, or panic), cognition (worrying and planning about the feared thing), and somatic functioning (sweating, dry mouth, shallow or rapid breathing, rapid pulse, increased blood pressure, throbbing in the head, and muscular tension). All of these somatic symptoms are consistent with short-term sympathetic activation of the autonomic nervous system, which is accomplished by means of the sympatho–adreno–medullary (SAM) axis, as discussed earlier. However, anxiety disorders can also lead to longer term autonomic changes; thus, they confront us with the mind–body problem in much the same manner as do depressive disorders. We may roughly distinguish between anxiety and depressive disorders by saying that someone with an anxiety disorder has a lower threshold for an acute stress response, which then remits, whereas someone with a depressive disorder is "stuck" in a chronic stress response. An influential conceptualization of the relation between anxiety and mood disorders is the tripartite model (Clark & Watson, 1991), in which there is a factor common to both kinds of disorders (i.e., negative affect or general distress) as well as factors specific to each (physiological hyperarousal in anxiety disorders, and anhedonia in mood disorders). As we will see, this common factor is genetically mediated, whereas there are environmental risk factors specific to each kind of disorder.

DSM-IV-TR distinguishes among anxiety disorders by first ruling out exogenous causes, such as substances or medical conditions. It then inquires about the presence of panic attacks (characteristic of panic disorder); anxiety about situations in which escape might be embarrassing, such as being in a crowd, or on a bus or train (characteristic of agoraphobia); fear of embarrassment in social or performance situations (characteristic of social phobia); or fear of a particular object or situation (characteristic of specific phobia). If neither these symptoms nor obsessive–compulsive or posttraumatic stress disorder are present, and the excessive anxiety has persisted for 6 months without an accompanying mood or psychotic disorder, then generalized anxiety disorder (GAD) is diagnosed. It is clear from this decision tree that GAD is a residual category. There is considerable controversy about the syndrome validity of GAD, because of both the low reliability of some definitions of this disorder and its high rate of comorbidity with other disorders (see discussion in Brown, 1999). Separation anxiety disorder (SAD) must have an onset before age 18 and last at least 4 weeks. It is characterized by developmentally inappropriate, excessive anxiety about separation from home or major attachment figures. As I discuss later in this chapter, children with SAD are at higher risk for anxiety disorders as adults.

Epidemiology

Anxiety disorders, the most common psychiatric illness in adults, with a lifetime prevalence of 25% (Kessler et al., 1994), are also among the most prevalent psychiatric disorders in children and adolescents (Bernstein & Borchardt, 1991). As is true for depressive disorders, rates of anxiety disorders are higher in adult females than in males. In general, their prevalence increases with age across these three age groups, the sole exception being SAD, which is much more common in children than in adolescents.

Development

Fears are common, even normative, in childhood, and there is a developmental progression of such fears, called the *ontogenetic* parade (Scarr & Salapatek, 1970). These fears include separation anxiety (6–22 months); stranger anxiety (6–24 months); fear of unfamiliar peers (20–29 months); fears of animals, darkness, and imaginary creatures (2–6 years); fear of school (3–6 years); and fear of physical harm and injury (8–16 years). Specific phobias and other anxiety disorders often emerge during the developmental period and may be viewed as an exaggeration of normal fears in terms of both intensity and persistence. For instance, SAD is characterized by the persistence or reemergence of a fear response that is developmentally normal at younger ages.

Developmental Continuity

There are no longitudinal follow-up studies of anxious children into adulthood, so we do not know for certain about long-term continuity of anxiety disorder, although family studies provide indirect evidence for developmental continuity, as will be discussed. Clear evidence of shorter term continuity from childhood to adolescence has been examined in several longitudinal epidemiological samples (reviewed in Costello & Angold, 1995). For any diagnosis, the proportion of children at time 1 who continue to have a diagnosis at time 2 as adolescents (on average, 4 years later) is roughly 50%. The continuity for specific diagnoses is less but significantly greater than chance for most disorders, including overanxious disorder, and that for internalizing disorders (either anxiety or depression) in girls was especially striking in data from the Dunedin study in New Zealand (McGee, Freehan, Williams, & Anderson, 1992). In this sample, on average, a girl with such a disorder at age 11 was 6.2 times more likely than a girl without an internalizing disorder at age 11 to have such a disorder at age 15. Some evidence for a developmental continuity in anxiety disorders is also provided by retrospective reports and by family risk data (reviewed below). For example, several studies have found that adults with agoraphobia recall excessive separation anxiety in childhood (reviewed in Bernstein & Borchardt, 1991), although these retrospective reports could be biased by subjects' current anxiety disorder.

Comorbidities

Among adults, anxiety disorders are comorbid with both each other, and major depression and substance abuse. For example, up to 65% of individuals with panic disorder also have major depression (DSM-IV-TR). Among children and adolescents, anxiety disorders are also comorbid with each other, major depression, and attention-deficit/hyperactivity disorder. For example, in epidemiological samples, about 12–17% of children and adolescents with anxiety disorders also had a depressive disorder (Bernstein & Borchardt, 1991), which is at least twice the rate expected by chance. Anxiety disorders also appear to be prodromal for later major depression in children (Kovacs, Gatsonis, Paulaskas, & Richards, 1989). In referred samples of children and adolescents with major depressive disorder, the rate of comorbid anxiety disorders exceeded 40% (Bernstein & Borchardt, 1991). These comorbidities are consistent with the hypothesis of shared risk factors among anxiety disorders and between anxiety and depressive disorders. As I discuss shortly, twin studies provide evidence for such shared genetic risk factors.

Etiology

There is clear evidence that anxiety disorders are familial and partly heritable. Consequently, both genetic and environmental risk factors must be involved in their etiology. The mode of transmission has not been clearly established. Linkage and association studies have yielded some preliminary positive results. In addition, some specific environmental risk factors have been identified.

Familiality

In terms of familiality, Knowles and colleagues (1999) have reviewed methodologically adequate studies of adults and provided the following relative risk (λ) estimates for first-degree relatives: 9.6 for panic disorder, 5.6 for GAD, 3.3 for specific phobia, 3.2 for social phobia, and 2.8 for agoraphobia.

Familiality for anxiety disorders extends to children and is bidirectional, supporting developmental continuity; that is, parents' anxiety disorders increase the risk for such a disorder in their children and children's anxiety disorders increase the risk in their parents. In terms of risk to children, Beidel and Turner (1997) found that children of parents with anxiety disorders are more likely to have anxiety disorders than children of parents with either depressive disorders or mixed anxiety and depression. In terms of risk to relatives of a child with an anxiety disorder, Last, Hersen, Kazden, Orvaschel, and Perrin (1991) found that the rates of anxiety disorders were significantly higher in the first-degree relatives of such children compared to the rates found in first-degree relatives of children with either attention-deficit/hyperactivity disorder or no disorder. Moreover, childhood onset of some anxiety disorders may be associated with a greater degree of familial risk. Goldstein, Wickramaratne, Horwath, and Weissman (1997) found that onset in a proband with panic disorder at or before age 20 was associated with much higher rates of panic disorder in relatives, more severe anxiety symptoms, and increased rates of agoraphobia, consistent with the hypothesis that earlier onset is due to a higher concentration of familial risk factors in the proband.

Besides bidirectional familiality, additional evidence for developmental continuity in anxiety is provided by studies of the families of children with behavioral inhibition. Behavioral inhibition, a somewhat longitudinally stable temperamental style indexed by a fearful response to strangers and novel play situations, is found in about 10–15% of young children (Kagan, Reznick, & Gibbons, 1989). Parents and siblings of inhibited toddlers were found to have higher rates of anxiety disorders than parents and siblings of noninhibited children (Rosenbaum, Biederman, Hirschfeld, Bolduc, & Chaloff, 1991a; Rosenbaum et al., 1991b). Conversely, children of parents with panic disorder with agoraphobia (PDAG) or PDAG with major depression had very high rates of behavioral inhibition, 85% and 70%, respectively. These rates are substantially higher than either the 10–15% population rate for this tempermental style or the 15% rate found in children of parents with a psychiatric disorder other than PDAG or major depression. Interestingly, the rate in children of parents with major depression by itself was intermediate, about 50% (Rosenbaum et al., 1988). However, children with behavioral inhibition but no family history of anxiety disorder are not at increased risk for anxiety disorders or other psychopathology (Biederman et al., 1993), so there appear to be subtypes of the phenotype of behavioral inhibition, with one subtype related to familial anxiety disorders. These studies nonetheless provide important evidence on the developmental course of anxiety disorders.

A third piece of evidence for developmental continuity is provided by a study that found a greater startle reflex in children of parents with anxiety disorders compared to children of either alcoholics or normal controls (Grillon, Dierker, & Merikangas, 1997). The children of alcoholics exhibited different alterations in the startle response, namely, impairments in both habituation and prepulse inhibition. Like the work on behavioral inhibition, this study suggests that the familial phenotype in anxiety disorders includes alterations in the stress response system that are detectable in childhood. Because there are animal models of the neuronal systems involved in modulation of the startle response, this kind of study may also help to elucidate the neuropsychology of anxiety disorders.

In summary, anxiety disorders are clearly familial in both adults and children, and childhood onset appears to increase familial risk, at least for panic disorder. Several lines of research suggesting that some of the familial risk factors for anxiety disorders are common across ages provide evidence for some developmental continuity in anxiety disorders.

Heritability

Twin studies indicate that some of these familial risk factors are genetic (e.g., Skre, Onstad, Torgersen, Lygren, & Kringlen, 1993). Heritability estimates for anxiety disorders range between 30% and 40% in the recent large-sample twin study by Kendler and colleagues (Kendler, Neale, Kessler, Heath, & Eaves, 1992a, 1992b, 1993b). These reports also support the hypothesis that the genetic influences on anxiety disorders are general rather than disorder-specific, which is consistent with the comorbidities among anxiety disorders discussed earlier. The one exception appears to be GAD, which is more related genetically to major depression than to panic disorder or phobia, which are genetically related (Kendler, Neale, Kessler, Heath, & Eaves, 1992c; Kendler et al., 1995). The genetic correlation between GAD and major depression is essentially 1.0, which means that all the genetic influences that act on either disorder also act on both disorders.

Interestingly, if we examine the genetic correlation between symptom measures of anxiety and depression in adult twins, the genetic correlation is also essentially 1.0, meaning that the genetic influences on these two symptom dimensions are completely shared (Kendler, Heath, Martin, & Eaves, 1987). The convergence of results from studies of both extreme and normal variations in depression and anxiety is consistent with a dimensional hypothesis, namely, that a common set of genetic influences underlies both extreme and normal variations in depression and some forms of anxiety. Of course, to prove this hypothesis, we would need molecular studies of both extreme and normal variations. At the same time, there must be at least partially distinct genetic influences acting on some anxiety disorders, such as panic disorder and phobia. In summary, twin studies are "recarving" the map of the anxiety disorders in ways that will eventually make it easier to trace developmental pathways.

The results of twin studies of symptoms of anxiety in child samples are generally convergent with the findings from adult studies, although methodological variations produce different results and more work is needed. One study did not find significant heritability for child-reported anxiety symptoms but did find a heritability of .59 for maternal reports of manifest anxiety (Thapar & McGuffin, 1995). Stevenson, Batten, and Cherner (1992) found a heritability of .29 for anxious symptoms in their sample. Similar to Thapar and McGuffin's results for child-reported symptoms, Stevenson and colleagues (1992) found that a substantial proportion of the variance was attributable to environmental influences shared by family members (c^2 = .59 and .49, respectively). Topolski and colleagues (1997) used self-reports collected in a semi-structured interview format from a very large sample of child and adolescent twins (around 600 pairs each of MZ and DZ twins) to examine the etiology of symptoms of manifest anxiety (MANX), overanxious disorder (OAD), and SAD. Because of the size of the sample, these researchers could test for both age and gender differences in the etiology of these three different measures of anxiety. The results for both etiology and age and gender differences varied by measure. There were no age or gender differences in the results for OAD or SAD, but they did differ in etiology. OAD was moderately heritable (h^2 = .37), with no significant shared environmental influence (c^2). In contrast, SAD was not significantly heritable, but c^2 (.40) was moderate and significant. In contrast to both OAD and SAD, the etiology for MANX varied by both age and gender. In females, heritabilities were significant and fairly stable across age groups, ranging from .42 to .57, whereas c^2 estimates were not significant. In males, heritabilities were lower and less stable across age groups (ranging from .23 to .45); the c^2 estimate of .44 approached significance (p = .06) for the 11- to 13-year-old age group. The gender difference was best explained by a model in which the same genes act in both genders but are more expressed in females than in males. Such a model would partly explain the higher rates of anxiety symptoms in females across all three measures in this study, as well as the female predominance of anxiety disorders.

Willcutt and Pennington (1997) found a heritability of .40 for self-reported symptoms of anxiety on a structured interview (Diagnostic Interview for Children and Adolescents) administered to 170 same-sex child and adolescent twin pairs, but no significant c^2. Both this study and that of Topolski and colleagues (1997) differed from the two earlier twin studies (Stevenson et al., 1992; Thapar & McGuffin, 1995) in using structured interviews as opposed to mailed questionnaires. The most striking result from the Willcutt and Pennington study was that the genetic correlation between symptom measures of anxiety and depression (child self-report on the Child Depression Inventory) was essentially 1.0, meaning there was complete overlap in the genetic influences on the two symptom measures. As discussed earlier, essentially the same result has been found in adult twin studies (Kendler et al., 1987, 1992c, 1995). Eley and Stevenson (1999) studied this same issue with self-report questionnaires of trait anxiety and depression (Child Depression Inventory) mailed to 395 same-sex twin pairs, but they added an important methodological refinement. Because symptom measures of anxiety and depression are fairly highly correlated (about .60), they used second-order factor analysis to derive less correlated (r = .27) anxiety and depression factors, and then tested the genetic correlation between these two factors. Even with these less correlated measures, the genetic correlation was again 1.0, making this a well-replicated result. As in the earlier two questionnaire studies, the c^2 (.36) for the anxiety factor was larger than the h^2 (.10), so it appears that how anxiety measures are collected in children and adolescents has a considerable effect on etiological estimates.

In summary, across adult and nonadult samples, most measures of anxiety are moderately heritable. The exceptions are symptoms of SAD and children's responses to mailed questionnaires. The results for SAD suggest there may be an etiological difference between extreme and normal variations, with extreme variations possibly being related to a genetic diathesis for agoraphobia and panic disorder (based on the family studies of behavioral inhibition reviewed earlier) and normal variations being due to environmental influences shared within families. Some measures of anxiety, such as panic disorder and phobia, show a stronger genetic relation with each other than they do with depression, whereas others exhibit a complete genetic correlation with measures of depression found for both extreme and normal variations. So the family and twin studies make predictions for what will be found in molecular studies: There will be genes that affect both extreme and normal variations in both depression and anxiety, but not panic disorder or normal variations in symptoms of SAD.

Since the genetic etiologies of depression and anxiety are completely shared, their differentiation into (partly) different syndromes at the symptom level must be due to different environmental influences. In particular, loss appears to be an environmental risk factor that is specific to depression, whereas threat events are specific to anxiety (Eley & Stevenson, 2000). So whether we treat major depression and GAD as separate syndromes depends on our goal. If we are phenotyping family members in a molecular genetic study, then we should lump these two disorders. However, if we are clinicians treating people with these disorders, then we would want to distinguish them.

Structure of Etiological Influences

B. Cox, Taylor, and Enns (1999) summarized results of numerous factor analyses of fear inventories, which find a hierarchical factor structure with multiple levels. At the top of the hierarchy is a single general factor, usually labeled neuroticism or negative affectivity, which is presumably similar to the neuroticism construct that has emerged from extensive research on personality inventories. This latter construct is essentially characterized by symptoms of anxiety and depression, and has been shown to be moderately heritable (Eaves, Eysenck, & Martin, 1989).

At the next level of the factor structure of self-reported fears are broad dimensions (social, injury, animal, and situational fears) that correspond roughly to the DSM-IV-TR categories of phobias. At lower levels, the fears are increasingly specific. Such a hierarchical structure means that lower-level factors have both unique and shared variance. So a fear of spiders shares some variance with the general trait of neuroticism and fears of animals generally, but it also has variance specific to itself.

An etiological model with a similar hierarchical structure would provide a parsimonious explanation of the structure of the phenotypic variance of self-reported fears. Moreover, genetic and environmental influences might act differently at different levels of the hierarchy. General genetic influences might be greater at the top of the hierarchy, and nonshared, specific environmental influences might be greater at lower levels. Kendler and colleagues' (1992a) multivariate twin results for phobias in adult women fit such a hierarchical model. In their results, a given anxiety disorder emerged from a combination of general and specific factors. All four groups of phobias were influenced by general genetic and environmental (i.e., nonshared) factors. Specific environmental factors were more important for animal and situational phobias. So, for example, an individual with animal phobia may inherit a mild genetic vulnerability for neuroticism and then suffer traumatic events in childhood that precipitate a specific phobia.

Gene Locations

I now turn to molecular studies of anxiety, which have mainly focused on polymorphisms of the serotonin transporter gene, originally found by Lesch and colleagues (1996) to be related to the personality dimension of neuroticism (which is composed of symptoms of anxiety and depression). One study (Hamilton et al., 1999) that used the haplotype relative risk method to test whether alleles of this gene were associated with panic disorder found no relation, a result consistent with the predictions just discussed. Six studies focusing on neuroticism generally, or on one of its components, harm avoidance, have now been conducted. Three studies (Katsuragi et al., 1999; Mazzanti et al., 1998; Ricketts et al., 1998) have replicated the findings of Lesch and colleagues (1996) and three have not (Ball et al., 1997; Ebstein et al., 1997; Gelernter, Kranzler, Coccaro, Siever, & New, 1998). A Japanese case–control association study (Ohara et al., 1999) found a relation between variants of this gene and two anxiety disorder diagnoses: GAD, a finding that also fits the predictions from twin studies, and obsessive–compulsive disorder.

Even when individuals with anxiety or other psychiatric disorders are excluded from the sample, the serotonin transporter allele is related to degree of anxiety evoked by an experimental challenge (Schmidt et al., 2000). In this study, four groups of nondisordered subjects were defined by crossing presence versus absence of the risk allele with high versus low scores on a personality measure of anxiety sensitivity. These four groups were then exposed to air delivered through a mouthpiece, both with and without added carbon dioxide (CO_2). Because the added CO_2 produces shortness of breath, it can trigger anxiety. (Moreover, as will be discussed later, suffocation false alarms are one theory of panic disorder.) The results supported both main and interaction effects of the risk allele. Subjects with the risk allele had a greater fearful response to the CO_2 challenge than those without the risk allele. Subjects who had *both* the risk allele and high anxiety sensitivity had even greater anxiety responses to the CO_2 challenge. The etiology of anxiety sensitivity was not explored in this study. If it were environmental, this study would provide a nice illustration of a gene × environment interaction effect on normal variations in anxiety.

Most other molecular studies have focused on panic disorder, which is the most familial of the anxiety disorders. Two genome scans that have largely excluded a major locus have been conducted. Association studies have examined several candidate genes, mostly genes for neurotransmitter receptors, but with no positive results as yet (see review in Knowles et al., 1999).

Finally, Rowe and colleagues (1998a) used a variety of association methods, including the transmission disequilibrium test, to examine the relation between alleles of the dopamine transporter 1 (DAT1) gene and symptoms of internalizing disorders, including social phobia and GAD. They found an association for symptoms of these two anxiety disorders even when controlling for attention-deficit/hyperactivity disorder, which has previously been found to be associated with DAT1. Given the complete genetic correlation between symptoms of anxiety and depression, it is puzzling that they did not also find an association with their depression measure. If replicated, this association would be one of the first to identify a fairly generic genetic risk factor for psycho-pathology, one that might help explain the comorbidity between anxiety disorders and attention-deficit/hyperactivity disorder.

Environmental Risk Factors

Since the heritabilities for anxiety disorders are modest, there must be environmental influences on their development. However, research aimed at identifying these environmental risk factors must face the same two conceptual challenges discussed earlier: Some apparent envi-ronmental correlates of anxiety disorders may be genetically mediated, and not all individuals exposed to the same environmental stressor de-velop an anxiety disorder.

Anxiety disorders in clinical samples of children and adolescents are correlated with perceptions of environmental stress (Bernstein, Garfinkel, & Hoberman, 1989; Kashani et al., 1990). This correlation is not just a referral artifact, because a correlation between anxious symp-toms and perceptions of environmental stress has also been found in a community sample (Kashani & Orvaschel, 1990). As we saw earlier, twin studies of self-reports of stressful life events find that some of the variance in such reports is genetically mediated. Because the correlation between anxiety and such self-reports has not been studied using a ge-netically sensitive design, we do not know how much of this correlation is environmentally mediated.

Experimental and quasi-experimental designs do demonstrate en-vironmental effects on anxiety. Mineka, Gunnar, and Champoux (1986) manipulated controllability of access to food, water, and treats in two groups of young rhesus monkeys. One group received these reinforcers contingently, whereas the other group received identical reinforcers noncontingently. The noncontingent group showed increased fear and reduced exploratory behavior in a novel environment. This experiment supports the view that lack of controllability is an important factor in the development of anxiety.

A quasi-experiment in humans supports the view that environmen-tal stress contributes to anxiety disorders, especially in persons with a previous history of such disorders. Russo, Vitaliano, Brewer, Katon, and Becker (1995) crossed previous history of anxiety disorders with the stress of caring for a spouse with Alzheimer's disease in a 2 × 2 design. About three-fourths of persons with both a previous history and the current stress had an anxiety disorder, which was about 3.5 times the rate in persons with just a previous history. Rates were much lower in the two groups without a previous history, about 5% and 3%, respectively, for those with and without the current stress.

So environmental risk factors play a role in the development of anxiety disorders, and stress and uncontrollability appear to be examples of such factors. Early trauma is another risk factor, as we see in the section on posttraumatic stress disorder. But more work is needed to identify which environmental risk factors at what ages and in which individuals are most important, as well as what protective factors can lessen the impact of such risk experiences.

Brain Mechanisms

Just as was the case for depression, some of our understanding of the brain mechanisms in anxiety began with a fortuitous pharmacological discovery. Another parallel is a gradual shift from single neurotransmitter theories to more complex theories.

Norepinephrine and the Acute Stress Response

A basic model for understanding anxiety disorders has been the acute stress response described earlier. Perception of threat triggers the fight-or-flight response: short-term autonomic arousal of multiple systems to facilitate dealing with the threat. One important control center for the acute stress response is the previously discussed locus ceruleus (LC) in the brainstem, which is the origin of most of the norepinephrine (NE) pathways in the brain. Perception of threat leads to intense firing of the LC and increased NE release, preparing both the brain and the body to deal with the threat. So overactivity of the LC in response to stress is a straightforward hypothesis to explain anxiety disorders.

The fortuitous discovery that benzodiazepines are effective in treating anxiety (hence, "anxiolytics") bolstered this simple model because of the mode of action of these drugs. Essentially, they increase inhibitory neurotransmission, which counters the arousal mediated in part by LC firing. It was found that benzodiazepines bind to the main gamma-aminobutyric acid (GABA) receptor in the brain, thereby increasing the receptor's affinity for binding to GABA. Hence, benzodiazepines are GABA agonists. Because GABA is the main inhibitory neurotransmitter in the brain, increasing its binding efficacy has a generalized inhibitory effect, countering the arousal mediated by NE release.

Beyond the Norepinephrine Theory

As was the case for depression, an early neurochemical theory of anxiety was an NE theory that eventually proved to be too simplistic. This shift in thinking occurred when it became clear that other medications, such as SSRIs, were effective in treating anxiety, and because of limitations in the acute stress response model. These limitations included the fact that anxiety lasts longer than the acute stress response and can occur without exposure to an external stimulus (Satcher, 1999). A broader model for anxiety disorders includes the amygdala and the HPA axis, and a wider set of neurotransmitters, including NE, serotonin, GABA, CRF (corticotropin-releasing factor), and cholecystokinin (CCK), which is a neuropeptide (Satcher, 1999). Administration of CCK can induce a panic attack in patients with panic disorder, as well as in some normal controls, especially those with higher prior levels of anxious symptoms (Cox & Taylor, 1999).

Suffocation False Alarms

Another physiological theory of anxiety disorder, specifically, panic disorder, is that the brain's suffocation monitor (which monitors CO_2 levels in the blood) has a low threshold in individuals with panic disorder, causing them to suffer suffocation false alarms. This model is supported by experimental manipulations of blood CO_2 levels through (1) slight increases of CO_2 levels in the air supply, (2) hyperventilation, or (3) sodium lactate injections (sodium lactate is converted into CO_2, thereby increasing blood CO_2 levels). In each case, the manipulation produced panic attacks in individuals with a history of panic disorder or their biological relatives, but not in controls (reviewed in Holmes, 1997). People with panic disorder also have shorter breath-holding times than those with other anxiety disorders or no anxiety disorder (Cox & Taylor, 1999).

However, as appealing as this simple physiological theory is, other evidence indicates that psychological factors also influence panic attacks. In the inhalation experiment, if individuals with panic disorder are led to (falsely) believe they can control CO_2 levels, their rate of panic attacks drops to the level seen in the absence of CO_2 (e.g., Sanderson, Rapee, & Barlow, 1989). In the sodium lactate experiment, a placebo injection also induces panic attacks (Goetz et al., 1993). This other evidence does not necessarily reject the suffocation false alarm theory; it just rejects it as a single-cause theory and shows that individuals' beliefs about controllability and threat also contribute to panic attacks.

Neuroimaging Studies

There have been fewer neuroimaging studies of anxiety disorders than of depression, but those that have been done find greater amygdala and right prefrontal activation in individuals with anxiety disorders compared to controls (see Davidson et al., 1999, for a review). One noteworthy study found reduction of benzodiazepine binding sites on GABA receptors throughout the brain in patients with panic disorder (Malizia et al., 1998). Whether this reduction is a cause, an effect, or a correlate of panic disorder is unknown.

Neuropsychology

As was true for depression, there are also conditioning and cognitive theories of anxiety disorders. These theories work better for some anxiety disorders (e.g., simple phobias) than others (panic disorder or GAD) and suffer from some of the same general criticisms reviewed earlier in the discussion of such theories of depression: (1) They do not account for individual differences in the susceptibility to anxiety disorders; (2) the cognitions related to anxiety disorders may be a *result* of anxiety rather than a cause; (3) they do not explain the somatic symptoms of anxiety disorders; and (4) they are not comprehensive; that is, they do not account for everything we know about anxiety disorders. As we will see shortly, by adding biological levels of analysis, these psychological theories can be modified to deal with these limitations.

Conditioning theories work best for phobias, which can be viewed as conditioned fear responses. Mowrer's (1939) two-factor model postulates that phobias are acquired by classical conditioning and maintained by operant conditioning. For example, say that a person received a painful bite from a dog. Classical conditioning of the fear response (one-trial learning) would cause him or her to fear dogs. Ordinarily, this fear would be extinguished by subsequent, repeated benign encounters with dogs. However, the second factor, avoidance of dogs, acts to prevent extinction from occurring.

Although this mechanism undoubtedly accounts for some phobias, it has three shortcomings: (1) Some phobias are acquired without conditioning; (2) there is a nonrandom distribution of feared objects; and (3) phobias do not form in some people even in very frightening situations (see discussion in Cox & Taylor, 1999). The first criticism may be partly addressed by adding observational learning as a mechanism by which phobias are formed. For instance, many people are phobic about airline travel but very few of them have experienced a plane crash firsthand. However, virtually all of them have had observational learning; they have heard about plane crashes or seen them on television. The second criticism has been dealt with by modifying Mowrer's (1939) classical conditioning account with evolutionary theory (see discussion in Öhman, 2000; Seligman et al., 2001). Specific phobias cluster around a small set of specific stimuli, including animals such as snakes and spiders; aspects of the natural environment, such as darkness, heights, or storms; blood and injury; or situations of confinement, such as elevators, tunnels, or airplanes. All these stimuli were at one point actually dangerous to our hunter–gatherer ancestors; therefore, evolution favored individuals who could readily develop a fear response to such stimuli.

This hypothesis of "evolutionarily prepared phobias" has been tested empirically (see review in Öhman, 2000) by comparing fear conditioning to such stimuli (e.g., snakes and spiders) and fear conditioning to nonprepared stimuli (e.g., houses and flowers). Stimuli were paired with an unconditioned aversive stimulus (a mild shock), and fear conditioning was measured by the galvanic skin response. Prepared stimuli produced fear conditioning in one trial compared to four or five trials for unprepared stimuli. Moreover, the conditioned fear response to the unprepared stimuli extinguished immediately, after they were no longer paired with shock, but persisted for the prepared stimuli.

Marks (1977) reported a case that dramatically illustrates this theory of evolutionarily prepared phobias. A 4-year-old girl walking through a park noticed a snake but reacted to it with much more interest than fear. Shortly thereafter, she accidentally injured her hand when the car door closed on it. Instead of developing a phobia to cars or doors, she developed a lifelong snake phobia!

The third criticism of the classical conditioning model, individual differences in the susceptibility to phobias, can be handled by positing partly heritable individual differences in evolutionary preparedness. Such genetic influences are consistent with the twin data reviewed earlier.

If we add what is known about the neuropsychology of the fear response, both conditioned and unconditioned, discussed earlier in the section on the Motivation System in Chapter 2, then we have the broad outlines of an integrated neuroscientific account of phobias. Recall that the amygdala (LaBar & LeDoux, 1997) is a critical structure in the conditioned fear response, which occurs rapidly and is resistant to extinction. It is also a central structure in the motivation system and regulates the physiological fear response through its connections to the hypothalamus. Add genetic influences on ease of fear conditioning to evolutionarily prepared stimuli, and the explanation is fairly complete. So this explanation of specific phobias began with a purely functional psychological analysis (based on classical conditioning). By adding biological levels of analysis (evolution, genetics, and neuropsychology), this functional explanation has been considerably refined.

Cognitive theories of anxiety disorders focus on distortions in information processing found in individuals with anxiety disorders (e.g., selective attention to dangerous events). While such cognitive processes have not been proved to cause anxiety disorders, they may be important in their maintenance. As we saw in the section on suffocation false alarms, a belief in controllability or uncontrollability of feared situations can play an important role in anxious symptoms.

Barlow (2002) proposed a theory of panic disorder that integrates biological and cognitive factors. On the biological side, he proposes that there are heritable individual differences in autonomic reactivity as well as anxiety sensitivity, the tendency to react to symptoms of anxiety. Having once experienced a panic attack in response to a real-life stressor, an individual becomes hypervigilant to cues and sensations associated with the panic attack, which are then more likely to trigger a second attack. Although this theory helps explain how expectations and beliefs can exacerbate panic attacks, it does not explain completely why the initial panic attack occurred. Combining Klein's (1993) suffocation false alarm theory with Barlow's theory might produce a more comprehensive explanation.

Öhman (2000) recently proposed such a comprehensive theory of panic and other anxiety disorders along lines that also integrate research on the evolution and neuropsychology of the fear response. In this theory, the anxiety response is an evolved, automatic, defensive response meant to deal with threats to survival (i.e., the classic fight-or-flight response). In the realistically threatening environment in which humans evolved, there was much more selection pressure against false negatives in the activation of this response (e.g., failing to run from a tiger) than against false positives (e.g., running from one's shadow). Consequently, part of our evolutionary heritage is an easily triggered anxiety response. This evolutionary perspective may help explain why anxiety disorders are the most common of all psychopathologies. This explanation is similar to the one offered earlier in this chapter for the high prevalence of depression.

Another requirement for such a response is that it detect potential threats quickly. Considerable empirical work by Öhman and others (reviewed in Öhman, 2000) using backward masking and divided attention paradigms, demonstrates rapid, nonconcious processing of threat stimuli, which is more pronounced in individuals with anxiety disorders. This preattentive, nonconscious processing of threat stimuli is consistent with LeDoux's model (LaBar & LeDoux, 1997) of amygdala functioning, in which certain threat stimuli reach the amygdala without first being processed by the cortex.

Hence, evolution has prepared us to be more anxious than we need to be, especially given the relative safety of modern life, and to rapidly and unconsciously process signs of threat. Genetically influenced individual differences in this evolved anxiety response mean that some people will be particularly prone to having the anxiety response triggered by the wrong context, as in phobias, or with too low a threshold, as in panic disorder (Öhman, 2000). Once such a false-positive anxiety response occurs, the quickness of fear conditioning, the misattribution of the sufferer (e.g., "I'm going to die"), and the avoidance of subsequent exposure all make a recurrence more likely.

Treatment

Both cognitive-behavioral and pharmacological therapies have been shown to be effective in the treatment of anxiety disorders. Different anxiety disorders respond best to different cognitive-behavioral approaches and to different drugs.

Phobias are probably the most treatable of all anxiety disorders, with about a 90% success rate using learning-based procedures such as systematic desensitization, and exposure and modeling procedures. Cognitive-behavioral approaches are somewhat less effective with GAD (see Nietzel, Speltz, McCauley, & Bernstein, 1998).

Barlow (2002) and others have developed cognitive-behavioral approaches for treating panic disorder that include (1) breathing retraining; (2) interoceptive exposure to anxiety cues, such as heart rate changes or dizziness, in order to reduce anxious reactions to such cues; and (3) cognitive restructuring. Such approaches have not only a high initial success rate but also a disappointingly high relapse rate (see review in Nietzel et al., 1998).

Drug treatments for anxiety disorders include (1) benzodiazepines, (2) antidepressants, and (3) buspirone (sold as Buspar). Benzodiazepines very effectively provide immediate relief from symptoms of anxiety, but they have the disadvantage of producing drug dependence, as well as side effects such as drowsiness. Therefore, benzodiazepines should be tapered after a few months. They can be combined with an antidepressant, which can be taken longer.

There is much less research on treatment efficacy in children and adolescents (see Satcher, 1999). For phobias, learning-based procedures have also been shown to be highly effective at younger ages. Cognitive-behavioral approaches for other anxiety disorders in children and adolescents have been evaluated as "probably efficacious." There is some preliminary evidence to suggest that SSRIs may be effective in the treatment of anxiety disorders in this age range.

Finally, in terms of *prevention*, promising results are emerging from an early intervention project in Australia (Dadds et al., 1999). A large sample ($N = 128$) of children (ages 9–14 years) at high risk for anxiety disorders (because of teacher nominations or self-reports of anxiety symptoms) were randomly assigned to either a cognitive-behavioral prevention course or an untreated control group. Six months after this intervention, the rates of anxiety disorders in the treated group (16%) were significantly lower than in the untreated group (54%). Although prevention effects were not evident at the 1-year follow-up, they reemerged at the 2-year follow-up.

POSTTRAUMATIC STRESS DISORDER

Posttraumatic stress disorder (PTSD) is usually classified as an anxiety disorder, but it is distinctive because it is defined etiologically and has a relation to dissociative disorders. It is also a more recently recognized disorder. Although "shell shock" and "battle fatigue" were described by clinicians working with soldiers in both World Wars, professional attention to these disorders waned after these wars were over. Pat Barker's (1994) historical novel, *The Eye in the Door,* provides a particularly vivid account of PTSD with dissociation in a World War I soldier. The novel also details the soldier's treatment by the real clinicians Sir Henry Head (1861–1940) and William H. R. Rivers (1864–1922), who were actually involved with such patients during the war and were also distinguished for their contributions to neurology and social anthropology, respectively. Despite this early work, the recognition of PTSD as a potentially chronic psychiatric disorder did not occur until much later. This recognition was prompted by the experiences of American veterans from the war in Vietnam, as well as case studies of disaster survivors. PTSD was first included in DSM-III (American Psychiatric Association, 1980). Earlier versions of the DSM considered stress-induced symptoms to be transient.

Definition

One of the central puzzles of PTSD is that it involves both heightened and decreased arousal, and both avoidance and intense reexperiencing of things connected with the traumatic event. An adequate theory of PTSD needs to explain these apparently contradictory symptoms.

PTSD is defined in DSM-IV-TR as the development of three types of persistent symptoms following exposure to an extreme traumatic stressor (death, serious injury, or other threat to bodily integrity), either as a victim, as a witness, or as a close confidant. The initial exposure must have produced intense fear, helplessness, or horror (or, in children, disorganization or agitation). Specifically, the three types of defining symptoms are reexperiencing, avoidance, and arousal symptoms; some symptoms of each type are necessary for the diagnosis. The symptoms also must last at least 1 month and interfere with adaptive functioning. Reexperiencing the traumatic event is indicated by recurrent recollections, dreams, flashbacks, and psychological and/or physiological arousal in reaction to cues related to the event. Avoidance symptoms include avoidance of trauma-related cues (even to the point of amnesia for aspects of the trauma) and generalized numbing of responsiveness, as evidenced by diminished interest in usual activities, a feeling of detachment, restricted range of affect, and sense of a foreshortened future. Arousal symptoms include difficulty falling or staying asleep, irritability or angry outbursts, problems with concentration, hypervigilance, and an exaggerated startle response.

There has been considerable discussion of what counts as a traumatic stressor. As we have seen, stressful life events are implicated in the etiology of most mood and anxiety disorders, so we need to distinguish stressors that increase the risk for PTSD specifically. As discussed in McNally (1999), the DSM-IV field trials provided some empirical evidence relevant to this question, as they found an extremely low rate (0.4%) of PTSD symptoms in individuals not exposed to life-threatening stressors such as combat, natural disasters, or rape. Exposure can include (1) being a victim of such stressors, (2) experiencing vicarious exposure, either as a witness or confidant, or (3) in some cases, perpetrating life-threatening violence on another person (e.g., a policeman or a soldier who shoots someone in the line of duty).

Epidemiology

The lifetime prevalence of PTSD in the National Comorbidity Study (NCS; Kessler, Sonnega, Bromet, Hughes, & Nelson, 1995) was 7.8%, with women (10.4%) affected about twice as often as men (5%). As we see later, males are somewhat more likely to be exposed to life-threatening trauma, so the female predominance of PTSD initially presents a paradox. The resolution of this paradox could be that women are more likely than men to perceive a physically dangerous situation as life threatening. Or it could be a difference in the kinds of trauma to which they are exposed. There is a much higher rate of exposure in females (13 times higher according to the NCS study) to the most traumatogenic stressor, rape. In one study, 80% of female rape victims developed PTSD, whereas only about 25% of those exposed to other forms of life-threatening trauma developed the disorder (Breslau, Davis, Andreski, & Peterson, 1991). Results of the NCS study (Kessler et al., 1995) indicate that after being raped, 46% of women and 65% of men developed PTSD, whereas overall rates of PTSD after any life-threatening trauma were 20% in females and 8% in males. So it is clear that the risk for PTSD after rape is several times higher than the risk after other forms of life-threatening trauma. Because females are much more likely to be rape victims, their overall rate of PTSD is higher than that of males.

Sociocultural Differences

In addition to the gender differences just discussed, it is well known that exposure to violence varies with both ethnicity and social class. Exposure to traumatic events is correlated with being male, black, and having less education (McNally, 1999).

Comorbidities

About 80% of adults with PTSD have a comorbid diagnosis, mainly alcohol abuse, depression, GAD, and panic disorder. Some of these conditions may precede PTSD and act as a risk factor for it; others may follow PTSD. This issue has not been thoroughly studied.

Etiology

Although it was originally believed that the cause of PTSD is completely environmental and that traumatic exposure is a sufficient, single cause of the disorder, it is now clear that there are individual differences in the response to trauma, some of which are genetically mediated. So PTSD, like most of the other disorders considered in this book, fits the general diathesis–stress model, although the exact nature of the diathesis has yet to be discovered.

Somewhat surprisingly, exposure to life-threatening trauma is more common than one might think. In the Breslau and colleagues (1991) study, 40% of the study sample had experienced such trauma. The rates in the NCS study (Kessler et al., 1995) were 61% in males and 51% in females. Since this rate of exposure is much higher than the rates of PTSD found in these studies, it is clear that trauma alone is rarely sufficient to cause PTSD. Other risk factors must be involved, some of which include lower IQ, lower social support, previous trauma (including childhood physical or sexual abuse), a preexisting mood or anxiety disorder, or a family history of such disorders (reviewed in McNally, 1999). Because some of these other risk factors are genetically influenced in part, it makes sense that individual differences in susceptibility to PTSD might be partly heritable. Another risk factor is the occurrence of dissociation (e.g., events happening in slow motion, feeling disconnected from one's body) at the time of the traumatic event (Foa & Riggs, 1995). Peritraumatic dissociation predicts later PTSD even after controlling for the intensity of the trauma (Shalev, Peri, Cannetti, & Schreiber, 1996).

Heritability

A large twin study of PTSD (with over 4,000 twin pairs) has been conducted using the Vietnam Era Twin Registry (Goldberg, True, Eisen, & Henderson, 1990; True et al., 1993). The results of this study have provided strong evidence of both environmental and genetic influences on PTSD. By examining MZ pairs discordant for heavy combat exposure, Goldberg and colleagues (1990) found that individuals with such exposure were *nine* times more likely to have PTSD than their co-twins who had not served in Vietnam. Because members of MZ pairs are genetically identical, this difference in rates of PTSD must be due to nonshared environmental experience (i.e., exposure to heavy combat). Unlike the methods used in many studies of putative environmental risk factors, this discordant MZ-pair design allows researchers to be sure that the risk factor is indeed environmental.

Interestingly, this study also found that for combat exposure the MZ concordance was higher than the DZ concordance, indicating some degree of genetic influence on the likelihood of being exposed to combat! Although such a finding at first seems counterintuitive (just as the heritability of divorce seems counterintuitive), it seems likely that combat exposure in Vietnam was correlated with individual cognitive and personality differences. To the extent that there are genetic influences on such individual differences, MZ pairs would be more likely than DZ pairs to be concordant for combat exposure.

Consequently, in examining the heritability of PTSD symptoms, it was important to control for combat exposure. When this was done, True and colleagues (1993) found modest heritabilities for each of the three types of PTSD symptoms: 13–30% for reexperiencing symptoms, 30–34% for avoidance symptoms, and 28–32% for arousal symptoms. We do not know exactly what the genetic diathesis for trauma is, although the evidence cited earlier suggests that some of it may overlap with genetic influences on mood and anxiety disorders.

Brain Mechanisms

Essentially the same neural circuits and animal models used to explain depression and anxiety have been applied to the explanation of PTSD, with one important addition, namely, the opiate system (see, e.g., van der Kolk & Greenberg, 1987; see reviews in Hollander, Simeon, and Gorman, 1999; McNally, 1999). These are the same neural circuits involved in the stress response system (i.e., orbitofrontal cortex, amygdala, HPA axis, and the noradrenergic projections from the LC); the animal models are those of conditioned fear, inescapable shock, and kindling. As we will see, there is certainly empirical support for these models from both autonomic and brain imaging studies of individuals with PTSD. However, something else is needed to construct a *specific* explanation of PTSD using these circuits and animal models. So the basic premise is that the stress response system is dysregulated in PTSD, which is also the basic premise in explanations of depression and other anxiety disorders. The added postulates that are specific to PTSD are that either extreme trauma produces an oscillation between noradrenergic overactivity and depletion and/or the stress response system interacts with the endogenous opiate system, again, because of the extremity of the trauma. Either the oscillation or the periodic release of endogenous opiates could help explain the paradoxical combination of overarousal and numbing found in PTSD. The kindling model has been used to explain reexperiencing symptoms (e.g., nightmares and flashbacks). The idea here is that such symptoms are spontaneous, intense discharges of memory circuits analogous to the spontaneous discharges of motor circuits in the kindling model of seizures, and that such discharges are kindled by repeated occurrences—a positive feedback loop. Although these ideas are illuminating, we still lack a definitive account of the brain mechanisms involved in PTSD and how they differ from the overlapping brain mechanisms involved in depression and other anxiety disorders.

Because trauma is rarely sufficient to produce PTSD, and because there are genetically influenced, individual differences in susceptibility, a brain theory of this disorder must also include an account of the neural basis of these individual differences. However, we currently know very little about brain differences that precede and predict the development of PTSD.

Instead, our empirical knowledge base consists of studies of brain mechanisms *after* the onset of PTSD. Studies document a number of findings consistent with a dysregulated stress response system, including greater autonomic arousal (measured by heart rate, facial electromyography [EMG], and skin conductance) to trauma cues, exaggerated startle responses, sleep abnormalities, and *decreased* cortisol levels, which distinguish PTSD from depression and other anxiety disorders (see reviews in Hollander et al., 1999; McNally, 1999).

Neuroimaging Studies

The main structural finding in PTSD is a reduction in hippocampal volumes, originally interpreted (see, e.g., Sapolsky, 1996) as a result of stress-induced cortisol release, since it is well established that cortisol can be toxic to hippocampal neurons. Such hippocampal damage could in turn provide an explanation of the amnesic symptoms in PTSD. However, this interpretation is contradicted by the consistent finding of decreased cortisol levels in PTSD. Two other hypotheses are that the hippocampal volume reduction is secondary to comorbid alcohol abuse or that it is a preexisting risk factor (see review in McNally, 1999).

Across three functional neuroimaging studies of PTSD (Rauch et al., 1996; Shin et al., 1997, 1999), exposure to auditory or visual trauma stimuli produced blood flow increases in limbic areas (including the amygdala), anterior cingulate, and orbitofrontal cortex, and a blood flow *decrease* in Broca's area. The increases are consistent with dysregulation of the stress response system; the decrease in Broca's area is unexplained.

Neuropsychology

The main psychological theories advanced to explain PTSD are learning and cognitive-behavioral theories, similar to those proposed to explain depression and other anxiety disorders. Hence, these theories, like the brain theories, face the problem of explaining PTSD *specifically*. In addition, they must also account for the paradoxical combination of symptoms that defines PTSD.

Mowrer's (1939) two-factor theory, discussed earlier as an explanation for phobias, has been applied to PTSD. In this view, PTSD is just a more intense conditioned fear response. Without additional postulates, this theory does not readily account for numbing, amnesia, or flashbacks.

Cognitive-behavioral theorists (e.g., Chemtob, Roitblatt, Hamada, Carlson, & Twentyman, 1988; Foa, Zinbarg, & Olasov-Rothbaum, 1992) have attempted to deal with these shortcomings in the learning theory by proposing a fear network theory of PTSD that integrates psychological and physiological aspects of this disorder. Their basic idea is that a traumatic experience strengthens the connections among widely distributed memory representations related to the traumatic event, including behavioral and physiological reactions to the trauma. Activation of any part of the network can thus reactivate the whole network, thereby explaining the three classes of PTSD symptoms: reexperiencing, avoidance, and arousal. While this theory is definitely a step in the right direction, further specification of the networks involved is needed.

Another important aspect of cognitive-behavioral theories of PTSD is their attempt to explain the altered views of both the self (e.g., as flawed or guilty) and the world (e.g., as unpredictable and unsafe) found in some individuals with persistent PTSD. These more general attributions are not readily dealt with by physiological theories and, once again, highlight the need for theories of psychopathology that incorporate both bottom-up (e.g., alterations in subcortical arousal circuits) and top-down influences (e.g., changes in expectations and beliefs). Such attributions turn out to be an important predictor of who recovers from PTSD and who does not (Dunmore, Clark, & Ehlers, 1999).

Treatment

As was true for depression and other anxiety disorders, both pharmacological and cognitive-behavioral therapies have been found to be useful in treating PTSD. There is no single, specific drug therapy for PTSD, but both antidepressants and beta-blockers (e.g., propranolol) are useful in reducing PTSD symptoms, although they do reduce all of them (e.g., numbing, alienation, and general anxiety persist). Treatment research on PTSD is fairly new, but there has been considerable progress in the last 10 years. A meta-analysis of 17 controlled treatment studies of PTSD (Sherman, 1998) found average improvement rates of 62% in the treated group versus 38% in controls.

Several cognitive-behavioral approaches are used to treat PTSD. One approach is direct exposure therapy, which, similar to the treatment of phobias, involves systematic desensitization. The fear network theory just discussed led to treatments of PTSD. One of these, developed by Foa, Steketee, and Olasov-Rathbaum (1989), involved activating the fear network and then providing experiences that are incompatible with it. Another approach, cognitive processing therapy (Resick & Schnicke, 1992), addressed the general attributions about self and world that can result from PTSD, and included writing about the traumatic event and challenging beliefs connected with it.

Particularly noteworthy is a *preventive* therapy for women who have been raped or physically assaulted (Foa, Hearst-Ikeda, & Perry, 1995). This preventive therapy includes four components: (1) education that PTSD symptoms in response to rape or assault are normal, (2) relaxation training, (3) reliving the experience through imagery, and (4) cognitive therapy to address negative general attributions. Two months after their trauma, the 10 women who received this therapy after a rape or physical assault had a much lower rate (10%) of PTSD than the rate observed (70%) in a matched group of 10 women who did not receive the treatment. Six months after trauma, there were still group differences in depression and reexperiencing symptoms. Although these results are quite promising, it is important to note the small sample size and the lack of random assignment to the treated and untreated conditions. The two groups were carefully matched on trauma and demographic variables, but it is still possible that the group was confounded with some other variable that contributed to the results.

In a follow-up prevention study, Foa and colleagues (1999) remedied these shortcomings by randomly assigning 96 female rape or assault victims to one of four treatment conditions: (1) prolonged exposure, (2) stress inoculation training, (3) a combination of 1 and 2, or (4) a wait-list control group. Groups 1, 2, and 3 had significantly less PTSD and depression after treatment and at a 1-year follow-up than group 4. The three active treatment groups did not differ significantly.

BIPOLAR DISORDER

Establishing the distinction between bipolar illness and schizophrenia on the one hand, and major depression on the other, was an important development in descriptive psychiatry. Nonetheless, there is some degree of etiological overlap between bipolar illness and major depression, the exact nature of which remains to be determined. Bipolar disorder has an intriguing relation to creativity, especially literary creativity. The old observation that "genius is to madness near allied" has found confirmation in work by Jamison (1993) and others documenting a much higher rate of bipolar illness among artists, especially poets. Consequently, the phenomenology of bipolar disorder has received a richer treatment in literature than perhaps any other psychiatric illness. For instance, Jamison illustrates the phenomenology of bipolar illness using passages from the English Romantic poets Byron, Shelley, Blake, and Coleridge. Jamison's (1995) autobiography, *An Unquiet Mind*, is a beautifully written, poignant account of her own struggle with bipolar illness. C. P. Snow's (1947) novel, *The Light and the Dark*, tells us about bipolar illness from the point of view of a close personal friend, who is unsuccessful in saving a talented young English airman from this disorder back in the days when there were no effective treatments for it.

Definition

DSM-IV-TR distinguishes three subtypes of bipolar illness. The main subtype, bipolar I disorder, is defined by the occurrence of one or more manic episodes, whereas the other two subtypes, bipolar II and cyclothymia, involve less severe manic symptoms. A manic episode is a "distinct period of abnormally and persistently elevated, expansive, or irritable mood" (American Psychiatric Association, 2000, p. 357) characterized by three of the following seven symptoms: exaggerated self-esteem or grandiosity, diminished need for sleep, increased talking or pressured speech, flight of ideas or feeling that thoughts are racing, disruptions in attention by unimportant or irrelevant details, increase in goal-directed activity or psychomotor retardation, and excessive pursuit of pleasure despite potential painful consequences (such as spending sprees, foolish investments, or sexual promiscuity). Whereas in major depression the predominant mood is anhedonia, the predominant mood in a manic episode is euphoria. The manic episode must cause a significant impairment in adaptive functioning and not be secondary to a substance or a general medical condition, such as hyperthyroidism.

The other two subtypes of bipolar disorder, bipolar II and cyclothymic disorder, both involve milder forms of mania called "hypomania" (literally, a reduced amount of mania). The definition of bipolar II disorder requires the presence of at least one major depressive episode and one hypomanic episode. The least severe subtype of bipolar illness, cyclothymic disorder, is defined by the presence of manic and depressive symptoms, without there having been a manic or major depressive episode (but there can have been a hypomanic episode). A hypomanic episode is defined very similarly to a manic episode except that it is less severe in its impact on adaptive functioning (does not cause marked impairment, require a hospitalization, and is not accompanied by psychotic symptoms) and may be briefer (at least 4 days as opposed to a week). So the occurrence of a manic episode, even without depressive symptoms, warrants the diagnosis of bipolar I, although the majority of patients with bipolar I disorder also have both depressive and recurring manic episodes. In contrast, the other two subtypes require the presence of both manic and depressive features. The final diagnostic consideration is the existence of what are called "mixed episodes," defined as cycling between a manic and a major depressive episode within the period of a day for most days of at least a week. Because a mixed episode involves a (brief) manic episode, it also warrants the diagnosis of bipolar I and excludes the diagnosis of the two less severe subtypes, bipolar II and cyclothymia.

It is increasingly appreciated that bipolar illness can occur in childhood (Carlson, 1990), with somewhat different symptom manifestations than seen in adults. However, a formal diagnostic definition of bipolar illness in childhood is not included in DSM-IV-TR.

Epidemiology

Bipolar illness is less prevalent than the other mood and anxiety disorders considered here. The lifetime prevalence of bipolar I disorder is usually stated to be around 1%, although the NCS study found a lifetime prevalence of 1.5% (Kessler et al., 1995). The lifetime prevalences for bipolar II and cyclothymic disorder are similarly low (0.5% and 0.4–1.0%, respectively; DSM-IV-TR). A minority of persons with the two milder subtypes eventually develop bipolar I disorder.

Unlike other mood and anxiety disorders, there is not a gender difference in the prevalence of the bipolar disorders. There are, however, gender differences in manifestation. The first episode is more likely to be a manic episode in males but a major depressive episode in females. Rapid cycling between episodes is more likely to occur in females.

Sociocultural Differences

Bipolar disorder is distinctive among most psychiatric illnesses in not exhibiting a correlation between prevalence and socioeconomic status (i.e., higher prevalence in lower socioeconomic groups). Indeed, some sources have reported a higher rate of bipolar illness in *higher* socioeconomic groups (Jamison, 1993), presumably because of the increased productivity and creativity associated with hypomania.

Comorbidities

There are increased rates of substance abuse in the bipolar disorders, which can be interpreted as attempts at self-medication or pleasure seeking, or both. Other comorbidities include eating disorders, social phobia, panic disorder, and attention-deficit/hyperactivity disorder. Distinguishing between attention-deficit/hyperactivity disorder and bipolar illness in childhood can present a diagnostic dilemma.

Etiology

Bipolar illness is one of the most familial and heritable of psychiatric illnesses, second only to autism. Considerable effort has been expended to find specific genes that influence bipolar illness.

Familiality

The relative risk (λ) for bipolar disorder to first-degree relatives of an individual with bipolar disorder is about 7 (Satcher, 1999). Family studies have also been used to examine the relation between bipolar and unipolar disorder, and the relations among subtypes of bipolar disorder.

If the familial etiology of bipolar and unipolar disorder were totally shared, then the relatives of a proband with either disorder should exhibit similar elevations in risk for either disorder. On the other hand, if the familial influences on the two disorders were totally separate, then the relatives of a unipolar proband should have no increase in risk for bipolar disorder, and, likewise, the relatives of a bipolar proband should have no increase in risk for unipolar depression. Neither of these extreme positions is supported by family data. Instead, some family data support a severity continuum in which only the more severe disorder (bipolar disorder) places relatives at increased risk for both disorders (e.g., Weissman, Gershon, & Kidd, 1984). Other family data find that the presence of either disorder in a proband increases the risk in relatives for the other disorder, but to a lesser extent (Merikangas & Kupfer, 1995). In other words, the rates of bipolar disorder among relatives of a unipolar proband are above population rates but below the rates found among relatives of a bipolar proband and vice versa. In either case, some degree of cofamiliality between unipolar and bipolar disorder is supported by existing data, consistent with partial overlap in the familial risk factors for the two disorders.

The familial relation among the three subtypes of bipolar disorder likewise supports the fact that subtypes "breed true" and exhibit partial familial overlap with other subtypes. Each subtype increases the risk in relatives for the other two subtypes but, again, to a lesser extent than the risk found when the proband and relative have the same subtype (Howland & Thase, 1999).

Heritability

The heritability of bipolar disorder is greater than that for major depression, because the difference between MZ and DZ concordance rates is greater for bipolar disorder. Across studies, the average MZ concordance for bipolar disorder is about 60%, whereas the average DZ concordance is about 12% (Kelsoe, 1997). Because the MZ concordance is less than 1.0, there must also be environmental influences on the development of bipolar illness.

Mode of Transmission

Although many families with bipolar disorder exhibit vertical transmission of the disorder across generations, suggestive of single, major gene transmission, more detailed analyses have not supported such a simple model. Instead, the mode of transmission appears to be complex and likely involves multiple interacting genes (Satcher, 1999).

Linkage Analyses

Early reports of linkage of bipolar disorder to chromosome 11p in Amish pedigrees or to the X chromosome, which generated considerable scientific excitement, were not replicated by subsequent studies. Quite a number of other studies have followed, but at this point no linkages have been consistently replicated, and no genes have been identified. The best replicated results are on chromosomes 18 (p and q) and 21q (Berrettini, 1998; Kelsoe, 1997; Satcher, 1999). The inconsistency across more recent studies could be due to phenotype definition or to the complex mode of transmission, which is thought to involve multiple interacting loci. The loci on chromosomes 18 and 21 could indeed be involved, but their effect size might be small, or they might only act as risk factors in a subset of families, resulting in inconsistent results (Satcher, 1999).

Some of the issues involved in finding genes that influence bipolar disorder are well illustrated by Berrettini and colleagues (1997), who found a weak susceptibility locus for bipolar disorder on chromosome 18, which, these authors note has been replicated in three other samples. Unlike the early linkage studies of bipolar disorder that attempted to find a single dominant gene that caused the disorder, methods in this study are based on the assumption of complex inheritance involving multiple susceptibility loci, possibly with only small effects. Berrettini and colleagues conducted a genome search of about half the genome in a large set ($N = 22$) of bipolar families with 365 individuals. Because a substantial region of chromosome 18 could not be excluded, they then conducted a more detailed, follow-up examination of this region. Their results depended on the phenotype examined, parental transmission, and the method of linkage analysis employed. Significant results for a susceptibility locus on chromosome 18 were found only in families with paternal transmission, and only with nonparametric (or model-free) sib-pair linkage methods. A broader phenotype that produced the strongest results included bipolar I and II disorders, schizoaffective illness (essentially a manic, mixed, or major depressive episode with psychotic features), and recurrent unipolar depression. This result would be consistent with familial data that indicate a partial overlap between familial risk factors for bipolar and unipolar disorder. The estimated effect size (λ = 1.5–2.0) of the susceptibility locus was weak, meaning that it would only be detected in large samples, and the linkage region was broad, including parts of both chromosomes 18 p and q.

Although this study varied the phenotype definition to include a spectrum of mood disorders, the phenotype employed was categorical rather than quantitative. As discussed earlier, there are powerful sib-pair linkage methods for analyzing quantitative phenotypes, but these methods have not been utilized in linkage studies of bipolar disorder.

In summary, the approximate locations of susceptibility loci that influence bipolar disorder and related conditions are beginning to be identified, and these results are generally consistent with what we have learned from family, twin, and segregation studies. But, clearly, more work is needed to define the relevant phenotypes and to identify conclusively which risk alleles influence them.

Environmental Risk Factors

Although twin studies indicate there are environmental influences on the development of bipolar disorder, these have for the most part not been clearly identified. There is evidence that psychological stress can affect the course of bipolar disorder (see review in Johnson & Roberts, 1995). A form of psychological stress that affects the course of the disorder, "expressed emotion," has been studied extensively in the families of individuals with bipolar disorder (Miklowitz & Goldstein, 1990). These studies have found a relation between the family's style of expressing and regulating emotion, and the probability of relapse in individuals with bipolar disorder.

Brain Mechanisms

An explanation of bipolar disorder must tell us why mood is unstable in this disorder, what brain systems are disrupted to give rise to mania, and how the transition from mania to depression occurs, especially the very rapid transitions seen in a mixed episode. While the terms "bipolar" and "unipolar" tempt us to think of major depression and mania as simply opposite extremes of the same underlying neurobiological mechanism, both the phenomenology and the physiology of the depression found in unipolar disorder differ somewhat from the depression found in bipolar disorder. In terms of phenomenology, bipolar depression typically includes excessive sleeping (hypersomnia), weight gain, and severe psychomotor retardation, whereas unipolar depression is typically associated with insomnia, anorexia, and psychomotor agitation (Kelley, 1987). The symptoms of bipolar depression fit with animal models of mesolimbic dopamine depletion (Depue & Iacono, 1989; Swerdlow & Koob, 1987), whereas the symptoms of unipolar depression are usually interpreted, as discussed earlier, as reflecting imbalances in NE and serotonin. To put it simply, the opposite of unipolar depression is relief from chronic stress and the return of a normal capacity for pleasure, whereas the opposite of bipolar depression is mania, which is an excessive pursuit and capacity for pleasure. So to understand mania, we must turn to the brain system involved in reward and goal-directed behavior.

This has been called the "behavioral facilitation" system (Depue & Iacono, 1989), which mobilizes approach behaviors to seek rewards and to remove obstacles to rewards. Depue and Iacono (1989) argue that most of the symptoms of mania can be viewed as exaggerated functioning of this system, whereas bipolar depression reflects reduced functioning. Neuroanatomically, the behavioral facilitation system corresponds to the main projection sites of the mesolimbic and mesocortical dopamine pathways, both of which originate in the ventral tegmental area. The mesocortical tract projects to the prefrontal cortex, whose function in action selection I have already discussed. The mesolimbic tract projects throughout the limbic system (e.g., to the amygdala and hippocampus), as well as to structures that might be considered part of a bridge between the limbic system and prefrontal cortex, such as the cingulate gyrus and nucleus accumbens. The cingulate gyrus appears to be an important part of an anterior attentional system. The nucleus accumbens may serve as a kind of gate for the flow of limbic motivational information into the brain structures involved in action selection (Depue & Iacono, 1989; Swerdlow & Koop, 1987). In other words, the mesolimbic tract helps provide an answer to the important question of how the motivation and action selection systems interact. Because the various neural structures in the behavioral facilitation system all receive dopamine projections, alterations in dopaminergic neurotransmission could either over- or underactivate this system, with opposite consequences for the level of goal-directed activity. Mania, characterized by extreme and maladaptive reward seeking, would thus represent extreme overactivity of this system, and bipolar depression, characterized by severe psychomotor depression, would represent extreme underactivity.

This brain theory of bipolar disorder is supported by studies of reward-seeking behaviors in animal models (reviewed in Depue & Iacono, 1989) and by evidence of alterations in dopamine neurotransmission in bipolar disorder (reviewed in Howland & Thase, 1999). Briefly, this evidence includes (1) increased dopamine metabolite (homovanillic acid) levels in cerebrospinal fluid taken from patients with mania; (2) upregulation of brain dopamine receptors (D2 receptors) in brain imaging studies of individuals with mania; (3) increased susceptibility of bipolar patients to dopamine agonists, which can trigger a manic episode; and (4) the fact that high doses of stimulant drugs that are dopamine agonists can produce mania in normal individuals.

While this is an appealing theory, it is important to point out that there are other neurotransmitter and neuroendocrine (i.e., HPA and HTA axis) abnormalities in bipolar disorder. For example, NE and NE metabolite (MHPG) levels vary systematically with mood transitions within bipolar patients studied longitudinally, and treatment with lithium reduces the rate of NE turnover in such patients (Howland & Thase, 1999). So alterations in NE levels are at least correlated with mood cycles in bipolar disorder and may play a causal role in the switch between cycles. There is also evidence of low levels of the main cortical inhibitory neurotransmitter (GABA) in bipolar disorder (Howland & Thase, 1999) and alterations in the so-called "second messenger" system, the chemical cascade that occurs in the postsynaptic neuron after a neurotransmitter binds to the synapse (Dubovsky & Buzan, 1999). In summary, just as was true for major depression, it is likely that multiple neurotransmitter systems are involved in the pathogenesis of bipolar disorder.

Neuroimaging Studies

Both structural and functional neuroimaging differences have been found in bipolar disorder. The two main structural findings—white matter hyperintensities and cortical atrophy (indicated by ventricular enlargement and sulcal widening)—both suggest a neurodegenerative process (see reviews in Dubovsky & Buzan, 1999; Howland & Thase, 1999). Unlike the situation in major depression, these findings are neither restricted to older patients nor accounted for by medication or

ECT; such findings are correlated with the severity and chronicity of the disorder, cortisol levels, and age (Howland & Thase, 1999). Because of these correlations, one possible explanation for these structural differences is that the physiological changes associated with episodes of mania and depression cause neurodegeneration.

Functional neuroimaging differences in bipolar disorder include (1) decreased frontal brain metabolism during a depressive episode, which is greater than that found in unipolar depression; (2) overall increases in brain metabolism, including the frontal lobes, with the switch to mania or hypomania; and (3) possible laterality differences in the frontal lobe metabolism between unipolar and bipolar disorder, with left-hemisphere decreases in the former and right-hemisphere decreases in the latter (reviewed in Howland & Thase, 1999). These differences in brain metabolism likely result from the underlying physiological changes that produce episodes of mania and depression, and are thus best conceptualized as state rather than trait markers.

In summary, available evidence strongly supports the view that bipolar disorder is a brain disorder, in that differences in neurochemistry, brain structure, and brain metabolism are found in individuals with this disorder. While the prevailing view is that the proximal brain cause of the disorder is neurochemical or neuroendocrine changes that in turn lead to the observed structural and metabolic changes, testing such causal hypotheses is difficult, and the pathophysiology of bipolar disorder remains unknown.

Neuropsychology

The brevity of this section reveals an important conceptual gap in our understanding of both bipolar disorder specifically and psychopathology generally. Current textbooks (e.g., Dubovsky & Buzan, 1999; Holmes, 1997; Nietzel et al., 1998) agree that there are essentially no modern psychological theories of bipolar disorder! The old psychoanalytic idea that mania is a flight from depression has obvious conceptual shortcomings (e.g., why is there no such flight in severe unipolar depression?) and has never been tested empirically. Setting aside some disorders as "biological," and thus outside the scope of psychological theory, just reveals the latent dualism discussed earlier and poses major problems for both biological and psychological theories of psychopathology. Any disorder of behavior, including neurological disorders such as Parkinson's and Alzheimer's diseases, requires a *functional* explanation (most likely at the neural network level). The behavioral facilitation model of bipolar disorder (Depue & Iacono, 1989) discussed earlier is an attempt at such a functional explanation, but it is striking that there have not been more recent attempts.

Treatment

The first-line treatment for bipolar disorder is pharmacological, but psychotherapy can be helpful to prevent relapses. ECT is also a useful treatment. I first consider pharmacological treatments, which can be divided into primary treatment aimed at stabilizing mood and adjunctive treatments for correlated symptoms, mainly agitation and psychosis. Three categories of mood stabilizers—lithium salts, anticonvulsants, and calcium channel blockers—have proven efficacy in both treating acute episodes and preventing relapses. The efficacy of all three types of mood stabilizers is about 60–80% (Dubovsky & Buzan, 1999), although more recent studies find a lower (40–50%) success rate for lithium, perhaps because of greater comorbid drug use, shorter hospital stays, or other changes in the samples studied (Satcher, 1999).

Lithium carbonate, an inorganic salt, was found to be effective for treating bipolar disorder in the late 1940s, but its exact mode of action is still unknown, although there is evidence that it influences intracellular calcium levels, as I discuss shortly. Because higher levels of lithium are toxic, especially to the liver and the kidneys, blood levels need to be monitored.

Anticonvulsants that effectively treat bipolar disorder include carbamazepine (Tegretol), valproic acid (Depakene), and valproate (Depakote). These medicines were first used to prevent seizures, which arise because of excessive neuronal firing. Thus, these anticonvulsants presumably act by stabilizing neuronal physiology, but their exact mode of action is unknown. One hypothesis is that they act by stabilizing neuronal membrane systems, including the cyclic AMP (adenosine 3, 5' = monophosphate) system (Satcher, 1999) that is part of the neuronal second messenger system (in which calcium ion influx plays an important role). Newer anticonvulsants—lamotrigine (Lamictal), gabapentin (Neurontin), and zonisamide (Zonegran)—have also proven useful in treating bipolar disorder (Dubovsky & Buzan, 1999).

The third category of drugs for bipolar disorder, calcium channel blockers, reduce calcium influx into neurons, thus altering the second messenger system and stabilizing neuronal physiology. *In vitro* studies have found elevations in intracellular calcium levels in blood platelets from affectively ill patients with bipolar disorder, but not in those from unipolar patients, normal controls, or successfully treated (euthymic) bipolar patients; lithium and carbamazepine lower calcium levels in platelets from such patients, but not in those from controls or euthymic patients (Dubovsky & Buzan, 1999).

Adjunctive drug treatments include neuroleptics for treating psychotic symptoms that sometimes accompany manic episodes and benzodiazepines for treating agitation and normalizing sleep.

ECT is also an effective treatment for bipolar disorder, both to end a current episode and to prevent recurrences. About 60% of bipolar patients who do not respond to medications benefit from ECT; there is about an 80% success rate of ECT for manic patients overall (Mukherjee, Sackeim, & Schnur, 1994).

Once an episode is terminated, maintenance drug therapy is important to prevent relapses, especially given the neurodegenerative changes that accompany the progression of this disorder. However, compliance with these maintenance therapies is a particular problem with bipolar patients, who may prefer hypomania to normal mood.

Psychotherapy has several important uses in the treatment of bipolar disorder, including (1) helping patients to stabilize their circadian rhythms, since sleep deprivation can trigger relapses; (2) reducing interpersonal and family stress; (3) improving medication compliance; and (4) helping the family understand and help in the treatment of this disorder. A form of psychotherapy called interpersonal and social rhythm therapy (IPSRT) has been developed to accomplish these goals. It has been shown to reduce the risk of relapse in bipolar disorder (Frank et al., 1997; Miklowitz & Goldstein, 1990).

Chapter 4

Disorders of Action Regulation

Five disorders are included in this chapter: (1) attention-deficit/hyperactivity disorder (ADHD), (2) conduct disorder (CD), (3) Tourette syndrome, (4) obsessive–compulsive disorder (OCD), and (5) schizophrenia. As discussed earlier, each disorder is characterized by disruptions in action and (thought) selection, though, admittedly, the first four disorders fit more neatly into this category than does schizophrenia. Schizophrenia also includes alterations in motivation, language, and aspects of memory, indicating a more pervasive impact on neuropsychological development.

ATTENTION-DEFICIT/HYPERACTIVITY DISORDER

A syndrome involving hyperactivity in children was first described over 150 years ago by a German physician, Heinrich Hoffman (1845), who wrote a humorous poem describing the antics of "fidgety Phil who couldn't sit still." Somewhat later, Still (1902) described the main problem in this syndrome as a deficiency in "volitional inhibition" or "a defect in moral control." Barkley (1996) points out that Still (1902) recognized several features of ADHD that have been validated by contemporary research: (1) It overlaps with oppositional and conduct problems; (2) it is familial; (3) it is cofamilial with conduct problems and alcoholism; (4) it has a male predominance of about 3:1; (5) it may also be caused by an acquired brain injury. As we will also see, problems with inhibition continue to be central to current conceptions of ADHD, although much more is now known about the brain bases of these problems.

Whether there is brain dysfunction in ADHD and how to characterize it have been confusing and controversial issues in the history of ADHD research. The notion that childhood hyperactivity is a brain disorder was also promoted by Strauss and Lehtinen (1947), based on similarities with the behavior of children who suffered brain damage because of encephalitis. Unfortunately, this analogy led to some muddled terminology, whereby children with hyperactivity were described as having "minimal brain damage" or "minimal brain dysfunction." These terms are misleading for several reasons: (1) The large majority of children with ADHD have a developmental disorder, not acquired brain damage; (2) the damage or dysfunction to the brain implied in these labels was not documented directly, but only inferred from behavioral symptoms that could have many different causes; (3) many children with acquired brain damage do not have hyperactivity (Rutter & Quinton, 1977); and (4) these terms were vague and overinclusive, and thus impeded progress in delineating distinct neuropsychological syndromes affecting learning and behavior in childhood. There is now much more direct evidence that ADHD is due to a specific kind of brain dysfunction that is substantially heritable.

Although ADHD is now more clearly defined and better understood than it once was, it remains a somewhat broad and controversial diagnosis. Over half of children who meet diagnostic criteria for ADHD qualify for a comorbid diagnosis (Biederman et al., 1992) and the list of comorbid disorders includes many of the other diagnoses in this book: CD, depression, anxiety, Tourette syndrome, dyslexia, and bipolar disorder. Moreover, children with autism and schizophrenia frequently exhibit the symptoms of ADHD, although DSM-IV-TR stipulates that their more serious primary diagnosis excludes an ADHD diagnosis. So more research is needed to understand the basis of these comorbidities and to define purer subtypes of ADHD.

ADHD is one of three "disruptive behavior disorders" (DBDs), the other two being CD and oppositional defiant disorder (ODD). The following section covers CD. There is not enough neuroscientific research on ODD to merit a separate section. However, since both comorbidity and shared etiological risk factors exist among all three DBDs, I do consider how ODD is related to both ADHD and CD.

Definition

DSM-IV-TR (American Psychiatric Association, 2000) defines ADHD with two distinct but correlated dimensions of symptoms, those involving *inattention* (e.g., making careless mistakes and not paying close attention to details, forgetfulness, difficulty organizing tasks and activities, and failure to begin or complete tasks that require sustained mental effort) and *hyperactivity–impulsivity* (e.g., excessive fidgeting, locomotion, or talking; interrupting or intruding in conversations, games, and other situations). With two dimensions, there are thus three possible subtypes of ADHD: inattentive, hyperactive–impulsive, or combined. Someone who meets the diagnostic cutoff (six of nine symptoms) for a single dimension qualifies for that subtype; someone who meets this cutoff on both dimensions qualifies for the combined subtype. Additional requirements for the diagnosis include that the symptoms must (1) cause a clinically significant impairment in adaptive functioning; (2) be inconsistent with developmental level (e.g., not just secondary to mental retardation); (3) have been present for at least 6 months, with an onset of some symptoms before age 7; (4) be present in two or more settings; and (5) not be better accounted for by another mental disorder (pervasive developmental disorder, psychosis, or a mood, anxiety, dissociative, or personality disorder). As we will see, there is better empirical support for the construct validity of the inattentive and combined subtypes than for the hyperactive–impulsive subtype.

Epidemiology

ADHD is one of the most common chronic disorders of childhood, with a 6-month prevalence of 3–5% among school-age children according to recent epidemiological studies (Satcher, 1999). Of course, prevalence depends on definition, and definitions vary in how pervasive they require the ADHD symptoms to be. In a careful epidemiological study that required pervasiveness across three different reporters—parents, teachers, and a physician—the prevalence was only 1.2% (Spreen, Tupper, Risser, Tuckko, & Edgell, 1984). Gender ratios in referred samples have been reported to be as high as 9:1 (males:females), but an epidemiological study found a gender ratio of 3:1 (Szatmari, Offord, &

Boyle, 1989). Thus, as in other disorders, such as reading disability, males are more likely to be referred than females. Because much of the research on ADHD has relied on referred samples, we know much more about ADHD in males than in females.

ADHD has been found across social classes and cultures, with higher rates of ADHD in lower social classes, but these differences are no longer found when comorbid conditions, such as CD, are controlled (see review in Barkley, 1996). Roughly comparable rates of ADHD have been found in studies in the United States, Japan, and India, with a somewhat higher rate in Germany (Barkley, 1996). There can be dramatic differences in prevalence even between very similar cultures (i.e., the United States and the United Kingdom). Such differences appear to be due to differences in diagnostic criteria and practice (Satcher, 1999) rather than representing true differences in prevalence.

In terms of natural history, the age of onset is usually in toddlerhood, with a peak "age of onset" between ages 3 and 4 (Palfrey et al., 1985). Symptoms of ADHD may appear earlier, even *in utero*. It is becoming clearer that ADHD is a chronic disorder across the lifespan (Gittelman, Mannuzza, Shenker, & Gonagura, 1985) and that many of the tasks of adult development are disrupted by ADHD, because sustained effort, planning, and organization are central to many adult responsibilities.

Etiology

Although the exact etiology of ADHD is still unknown, we know more about its etiology and pathogenesis than any other psychopathology reviewed in this book. Thus, ADHD represents a fairly clear success story for a neuroscientific approach to understanding psychopathology. In this section, I review environmental influences on ADHD and evidence that ADHD is familial, moderately heritable, and influenced by two genes that affect dopamine neurotransmission.

Familiality

The rate of ADHD in families of male probands has been found to be over seven times the rate of the disorder in nonpsychiatric control families (Biederman, Faraone, Keenan, Knee, & Tsuang, 1990); a later study has reported a similar increase in risk among relatives of female probands (Faraone, Biederman, Keenan, & Tsuang, 1991; Faraone et al., 1992).

Heritability

Stevenson (1992) found a heritability of .76 for ADHD in his twin study, and numerous other twin studies have found similar results, both for the diagnosis of ADHD and individual differences in ADHD symptomatology (Eaves et al., 1997; Gillis, Gilger, Pennington, & DeFries, 1992; Gjane, Stevenson, & Sundet, 1996; Levy, Hay, McStephen, Wood, & Waldman, 1997; Sherman, Iacono, & McGue, 1997; Thapar, Hervas, & McGuffin, 1995; Willcutt, Pennington, & DeFries, 2000b; Willerman, 1973). Although extreme scores on both the defining dimensions of ADHD, inattention and hyperactivity–impulsivity (HI), are moderately heritable, this appears to *not* be the case for the HI dimension once the correlation between the two dimensions is accounted for (Willcutt et al., 2000a); that is, extreme scores on the inattention dimension are moderately heritable regardless of the level of HI symptoms in the proband (i.e., both the inattentive and combined subtypes of ADHD are moderately heritable). However, extreme scores on the HI dimension were *not* significantly heritable ($h^2_g = .08$) when probands were not also extreme on the inattention dimension. These results suggest that the etiology of the HI subtype is largely nongenetic and differs from the etiology of the other two subtypes.

Mode of Transmission

One segregation analysis of ADHD (Faraone et al., 1992) found autosomal dominant transmission, with considerably reduced penetrance of the hypothesized major gene. Although this suggests there may be loci of sizable effect, the genetic etiology of ADHD is very unlikely to be due to just one gene.

Gene Locations

Efforts to identify specific genes influencing ADHD illustrate the potential power of the candidate gene association approach. As discussed earlier, this approach usually depends on a hypothesis derived from an understanding of the neurobiology of the disorder. We know that the primary drug used to treat ADHD, methylphenidate (Ritalin), is a dopamine agonist, and that it achieves this effect by blocking the dopamine transporter, a receptor on the presynaptic neuron involved in the reuptake of dopamine in the synapse. Hence, blocking reuptake increases the dopamine available in the synapse. Since receptors are coded for by genes, a gene for a dopamine transporter or genes for other dopamine receptors are reasonable candidate genes in ADHD.

Molecular genetic research on ADHD has focused on dopamine genes, particularly a dopamine transporter gene (DAT1) and one of the dopamine receptors, DRD4. Since both of these dopamine genes are polymorphic (they have frequently occurring allelic variations), they could be tested as candidates in association studies.

The 10 copy allele of DAT1 was significantly associated with ADHD in a study of 53 families (Cook et al., 1995). This finding has now been replicated in two separate samples (Gill, Daly, Heron, Hawi, & Fitzgerald, 1997; Waldman et al., 1996), although it is not significant in all samples (Asherson et al., 1998; LaHoste et al., 1995; Poulton et al., 1998).

An allele of the DRD4 gene that contains a 7-repeat base pair sequence was shown to be significantly associated with novelty-seeking behavior, which prompted the hypothesis that it might also be linked to impulsive behavior seen in ADHD (Benjamin, Patterson, Greenberg, Murphy, & Hamer, 1996; Ebstein et al., 1996). Indeed, numerous studies have now found an association between the DRD4 allele and ADHD (Faraone et al., 1999a; La Hoste et al., 1995; Rowe et al., 1998b; Smalley et al., 1998; Swanson et al., 1998), although, again, this result is not significant in all studies (Asherson et al., 1998; Castellanos et al., 1998).

Although these are exciting findings, there are complications that still need to be resolved. First, counterintuitively, the risk allele of the DAT1 gene is *more* frequent than the nonrisk allele in the general population, a result that may well hold for many alleles associated with psychopathology. Second, the effect size of each of these risk alleles is small. Finally, as I discuss later, one study (Swanson et al., 2000) found that presence of the DRD4 risk allele was *not* associated with the neuropsychological deficits that characterize ADHD.

In summary, there will likely be other risk alleles that influence ADHD, and this influence may vary by ADHD subtype, whether these be DSM-IV-TR subtypes or those defined by comorbidities. In the Dyslexia section in Chapter 5, I discuss evidence that the subtype of ADHD comorbid with dyslexia is influenced by the dyslexia locus on chromosome 6, and not by these two dopamine alleles.

Other evidence for genetic influence on ADHD or its symptoms comes from the association with known genetic syndromes, including Turner's syndrome (45, X) in females and (47, XYY) in males; fragile X syndrome, neurofibromatosis, and early-treated phenylketonuria (reviewed in Pennington, 1991).

Environmental Risk Factors

There are several known bioenvironmental correlates of ADHD, including fetal alcohol exposure, environmental lead poisoning, and pediatric head injury (reviewed in Pennington, 1991). Since that review, it has become clear that maternal smoking in pregnancy is associated with an increased risk of ADHD in offspring (see review in Barkley, 1996). However, exposure to these bioenvironmental risk factors is not randomly assigned and so exposure to them could be correlated with ADHD in the parent or child, which may be genetically mediated. At the same time, it seems implausible that the dramatic ADHD symptoms observed clinically in fetal alcohol syndrome or pediatric head injury can be entirely explained by such a confound. Instead, it might be better to conceptualize at least some of these bioenvironmental risk factors as examples of gene–environment correlations: The presence of the ADHD genotype increases exposure to environmental risk factors that exacerbate the ADHD phenotype.

We do not have evidence that the social environment, particularly parenting practices, can directly cause ADHD. At the same time, there is no doubt that the social environment influences the course of ADHD, particularly whether ADHD develops into another DBD. This evidence is reviewed in the section on Conduct Disorder.

Brain Mechanisms

The hypothesis of frontal lobe dysfunction in ADHD has been advanced by several researchers (Gualtieri & Hicks, 1985; Mattes, 1989; Pontius, 1973; Rosenthal & Allen, 1978; Stamm & Kreder, 1979; Zametkin & Rapoport, 1986), based on the observation that frontal lesions in both experimental animals and human patients sometimes produce hyperactivity, distractibility, or impulsivity, separately or in combination (Fuster, 1989; Levin, Eisenberg, & Benton, 1991; Stuss & Benson, 1986). Of course, lesions in other parts of the brain can also produce these symptoms. In the following section, I review evidence that supports frontal–striatal dysfunction in ADHD.

Structural Neuroimaging Studies

With regard to brain structure, earlier researchers (Harcherick et al., 1985; Shaywitz, Shaywitz, Cohen, & Young, 1983) found no evidence of structural differences in computed tomography scan studies of children with ADHD. Hynd, Semrud-Clikeman, Lorys, Novey, and Elio-pulas (1990), however, did find an absence of the usual right > left frontal asymmetry in children with ADHD using MRI scans. They con-trasted subjects with ADHD and both subjects with dyslexia and con-trols; the frontal finding was present in both clinical groups but did not differentiate between them, even though the group with dyslexia was selected to be non-ADHD. There is an association between the right frontal lobe and measures of sustained attention, a neuroanatomical dif-ference that has theoretical relevance to ADHD. This lack of frontal asymmetry in ADHD has been replicated in two other studies (Castel-lanos et al., 1996; Filipek et al., 1997). Abnormalities of caudate volume have also been found across numerous studies of ADHD (Castellanos et al., 1996; Filipek et al., 1997; Hynd et al., 1993; Mataro, Garcia-Sanchez, Junque, Estevez-Gonzales, & Pujol, 1997). In addition, the globus pallidus has been found to be significantly smaller in subjects with ADHD (Aylward et al., 1996; Castellanos et al., 1996; Singer et al., 1993). These structural studies support developmental differences in frontal–striatal structures known to be important in action selection.

The hypothesis that these structural differences are related to defi-cits in action selection was tested in a study by Casey and colleagues (1997), who correlated performance on three separate inhibition tasks with measures of prefrontal cortex and basal ganglia volume. Perfor-mance on the three inhibition tasks, designed to tap response inhibition at different stages of attentional processing, was impaired in the chil-dren with ADHD compared to controls. Furthermore, prefrontal cortex, caudate, and globus pallidus volumes correlated significantly with task performance. Of course, this correlation does not prove cause. As dis-cussed earlier, such a finding could be a *result* or just a correlate of ADHD.

However, brain structure differences in ADHD are not restricted ex-clusively to the prefrontal cortex and basal ganglia. In addition, in sev-eral studies, decreased areas in different regions of the corpus callosum have been observed (Baumgardner et al., 1996; Castellanos et al., 1996; Giedd, Castellanos, Casey, Kozuch, & King, 1994; Hynd et al., 1991; Semrud-Clikeman et al., 1994), as well as less total cerebral volume and a smaller cerebellum (Castellanos et al., 1996).

Functional Neuroimaging Studies

In terms of brain function, electrophysiological measures have sup-ported the hypothesis of central nervous system underarousal in at least a subgroup of hyperactive children (Ferguson & Rappaport, 1983). Likewise, in children with ADHD, Lou, Henricksen, and Bruhn (1984), using regional cerebral blood flow, found that decreased blood flow to the frontal lobes increased after the children received Ritalin. Ritalin treatment also decreased blood flow to the motor cortex and primary sensory cortex, "suggesting an inhibition of function of these structures, seen clinically as less distractibility and decreased motor activity during treatment" (p. 829). These investigators have replicated this result in an expanded sample (Lou, Henricksen, & Bruhn, 1989); in this second report, they emphasize the basal ganglia as the locus of reduced blood flow in ADHD. Zametkin and colleagues (1990) used positron emission tomography scanning to study the parents of children with ADHD, who themselves had residual-type ADHD, and found an overall reduction in cerebral glucose utilization, particularly in right frontal areas, but increased utilization in posterior medial–orbital areas. A second study by this group (Zametkin et al., 1993) investigating teenagers with ADHD replicated some but not all of those findings and found significant reductions in the group with ADHD in normalized glucose metabolism in 6 of 60 brain regions, including the left anterior frontal lobe. Metabolism in that region correlated inversely with ADHD symptom severity across the combined sample of patients and controls. Because hyperfrontality of blood flow is characteristic of the normal brain, in ADHD, it could explain the low central arousal found in the electrophysiological studies.

Other studies have demonstrated decreased blood flow in ADHD subjects, both in prefrontal regions and the striatum (Amen, Paldi, & Thisted, 1993). More recently, functional magnetic resonance imaging (fMRI) techniques have demonstrated similar results, showing hypoperfusion in the right caudate nucleus that was ameliorated after treatment with Ritalin (Teicher et al., 1996).

Neurochemical Studies

In terms of brain biochemistry, Shaywitz, Cohen, and Bowers (1977) found lower levels of homovanillic acid (HVA; the main dopamine metabolite) in the cerebrospinal fluid of children with ADHD compared to controls. Dopamine has a preponderant distribution in the frontal regions of the cortex. Moreover, a well-validated animal model of ADHD involves dopamine depletion (Shaywitz et al., 1983).

In summary, one plausible theory of brain mechanisms in ADHD is that symptoms are caused by functional hypofrontality, which in turn is caused by structural and/or biochemical changes in the prefrontal lobes and striatum, and is detectable as reduced frontal blood flow. Biochemically, the cause would be low dopamine levels, which are reversed, at least in part, by Ritalin treatment.

Unfortunately, the story is not that simple. One study found that certain dopamine *antagonists* have unexpected beneficial effects in children with ADHD (Zametkin & Rapoport, 1986). This result is the opposite of what was predicted by the dopamine depletion hypothesis. Zametkin and Rapoport (1986) argued that no single neurotransmitter is exclusively involved in the pathogenesis of ADHD, because stimulant medications always affect more than one neurotransmitter, and because of the multiple interrelations among specific catecholamines and their precursors and metabolites. They, along with Oades (1987), argued that the combined action of dopaminergic and noradrenergic systems should be considered in the biology of ADHD. So the neurochemical mechanisms may be more complex, although the ubiquitous problem of heterogeneity in ADHD samples is another explanation.

Obviously, much more research is needed, preferably using familial samples that are as phenotypically homogeneous as possible. The associations between ADHD and the DAT1 and DRD4 alleles would allow neurobiological research to focus on genetic subtypes of ADHD.

Neuropsychology

A fairly extensive literature on cognitive processes in ADHD has become more explicitly neuropsychological in the hypotheses tested. Virginia Douglas (1988), a pioneer in this area, has established that there is a distinctive cognitive phenotype in ADHD that needs to be explained. She and others have found that children with ADHD are impaired on tasks requiring vigilance, systematic search, and motor control and inhibition, but are unimpaired on tasks tapping basic verbal and nonverbal memory functions.

Neuropsychological studies of ADHD have focused mainly on the frontal lobe or executive function (EF) hypothesis for reasons discussed earlier. A number of researchers have proposed an EF deficit theory of ADHD (Barkley, 1997, 1998; Conners & Wells, 1986; Douglas, 1983; Pennington, 1991; Schachar, Tannock, & Logan, 1993).

We recently reviewed published studies of EFs in ADHD (Pennington & Ozonoff, 1996) and found that 15 of 18 studies found a significant difference between ADHD subjects and controls on one or more EF measures. In a total of 60 EF measures used across studies, 40 of these (67%) revealed significantly poorer performance in the ADHD group. In contrast, *none* of the 60 measures was significantly better in the ADHD group. The most consistently impaired domain of EF was inhibition; in contrast, children with ADHD were less likely to have impaired set-shifting or working memory.

In addition, children with ADHD in these studies were generally unimpaired on measures of verbal memory, other verbal processes, or visuospatial processing. They were fairly consistently impaired on measures of vigilance (Gordon Diagnostic System) and perceptual speed, but these measures would expectedly be influenced by an inhibitory deficit.

Although the term "inhibition" has many different meanings within psychology, inhibition in this case is "intentional motor inhibition" (Nigg, 2000), which requires conscious restraint of a dominant or prepotent motor response. This inhibitory process is thought to be primarily mediated by higher cognitive processes and is thus thought to require prefrontally mediated EF.

The most widely researched measure of this type of inhibition in the domain of ADHD is the stop signal paradigm (Logan, Cowan, & Davis, 1984; Logan Shachar, & Tannock, 1997), in which a subject is taught a particular response and then later is told to inhibit the very same response on the subset of trials signaled by a beep. The paradigm allows for the computation of the stop signal reaction time (SSRT), or the time it takes to inhibit a response. In a recent meta-analysis of studies using the Stop Task (Oosterlaan & Sergeant, 1998), consistent deficits were demonstrated in groups with ADHD, providing evidence that children with ADHD are impaired in their ability for response inhibition. Nigg (1999) also recently demonstrated inhibitory deficits in children with ADHD, combined type, using the stop signal paradigm. Deficits on the task were specific to ADHD and not associated with comorbid reading or behavior problems. Furthermore, a study by Aman, Roberts, and Pennington (1998) demonstrated that deficits of children with ADHD on the Stop Task were normalized when the children had taken methylphenidate.

These findings that children with ADHD consistently have slower SSRTs than control children, that this deficit is specific to ADHD, and that it is reversed by stimulant medication are all consistent with the hypothesis that ADHD is caused by a slow inhibitory process. However, this interpretation is clouded by the fact that children with ADHD often have slower "go" reaction times as well. Swanson (personal communication, July 10, 1999) suggests that, rather than a specific inhibitory deficit, ADHD is characterized by slower and more variable reaction times, which would produce the pattern of performance observed in groups with ADHD on the Stop Task and a variety of other tasks.

More generally, although the executive or inhibitory deficit theory of ADHD has considerable support, there are nonetheless several important threats to its validity. Perhaps the most important threat is the amount of variance in ADHD symptoms for which EF measures can account. The most sensitive measures of EF with regard to ADHD, as discussed previously, tend to be those that tap inhibition, such as the Stop Task and continuous performance tasks (Barkley, Grodzinsky, & DuPaul, 1992; Halperin et al., 1988; Losier, McGrath, & Klein, 1996). However, when comparing performance of children with ADHD and controls, even these measures produce effect sizes that are relatively small, ranging from about 0.5 to 1.5 (Chhabildas, Pennington, & Willcutt, in press; Nigg, 1999; Pennington & Ozonoff, 1996). This is much smaller than the effect size of the typical difference in symptoms of ADHD between the two groups, which is usually in the range of 2.5 to 3.5. In addition, correlations between EF measures and behavior ratings of attention/impulsivity are typically in the .15 to .30 range (Nigg, Hinshaw, Carte, & Treuting, 1998). These limited correlations mean that an EF deficit, as currently measured, cannot totally account for the symptoms that define the disorder.

There are several competing explanations to account for these relatively small effect sizes. One possibility is that children with ADHD are a substantially heterogeneous group, and some, but not all, have primary deficits in inhibition. In addition, differences within or among samples in ADHD subtype, age, gender, and prevalence of comorbid disorders could also impact the findings. A second possibility is that EF deficits are not the primary deficit in ADHD but are instead just a correlate of the actual, underlying deficit. A number of competing motivational and arousal theories of ADHD argue that the primary deficit in ADHD is not a cognitive one. For example, Sonuga-Barke, Taylor, Sembi, and Smith (1992) argue that the underlying difference in ADHD is not a deficit of inhibition, but rather a preference to shorten delay. Other, competing theories of ADHD argue that regulation of arousal or motivation may truly be the critical deficit in children with ADHD

(Borger et al., 1999; Douglas, 1989; Sanders, 1983; Sergeant & van der Meere, 1990). These authors view the inhibition deficit as secondary to a more primary difficulty in another area. Therefore, in the appropriate circumstances, children with ADHD should be able to inhibit responses. Recent studies by Kuntsi and colleagues (Kuntsi, Osterlaan, & Stevenson, 2001; Kuntsi & Stevenson, 2001) have found a stronger phenotypic and genetic relation between ADHD and a state regulation variable (variability in speed of responding) than with inhibition or working memory measures. Yet another possibility is that two (or more) primary deficits in ADHD may interact. In this case, each deficit, by itself, would account for a relatively small proportion of the variance in ADHD symptoms.

Another threat to the validity of an EF theory of ADHD comes from a recent study relating molecular measures to executive measures in ADHD (Swanson et al., 2000). Because the 7-repeat allele of the DRD4 receptor is significantly associated with ADHD, the next link in an EF theory of ADHD would be to test whether this gene is linked to the underlying psychological deficit in ADHD, an EF deficit. Such a finding would provide a comprehensive explanation of symptom presentation in ADHD using an EF framework: Variations in dopamine genes lead to reduced dopaminergic function in the prefrontal cortex and basal ganglia, thereby impairing EFs, particularly inhibition, thus producing the behavioral symptoms of ADHD. So, from an EF framework, the presence of the 7-repeat allele should be significantly associated not only with ADHD but also with EF deficits.

To test this theory, Swanson and colleagues compared subgroups of children with ADHD with and without the 7-repeat allele, on a series of EF tasks. Directly *opposite* to prediction, only children in the 7-absent group were impaired on EF tasks, whereas those with the DRD4 risk allele performed very similarly to controls on all EF measures in the study. This finding is inconsistent with an EF theory of ADHD, or at least inconsistent with the hypothesis that the DRD4 receptor mediates the EF deficits.

However, this study had a relatively small sample size (with 13 children in the 7-present group and 19 children in the 7-absent group) and needs to be replicated. In addition, the presence of the DRD4 7-repeat allele is not necessary for a diagnosis of ADHD and is clearly not the only genetic locus contributing to the phenotype of ADHD. It is possible that EF deficits in ADHD are instead related to another genetic locus, such as the DAT1 allele, or to an interaction among several alleles. It is also possible that the DRD4 receptor is significantly related only to a particular subtype of ADHD, the inattentive subtype. A recent study (Rowe et al., 1998b) found that the 7-repeat allele of DRD4 is associated more strongly with the predominantly inattentive subtype than the combined subtype of ADHD. In the Swanson and colleagues (2000) study, however, only children with the combined subtype of ADHD were studied.

In summary, despite converging evidence in support of an EF theory of ADHD, there are several important threats to the validity of this theory, including the low effect sizes obtained in studies using inhibition paradigms, competing explanations for the underlying deficit (such as motivational, delay aversion, and arousal perspectives), and the inconsistent DRD4 findings by Swanson and colleagues (2000).

Treatment

The treatment of ADHD has been recently reviewed (Satcher, 1999). Here, I summarize the main points of that review. The use of psychostimulant drugs, such as methylphenidate (Ritalin), dextroamphetamine (Dexadrine), and pemoline (Cylert), to treat ADHD is the most thoroughly researched application of psychopharmacology in child psychiatry. The efficacy and safety of these drugs in treating ADHD have now been well established. About 75–90% of children with ADHD show a favorable treatment response with psychostimulant medication.

The side effects of psychostimulants are generally mild, especially compared to other psychopharmacological treatments, and usually abate with time and changes in dose. These side effects include decreased sleep and appetite, jitteriness, stomachaches, and headaches. Earlier concerns about growth retardation, precipitation of a tic disorder, psychostimulants becoming drugs of abuse, overdiagnosis of ADHD, or overprescription of psychostimulant drugs are not supported by research. There is nonetheless valid concern about the misdiagnosis of ADHD. Not all practitioners prescribing stimulant medication for ADHD have the time or the training to make this demanding differential diagnosis accurately.

Psychosocial treatments for ADHD consist mainly of behavioral intervention techniques to help parents and teachers better manage these children, who can be very disruptive in a classroom or family. Such treatments are particularly important for children who do not respond to medication or for those whose parents prefer not to use medication.

In general, the efficacy of psychosocial treatments for improving ADHD symptoms is less than that of psychostimulants (Pelham, Wheeler, & Chronis, 1998), and greater for teachers than parents.

The question naturally arises as to whether the combination of psychostimulant and behavioral interventions would be more efficacious than either alone. A recent large study funded by the National Institutes of Mental Health (NIMH) addressed this question. This 3-year study on multimodal treatment of ADHD (MTA Cooperative Group, 1999) compared four treatment conditions: medication alone, behavioral intervention alone, a combination of the two, and no treatment beyond that typically provided in the community. The behavioral intervention was intensive, involving parent training, school intervention, and summer treatment in a camp setting. The medication management was more intensive than that typically provided in a community setting. Subjects were randomly assigned to one of the four conditions, treated for 14 months, and followed for 22 months. There was a large main effect of medication treatment on ADHD symptoms, for which the addition of the behavioral intervention produced no added benefit. The behavioral intervention did improve outcome in some nonsymptom areas.

Several nonconventional therapies for ADHD, including the Feingold diet and EEG biofeedback, have not been supported by careful treatment studies.

CONDUCT DISORDER

Although all psychopathologies have high social costs, those associated with conduct disorder (CD) are immediately salient, because CD, by definition, involves harm to others. At a time when rates of incarceration in the United States are the highest they have ever been, and there is an epidemic of gun violence, understanding and preventing CD is a top social priority.

CD also confronts us immediately with difficult conceptual issues concerning the relations among legal, moral, and psychological views of behavior. Inherent to legal and moral perspectives are the folk psychological notions of intentional agents, with some degree of free will, that make autonomous choices about their behavior. An illegal or immoral act is thus a bad decision, but a decision and a free choice nonetheless. Psychological and neuroscientific views threaten the notion of free will because they aspire to a deterministic explanation of behavior. A scientific explanation of a moral or immoral behavior is not very satisfying if, at its heart, it depends on a homunculus with free will!

Another important, related issue for a scientific account of moral development concerns moral behavior in other species. For some, the phrase "moral behavior in other species" is an oxymoron. Traditional views have limited morality to humans, because it was thought that only humans have free will and are capable of moral decisions. From an evolutionary perspective, however, it is very likely that human moral behavior has its roots in the social behavior of other animals, which are not usually credited with having free will. Two such possible roots, attachment and altruism, are clearly present in other animals.

Evolutionary and developmental perspectives on moral behavior may help to solve a problem faced by traditional psychological theories in accounting for moral behavior. These traditional theories, such as psychoanalytic and learning theories, have a hard time accounting for moral behavior, because they assume the inherent selfishness of individuals (Wallach & Wallach, 1983). But moral behavior does not arise just out of fear of punishment and increasingly sophisticated calculations about long-term negative consequences of yielding to a current impulse. Healthy humans are spontaneously prosocial and avoid immoral acts because they "feel" bad, not just because of a calculation about future punishments.

So how does moral behavior develop, why does this development sometimes go wrong, and how may we think about these questions neuroscientifically? Human moral behavior is clearly not innate. Instead, its "core" develops early and depends crucially on the social stimulation provided by a nurturant caregiver. One of the important foundations of human moral behavior, empathy, detectable early in life, is notably reduced in children who have had abusive or neglectful caregivers (Feshbach, 1989). Empathy is one aspect of intersubjectivity, which develops out of reciprocal imitative exchanges of attention, intention, and affect (Stern, 1985). "Intersubjectivity," defined as the ability to infer quickly what others are thinking and feeling, or *will* think and feel in a given context, is a cornerstone of human moral behavior.

In summary, the development of CD touches on several profound questions about the human condition: How did moral behavior evolve, how does it develop, and what brain systems does it depend on? The study of CD also nicely illustrates several key issues in developmental psychopathology, including (1) how tests of external validity can lead to the division of a broader syndrome into distinct subtypes, (2) the inter-action between genetic and environmental risk factors, (3) how envi-ronmental influences shared by siblings can influence the development of a disorder, (4) the boundaries of psychopathology, specifically, how the developmental and cultural context can influence whether a given set of behaviors is considered to be psychopathology, and (5) the conti-nuity of child disorders into adulthood.

I briefly summarize what has been learned about these five issues. First, considerable evidence supports the validity of two subtypes of CD: a life-course-persistent and an adolescence-limited subtype (Moffitt, 1993). Second, the first subtype is more heritable and provides one of the clearest examples of an interaction between genetic and environ-mental risk. Third, the second subtype is much less heritable and more influenced by environmental factors shared by siblings. Fourth, adoles-cent males, especially in certain cultural contexts, have such high rates of delinquent behavior that it is virtually normative and hence difficult to characterize as psychopathology. Fifth, CD provided one of the earli-est and strongest examples of the continuity of a disorder from child-hood to adulthood (Robins, 1966).

Definition

DSM-IV-TR (American Psychiatric Association, 2000, p. 93) defines conduct disorder (CD) as a "repetitive and persistent pattern of behav-ior in which the basic rights of others or major age-appropriate societal norms or rules are violated." This definition is operationalized as the presence of three or more such behaviors (out of a list of 15) in the past 12 months, with at least one occurring in the past 6 months. Similar to other DSM diagnoses, this pattern of behavior must cause clinically sig-nificant impairment in social, academic, or occupational functioning. If the patient is 18 or older and meets the criteria for antisocial personality disorder, then the CD diagnosis cannot be given.

The 15 behavioral criteria are divided into four categories: (1) ag-gression toward people and animals (seven criteria: bullying, fighting, use of a weapon, physical cruelty to people or animals, theft involving direct confrontation, and sexual coercion); (2) destruction of property (two criteria: intentionally destructive fire setting or other deliberate destruction of another's property); (3) deceitfulness or theft (three crite-ria: breaking and entering, conning others, and theft without confronta-tion); and (4) serious violations of rules (three criteria: staying out at night without permission before age 13, running away from home over-night, or school truancy before age 13).

Because only three behaviors out of this list of 15 are required for the diagnosis of CD, it is readily apparent that this definition will iden-tify subtypes of CD with no overlap in their symptoms. This lack of symptom overlap would not be problematic for syndrome validity if such symptomatic subtypes did not differ in criteria for external valid-ity, such as etiology, brain mechanisms, and response to treatment. However, this list of 15 behaviors includes two distinct dimensions of antisocial behavior, one involving overt aggression (the first two catego-ries) and the other involving nonaggressive, covert actions (the last two categories), which research has shown to have discriminant validity on external criteria. Another externally valid distinction, which is partly correlated with the overt versus covert distinction, is that between "undersocialized," solitary aggressive behaviors and "socialized," anti-social behaviors, both aggressive and nonaggressive, committed by a group (see Hinshaw & Anderson, 1996, for a review of these distinc-tions). Yet another partly overlapping distinction is that between impul-sive, reactive aggression (more likely to be associated with ADHD) and the instrumental aggression associated with psychopathy, which is also associated with physiological underarousal and sensation seeking. Con-sequently, to an extent probably greater than that for the other diagno-ses considered in this book, it is inevitable that the broad list of criteria that define CD will identify distinct subtypes of individuals. DSM-IV-TR partly acknowledges this problem by distinguishing two subtypes of CD based on age of onset (before or after age 10).

A second, definitional problem concerns the relation between CD and oppositional defiant disorder (ODD). ODD symptoms include fre-quent temper outbursts, arguing with or defying adults, annoyance with or blaming others, touchiness, anger, resentment, spitefulness, or vin-dictiveness. Some authors consider ODD to be an earlier form of CD or a variant of ADHD, and hence lacking in external validity.

Epidemiology

Prevalences depend on the definition utilized and the population stud-ied. The definitions of CD have changed across versions of the DSM, and rates of CD are usually higher in urban than in rural communities (American Psychiatric Association, 2000). Moreover, most epidemio-logical surveys have not distinguished the two age-of-onset subtypes discussed earlier. Including individuals with the adolescence-limited subtype will inflate the prevalence. A Canadian epidemiological study of children and adolescents using DSM-III criteria (Offord, Alder, & Boyle, 1986) found CD in 8.1% of males and 2.8% of females, for an overall CD rate of 5.5%. Hence, the male:female gender ratio was close to 3:1; a male predominance of about this magnitude is a consistent finding, especially for the childhood-onset subtype. Gender ratios are closer to equal for the adolescent-onset subtype (Hinshaw & Anderson, 1996).

Longitudinal designs are needed to measure the prevalence of life-course-persistent CD. One such study (of males from ages 3 to 15) that could examine age of onset found a somewhat lower 5.9% rate of persistent CD, defined as being present at all seven measurement points and pervasive across raters. In contrast, an additional two-thirds of the *entire* sample of males in this study was rated as highly antisocial, either at a single age or by a single reporter (see Caspi & Moffitt, 1995, for a review). So some degree of antisocial behavior is common in males, but persistent CD is restricted to a much smaller group.

Other studies also find that the majority of adolescent males self-report some illegal behavior. Police records concur; males' lifetime prevalences of being arrested (33%) and of police contact for a minor infringement (80%) are similarly high. Hence, epidemiological studies support the validity of childhood-onset CD as a disorder, because of its persistence and pervasiveness, but not the validity of adolescence-limited CD.

Life-course-persistent CD is comorbid with ADHD, ODD, depression and anxiety, and academic underachievement (Hinshaw & Anderson, 1996). I next review the basis of the comorbidities with ADHD and ODD.

Etiology

Familiality

Several disorders in parents increase the risk for CD in their offspring, including antisocial personality disorder, especially in fathers; alcohol dependence; schizophrenia; and depression, especially in mothers (American Psychiatric Association, 2000; Hinshaw & Anderson, 1996). Interestingly, parental histories of CD, ADHD, and aggression in childhood are also associated with higher rates of CD in offspring (DSM-IV-TR,

2000; Hinshaw & Anderson, 1996). Across these different parental diagnoses, the pathways to CD in offspring likely differ. Some may involve mainly the environmental effect of harsh or disrupted parenting; others may involve gene × environment interactions or correlations (a child with genes for ADHD raised in a harsh or chaotic household), and perhaps still others may represent genetic main effects. More work is needed to sort this out.

Heritability

The heritability of adult criminality is much higher than that for juvenile delinquency, which shows a considerable shared environmental effect. In a review of existing twin studies, DiLalla and Gottesman (1989) found only a small difference between MZ (87%) and DZ (72%) concordances for juvenile delinquency, but a much larger difference for adult criminality (51% vs. 22%, respectively). Hence, for juvenile delinquency, there is only a small genetic effect and a very sizable shared environment effect. In contrast, there is a larger genetic effect on adult criminality, as well as a very sizable nonshared environmental effect. These results indirectly support the external validity of the distinction between the life-course-persistent and adolescence-limited subtypes of CD, if we can assume that those subtypes largely overlap with adult criminality and juvenile delinquency, respectively. Of course, a better test would come from a twin study of those two subtypes, which, to my knowledge, has not been conducted.

There have been recent twin studies of DBDs in child and adolescent samples, some of which have tested whether the heritability of CD differs significantly across these two age groups. These studies also indirectly test Moffitt's (1993) theory, which would predict a higher heritability for CD in childhood than in adolescence, because the child samples should contain a much higher proportion of the life-course-persistent subtype than the adolescent samples, in which the adolescence-limited subtype should predominate. Nadder, Silberg, Eaves, Maes, and Meyer (1998) found moderate heritability for the combined diagnoses of CD and ODD in childhood in both boys ($h^2 = .65$) and girls ($h^2 = .53$). Since these heritabilities are considerably higher than those for juvenile delinquency in the DiLalla and Gottesman (1989) review, these results are consistent with the predictions of Moffitt's theory. Silberg and colleagues (1996) studied the symptoms of CD in two groups of twins, ages 8–11 and 12–16. Contrary to Moffitt's theory, heritabilities of CD symptoms were slightly greater in older than in younger males (h^2 = .66 and .57, respectively) and significantly greater in older than in younger females (h^2 = .48 and .24, respectively).

This discrepancy might be a function of how CD symptoms were defined. As discussed earlier, the symptoms that define CD are quite broad and include both overt and covert, and aggressive and non-aggressive antisocial actions. Eley, Lichtenstein, and Stevenson (1999b) examined age and gender effects on the heritability of the aggression and delinquency subscales of the Child Behavior Checklist. Consistent with earlier studies, and with Moffitt's (1993) theory, delinquency in both females and males, respectively, was considerably less heritable (h^2 = .00 and .47, respectively) than aggression (h^2 = .69 and .70, respectively). As can be seen, delinquency was considerably more heritable in females than in males, but aggression was similarly heritable in both genders. Also consistent with Moffitt's (1993) theory, delinquency was more heritable in children (h^2 = .36) than in adolescents (h^2 = .12). In summary, existing twin studies generally support Moffitt's theory, but recent results emphasize the importance of differentiating the broad CD phenotype and testing for gender effects.

Recent twin studies have also examined the etiological relations among all three DBDs, with the general result that there is a large genetic overlap among all three DBDs, especially in childhood (Nadder et al., 1998; Silberg et al., 1996; Waldman, Rhee, Levy, & Hay, 2001). Waldman and colleagues (2001) found that 93% of the phenotypic overlap between ADHD and either ODD or CD, and 79% of the phenotypic overlap between ODD and CD, was attributable to genes common to both disorders in the pair. So the comorbidity among these three disorders is largely due to shared genes. Nonetheless, these shared genes might be a small proportion of all the genes acting on the disorders considered separately; that is, genes might account for most of their phenotypic overlap, but many other genes could be acting on the nonoverlapping portions of each disorder. To address the degree of genetic overlap between two disorders, a different statistic is needed, namely, the genetic correlation. As discussed earlier, the genetic correlation tells us what proportion of the genetic influences that act on either disorder also act on both disorders. Waldman and colleagues also found high genetic correlations among all three pairs of DBDs, ranging from .73 to .82, indicating a high degree of genetic overlap. Consistent with these results, Silberg and colleagues (1996) found a genetic correlation of 1.0 between ADHD and CD in both boys and girls in their child sample. In their adolescent sample, the genetic correlations were lower, .58 and .46, respectively, for males and females. Nadder and colleagues (1998) found a lower genetic correlation (.50) between ADHD and ODD/CD symptomatology in a mostly child sample (ages 7–13) than in either of the other two studies.

In summary, the genetic risk factors that act on the development of the DBDs, especially in childhood, appear to be largely shared. Thus, the environment must act to differentiate individuals with a similar genetic risk into different DBDs. Other research, to be considered shortly, strongly implicates parenting effects on this differentiation. With optimal parenting, a child with this genetic risk profile will develop ADHD only. With harsh parenting, the same child will also develop comorbid ODD or CD, whereas a child without this genetic risk profile in the same family might attract less harsh parenting and nonetheless develop different symptoms if he or she did receive similar parenting. In other words, there are likely to be both gene–environment correlations and gene × environment interactions in the etiology of life-course-persistent CD (see Rutter, 1997, for a review). For adolescence-limited CD, there appears to be a much smaller contribution of genetic risk, and if Moffitt's theory (1993) is correct, there should be very little association with earlier ADHD or CD. Instead, her theory proposes that peer-group and other neighborhood influences induce a substantial proportion of otherwise normal adolescents to engage temporarily in some antisocial behaviors, and to desist in young adulthood.

As mentioned earlier, there is also strong direct evidence for gene × environment interactions in the etiology of CD, which mainly comes from adoption studies (Cadoret, Yates, Troughton, Woodworth, & Stewart, 1995; Cloninger, Sigvardsson, Bohman, & von Knorring, 1982; Mednick, Gabrielli, & Hutchings, 1983). Each of these studies utilized a cross-fostering design in which presence or absence of criminality in the biological parents was crossed with presence or absence of criminality in the adoptive parents (in Cadoret et al., 1995, risk in the adoptive parents was more broadly defined and included marital, legal, or psychiatric difficulties). If a gene × environment interaction is present, then the risk for criminal behavior in adopted offspring who have both genetic and environmental risk factors should be greater than the simple sum of the increased risk associated with each of these risk factors in isolation. That pattern was found in all three studies. For instance, Cloninger and colleagues (1982) found that the incidence of petty criminality in adult male adoptees was 2.9% when neither risk factor was present, was doubled (6.7%) when only the adoptive parents had criminal histories (environmental risk only), was quadrupled (12.1%) when only the biological parents had such histories (genetic risk only), but reached 40% when both risk factors were present. This is a fairly dramatic example of an interaction effect, because, if the genetic and environmental risk factors acted independently, the expected risk with both present would only be about 15%. As Rutter (1997) points out, gene × environment interaction effects of this magnitude are very important for understanding the development of individuals with extreme phenotypes, such as CD, even though they will only make small contributions to the overall population variance.

A later study by Ge and colleagues (1996) investigated this interaction using an adoption design. Biological offspring of antisocial parents provoked greater harshness and less nurturance from adoptive parents than did biological offspring of nonantisocial parents. Adoptive parents' marital warmth independently predicted their parenting practices. These results suggest a complex interplay between nature and nurture in the development of CD.

The results of these adoption studies also document that there are main effects of genetic and environmental risk factors acting in isolation, consistent with the results of the twin studies discussed earlier. This is important information, because many of the environmental correlates of CD have been found in study designs that confound genetic and environmental influences.

Raine, Brennan, and Mednick (1997) found a similar interaction between a biological risk factor (perinatal risk) and an environmental risk factor (lack of maternal warmth) in the etiology of CD. Again, the presence of both risk factors produced a much higher rate of CD than that expected if each risk factor acted independently.

In summary, the etiology of CD presents us with a clear example of the diathesis–stress model. Genetic or other biological risk factors (mainly for ADHD) interact with the environmental stress of a nonoptimal parenting environment to increase greatly the risk for CD.

Gene Locations

Because the majority of individuals with life-course-persistent CD have comorbid ADHD, genes that affect ADHD, such as the DAT1 and DRD4 alleles, discussed earlier in the section on ADHD, are also risk factors for this form of CD. So molecular genetic studies of ADHD will also advance our understanding of the genetics of both ODD and CD, because of the high genetic correlation among the DBDs. Once we know which genes account for the shared genetic influence on the DBDs, it will be easier to identify any genetic influences specific to a given DBD.

Two other identified genes influence CD, both of which alter neurotransmission. Brunner, Nelen, Breakfield, Ropers, and Van Oost (1993) found a family with a rare, X-linked, single-gene disorder that caused both violent outbursts and mental retardation. The gene in question codes for the enzyme monoamine oxidase A (MAOA). Monoamine oxidases act to degrade monoamine neurotransmitters (such as norepinephrine, serotonin, and dopamine) in the presynaptic neuron and thus help regulate neurotransmission. The mutation in this family prevented the synthesis of MAOA, thus destabilizing neurotransmission and altering cognitive and behavioral development.

The second gene codes for tryptophan hydroxylase (TPH). Tryptophan, a basic amino acid derived from food, is the necessary precursor for the synthesis of serotonin. TPH is the rate-limiting enzyme in this synthesis, so mutations in the gene for this enzyme could change central serotonin levels. Considerable other research, discussed next, has found a relation between low serotonin levels and aggressive behavior. Nielsen and colleagues (1994) found an association between an allele of the TPH gene and measures of aggression. Since such an association could be due to an artifact, such as population stratification, a follow-up study (Manuck et al., 1999) both replicated this association and tested it further, with a pharmacological challenge (administration of the serotonin agonist fenfluramine, which acts on the hypothalamus to produce an elevation of the hormone prolactin in the blood). Males with the risk allele of the TPH gene had a blunted prolactin response to the pharmacological challenge, providing evidence that the risk allele alters serotonergic functioning. While intriguing, this association needs to be replicated using within-family association methods, since it still could be an artifact; that is, whereas the effect of the risk allele on serotonin could be real, the association with aggression could still be an artifact.

Environmental Risk Factors

What else do we know about environmental risk factors for CD besides the factors discussed earlier? Some of these have been reviewed by Caspi and Moffitt (1995), Hinshaw and Anderson (1996), and Rutter (1997). In thinking about environmental risk factors for CD, it is important to appreciate that environmental stressors acting to increase the rate and persistence of CD are mainly not randomly assigned but may be evoked or self-selected by the individual with a tempermental or cognitive risk for CD. Thus, across development, there are likely to be complex chains of transactions (positive feedback loops) between biologically at-risk individuals and their environment that act to increase the rate and persistence of antisocial behaviors. Implicit in this view is the assumption of both the developmental continuity and different developmental pathways in CD.

With regard to developmental continuity, although the overt form of problematic behavior will change with stage of development, problematic behaviors at one stage will substantially predict those of the next stage (i.e., heterotypic continuity). For example, overactive and irritable infants are more likely to display argumentative and defiant behaviors in preschool and early childhood; these ODD behaviors predict physical aggression and stealing in later childhood, which in turn predict antisocial behavior in adolescence and adulthood (Hinshaw & Anderson, 1996). Yet at every age, there is desistance. Thus, while virtually every case of childhood CD had earlier ODD, the majority of those with earlier ODD do not develop CD. Similarly, virtually every case of adult antisocial personality disorder (APD) had CD in youth but, again, the majority of those with earlier CD do not develop APD as adults. Hinshaw and Anderson (1996) estimate that about 10% of children with ODD remain on the developmental pathway that eventuates in adult APD.

In addition, there are distinct developmental pathways characterized by different antisocial behaviors. Loeber (1990) and colleagues (Loeber et al., 1993) have developed novel longitudinal methods to elucidate such distinct pathways in CD. Their research has validated the distinction between overt (aggressive) and covert (theft and property crime) antisocial behaviors. Persistence in a pathway is predicted by earlier initiation of antisocial behaviors; those who persist are more likely to diversify the range of antisocial behaviors in which they engage. For instance, while Loeber and colleagues have identified an exclusive substance use pathway, individuals on the overt and covert pathways are also at risk for adolescent substance use. In turn, as has been well-documented, substance use increases the probability of impulsive criminal behavior. In other words, remaining on these pathways is partly due to the increased exposure to environmental risk factors that potentiate antisocial behavior: a vicious circle.

What are some of the other environmental risks that enter into such feedback loops affecting CD? Robins (1966) conducted a classic, long-term follow-up study of antisocial boys into middle adulthood, comparing their adult outcomes to those of control boys who lived in the same neighborhood in childhood. The antisocial group, as adults, was more likely to have experienced multiple divorces and job changes, to be unemployed or in a low-status job, and to have no friends. Longitudinal studies that have controlled for the autocorrelation between prior and later behavior and environmental circumstances have found incremental validity for the environmental stressors of marital quality, unemployment, and alcohol abuse in the prediction of the persistence of adult antisocial behavior (Rutter, 1997).

Although both CD and APD are correlated with poverty and neighborhood characteristics, again, the influences are bidirectional and transactional (see Caspi & Moffitt, 1995, for a review). Adults with APD, partly because of their employment and marital difficulties, are more likely to move to certain less desirable neighborhoods and are less likely to leave them. Once there, their behavior further worsens the neighborhood environment, which in turn increases their own risk and the risk of their children for antisocial behavior. Poverty by itself does not consign a neighborhood to high crime rates. Equating for poverty, neighborhoods vary in rates of CD in their youth as a function of both neighborhood cohesion (as indexed by local friendship networks and voluntary community organizations) and the extent to which adults help monitor and supervise the behavior of the neighborhood's adolescents. So both family and neighborhood characteristics can act either as risk or protective factors in the development of CD.

Within the family, it is clear that both abuse and harsh parenting increase the risk for CD in children. Dodge, Bates, and Pettit (1990) found that early physical abuse predicts later aggressive behavior at school, even after controlling for child temperament and family variables other than abuse. The microanalysis of family interactions conducted by Patterson and colleagues (see Dishion, French, & Patterson, 1995, for a review) has elegantly demonstrated how coercive but inconsistent parenting can set in motion a vicious circle that potentiates the development of CD behaviors in children. The occasional success of harsh and coercive discipline in reducing the child's aggressive and demanding behavior reinforces the use of these disciplinary practices by parents. Such practices also teach the child that coercion is an acceptable means for reaching goals, and that regard for another's feelings (i.e., empathy) is at best a secondary priority in interpersonal conflicts. Since few parents can be consistently harsh and coercive, their occasional capitulation to the child's coercion reinforces that interpersonal strategy in the child. As I discuss later, this group of researchers has also demonstrated that reducing such coercive exchanges is an effective treatment for CD.

Bioenvironmental variables (such as perinatal risk, environmental lead, closed head injury, and maternal smoking during pregnancy) also likely contribute to the development of CD. Most plausibly, these risk factors would act by increasing the risk for ADHD and other neuropsychological deficits, such as language delay and lower IQ, which have been shown to be risk factors for CD. As discussed later, certain forms of acquired brain damage (to the orbitofrontal and ventromedial prefrontal cortices) appear to act more directly to produce antisocial behavior in both adults and children (see Pennington & Bennetto, 1993, for a review).

Brain Mechanisms

A circuit including orbitofrontal and ventromedial prefrontal cortex and the amygdala, as well as other structures, is an important contributor to socially appropriate behavior (Damasio, 1994; Davidson, Putnam, & Larson, 2000). In Damasio's "somatic marker" hypothesis, as discussed earlier, these portions of cortex guide everyday behavior by computing and representing the emotional consequences (somatic markers) of candidate actions. We quickly know which possible actions do not "feel right" without complete cognitive explication of why they are "bad" choices, and part of that "feeling" involves the autonomic system. After learning, presentation of the "bad" choice generates autonomic arousal in a normal individual, whereas such arousal and avoidance of risky choices is missing in patients with lesions in these portions of cortex.

Davidson and colleagues (2000) focus on a particular antisocial behavior, impulsive aggression, and propose that the relevant neural circuit includes orbitofrontal and ventromedial prefrontal cortex and the amygdala, as well as the hippocampus, hypothalamus, anterior cingulate cortex, insular cortex, and ventral striatum. Based on their evidence, they view impulsive aggression as a failure of emotion regulation. In their theory, the amygdala is important in generating emotional responses, particularly fear in response to threatening stimuli, and prefrontal structures, through inhibitory connections, regulate this negative emotional arousal. A failure of inhibition leads to an aggressive outburst in response to negative emotional arousal.

We can think about both these theories in the context of the functions of the motivation and action selection systems, and their interaction. As discussed earlier, the prefrontal cortex computes representations of the current adaptive context and holds these in active or working memory to guide action selection. These active representations of the current context also serve to inhibit or deselect prepotent responses that are inappropriate for the context. As discussed in Roberts and Pennington (1996), the probability that a prepotent response will escape inhibition is a joint function of the strength of the prepotency and the degree of demand placed on working memory. The orbitofrontal cortex (OFC) implements this general prefrontal function in the domain of emotional and social behavior. The amygdala and other limbic and subcortical structures can be thought of a source of prepotent emotional responses, some of which will be inappropriate to the current context, which is represented by the OFC. If the prepotency is too strong, or if the representation of the social context is too weak, a prepotent but inappropriate response will be selected. So factors that either (1) increase the prepotency of bottom-up activation from the amygdala and other structures, or (2) decrease working memory capacity of OFC could lead to conduct problems. These factors could be early social or emotional experience, acquired damage to these structures, or genetic variations that affect their development.

The theories of Damasio (1994) and Davidson and colleagues (2000) were based in part on the biological correlates of CD and APD, including neuroimaging results in those populations. Davidson and colleagues review these neuroimaging results, which include sizable prefrontal volume reductions (11–17%) in structural MRI studies, and prefrontal hypoactivity coupled with right-sided hyperactivation in the amygdala and related subcortical structures in PET studies. Other, well-replicated biological correlates of CD and APD include (1) low autonomic arousal, as indexed by heart rate and skin conductance, and (2) low serotonin levels (see Raine, 1993, for a review). There is also some evidence of elevated testosterone levels. However, the causal relation between these correlates and CD behavior is far from clear. It is possible, for example, that an aggressive or antisocial lifestyle could produce these biological differences, instead of the reverse.

As discussed earlier, autonomic arousal is related to the short- and long-term stress response. An individual with low autonomic arousal could thus be thought of as experiencing less stress in the face of threatening cues and thus be less likely to avoid aggressive encounters or punishment. By the same logic, individuals with high levels of autonomic arousal (such as anxious individuals) might be expected to be more likely to avoid such encounters. In fact, two studies (Brennan et al., 1997; Kerr, Tremblay, Pagani, & Vitaro, 1997) document the fact that higher levels of autonomic arousal are associated with lower rates of CD. There is considerable evidence, using a variety of paradigms, of decreased autonomic arousal in adults with APD (e.g., Hare, 1965, 1982; Hare, Frazelle, & Cox, 1978; Lykken, 1957; Patrick, Cuthbert, & Lang, 1994). Similar results have been found in children and adolescents with CD (e.g., Raine & Jones, 1987; Raine, Venebles, & Williams, 1990). The Raine and colleagues (1990) study is of particular interest. In this longitudinal study documenting the predictive value of low autonomic arousal for later criminality, heart rate and skin conductance were measured in 101 fifteen-year-old English boys whose court records were examined 10 years later. Subjects with a later criminal history had significantly lower autonomic arousal on both measures at age 15 than those without a later criminal record. Although such a predictive finding is consistent with a causal role for low autonomic arousal given what we have learned about the life course of CD and APD, it is quite likely that CD was already present at age 15 in subjects who had later criminal records.

While the usual theory relating low autonomic arousal to CD posits decreased aversive conditioning, it is known that the development of prosocial behavior depends more on the development of empathy than on punishment. Indeed, as discussed earlier, harsh or coercive parenting is a risk, not a protective, factor for the development of CD. Based on these considerations, Blair (1995) developed a theory of psychopathy in which a deficit in the ability to respond to distress cues in others (an empathetic failure) produces a failure to inhibit aggressive behavior toward them. Blair proposes that instead of terminating aggressive behavior when the opponent produces submission cues, such as distress, as do most humans and other social animals, psychopaths persist because they are insensitive to such cues. This theory predicts that such individuals should exhibit low autonomic arousal in response to distress cues. Blair, Jones, Clark, and Smith (1997) tested this prediction by measuring electrodermal responses of psychopaths and controls to slides of three types of stimuli: neutral objects (a book), threat cues (a pointed gun), or distress cues (a person crying). Consistent with the hypothesis, the groups differed only in their electrodermal response in the distress condition; autonomic arousal was lower in the psychopaths than in controls in that condition.

While these findings in regard to autonomic arousal are important, such measures are several steps away from the relevant brain variables. For instance, is the observed PET scan profile of frontal hypoactivation and amygdala hyperactivation, discussed earlier, consistent with low autonomic arousal? One might expect an overactive amygdala to produce high autonomic arousal. So a neuroscientific explanation of CD will need to specify the brain changes that lead to lower autonomic arousal in CD.

Another biological correlate of antisocial behavior is a low serotonin level. As already reviewed in Chapter 3, in the section on Depression, serotonin contributes to emotional stability, so low serotonin levels would lead to a problem with emotion regulation, which in turn, according to the theory of Davidson and colleagues (2000), increases the risk for impulsive aggression. Although low serotonin may contribute to certain kinds of impulsive aggression in depression (i.e., suicide), we still need to understand how low serotonin leads to depression in some people and aggression in others. In other words, we have a discriminant validity problem. The solution may lie in there being different brain locations for the serotonin deficiency in depression versus CD. Davidson and colleagues reviewed evidence indicating a high density of serotonin 2 receptors in the prefrontal cortex, as well as increases in prefrontal metabolism (as measured by PET) after a fenfluramine challenge in normals. Other PET studies of aggressive adults with APD indicated a blunted or absent prefrontal response to such a challenge. They hypothesized that, in individuals with impulsive aggression, the serotonin deficit is in the prefrontal cortex. A finding that the serotonin deficit in depression is elsewhere, such as the amygdala or HPA axis, might provide a solution to the discriminant validity problem.

The evidence for a causal link between low serotonin and increased risk for aggression is fairly impressive and includes both prospective and experimental studies. First of all, as reviewed by Davidson and colleagues (2000) and others (e.g., Holmes, 1997), there are replicated reductions of the serotonin metabolite 5-HIAA in aggressive antisocial adults and youths with CD across several studies. This correlation is not restricted to clinical samples. Brown, Goodwin, and Ballenger (1979) found that serotonin metabolite levels accounted for 80% of the variance in levels of aggression in a sample of young males in the military.

In a community sample, Manuck and colleagues (1998) found a correlation between aggressive traits and a lower prolactin response to a fenfluramine challenge. Second, this relation between low serotonin and aggression is predictive. In a prospective study, Kruesi and colleagues (1992) found that 5-HIAA levels substantially predicted aggression ($r = -.72$) 2 to 3 years later in boys with CD. Finally, experimentally depleting serotonin increases aggressive behavior. As discussed earlier, the monoamine precursor for the synthesis of serotonin, tryptophan, is obtained from food. Consequently, serotonin levels can be manipulated by dietary changes. As reviewed in Davidson and colleagues, a dietary depletion of tryptophan increased laboratory aggression in two studies of normal men and in a study of monkeys. These last studies, unlike the others, indicated that the direction of causality is from low serotonin to aggression, and not some other relation.

The third possible biological correlate of CD, a high level of testosterone, is correlated with aggression in animal studies and some human studies (e.g., Ehrenkranz, Bliss, & Sheard, 1974). But we do not know whether elevated testosterone is a cause or a consequence of an aggressive lifestyle (Robins, 1991).

In summary, the studies reviewed here support the general view that overt or aggressive CD represents a deficit in a particular aspect of the prefrontally mediated action selection system. Unlike the action selection deficit in ADHD, which may involve dysfunction in a prefrontal–striatal circuit, that in CD may involve an OFC–limbic circuit. It is not clear from these reviews exactly how ADHD increases the risk for CD at the brain level, although it is likely that these two circuits interact in action selection. A genetically mediated ADHD deficit in the prefrontal–striatal circuit could interact with a socially influenced deficit (e.g., in empathy or emotion regulation) mediated by the OFC–limbic circuit.

Neuropsychology

There are several well-documented neuropsychological correlates of life-course-persistent CD, some of which precede later CD behavior (see reviews in Caspi & Moffitt, 1995, and Pennington & Ozonoff, 1996). First, about a one-half standard deviation decrement in overall IQ precedes the onset of CD. This IQ deficit is not simply a socioeconomic or ethnic confound (Caspi & Moffitt, 1995), which it could be, given that both lower IQ and higher rates of CD are associated with lower socioeconomic status. Second, there is some specificity to the IQ profile in CD, with verbal IQ on average being more depressed than performance IQ (Caspi & Moffitt, 1995). So some of the deficit in overall IQ is attributable to a verbal deficit, although we do not know exactly how a verbal deficit is related or how it might contribute to CD development. Third, the other neuropsychological domain that is consistently impaired in CD samples is executive function (EF). EF deficits may also contribute to lower overall IQ in CD and are both consistent with the structural and functional neuroimaging findings just reviewed and have face validity as contributors to deficits in impulse control. The association between EF deficits and CD is clearest in samples with both CD and ADHD (Pennington & Ozonoff, 1996). EF deficits, along with ADHD, contribute to early onset and persistence of CD behavior (Caspi & Moffitt, 1995).

It is also important to mention the work of Dodge and colleagues (reviewed in Crick & Dodge, 1994, and in Hinshaw & Anderson, 1996), who have documented a cluster of psychological correlates of CD that, while not strictly neuropsychological, need to be accounted for in a neuroscientific theory of CD. This cluster involves social information-processing deficits, including underutilization of relevant social cues, misattribution of hostile intent in ambiguous social interactions, failure to generate assertive (but nonaggressive) solutions to interpersonal problems, and the expectation that aggressive solutions will work. These deficits are found in both clinical and community samples, and may be related to harsh parenting. The first two deficits, underutilization of social cues and misattribution of hostile intent, appear to be specific to an aggressive subtype of CD with comorbid ADHD (essentially the life-course-persistent subtype).

This work and the previously discussed work of Blair (1995) raise a now-familiar issue in constructing integrated explanations of psychopathology—the need to understand the interactions between "bottom-up" biological influences, such as genes that affect prefrontal functions, and "top-down" social-cognitive influences, such as cognitive distortions (in depression) and these social information-processing deficits in CD that partly derive from experience. Social-cognitive theories of psychopathology are incomplete in that they do not explain why some people have such social-cognitive deficits and others do not. Bottom-up neuroscientific theories can provide powerful insights about the origin of individual differences but are incomplete, because they tell us little about how risk is mediated in moment-to-moment social interactions. Because a certain kind of adverse socialization (harsh or abusive parenting) is clearly important in the development of CD, we need to understand better how such parenting leads to social-cognitive deficits, especially in biologically vulnerable individuals, and how these deficits can be explained neuropsychologically.

Hence, the further development of the neuropsychology of CD will benefit from not only the recent brain research and theories just reviewed but also the attempt to ground constructs such as empathy, social cognition, and emotion regulation in neuropsychological theory. Both neurocomputational models of CD and new neuropsychological measures based on this attempted integration are needed.

Treatment

Treatment has focused on psychosocial interventions, especially preventive interventions. There is no pharmacological intervention for CD that has well-documented efficacy (Satcher, 1999), although comorbid ADHD can be effectively treated with psychostimulant medication.

There are two psychosocial interventions for CD that meet American Psychological Association criteria for a well-established treatment (see Brestan & Eyberg, 1998; Satcher, 1999), both of which are parent training programs. The previously discussed pioneering treatment approach of Patterson and colleagues, designed to reduce the vicious cycle of coercive parent–child interactions, has also demonstrated treatment efficacy (Dishion, Patterson, & Kavanagh, 1992).

Because the impaired social-cognitive skills in CD develop so early, considerable recent work has focused on the prevention of CD. Although not specifically designed for this purpose, the early intervention provided by Head Start appears on follow-up to reduce CD behaviors (Satcher, 1999). A much earlier intervention provided by the Elmira Prenatal/Early Infancy project conducted by Olds and colleagues (1998) involved nurse home visits to high-risk women bearing their first child, as well as developmental screening and transportation to health care facilities. Women were randomly assigned to four treatment groups, only two of which included nurse home visits, that continued in the most intensively treated group until the infant was 2 years old. Fifteen years later, the children from that group (who are now adolescents) have significantly reduced rates of CD behaviors, including less running away, fewer arrests and convictions, and less substance use and promiscuity. Another recent preventive intervention with documented efficacy is project FastTrack, which was designed specifically to prevent CD.

The results of these psychosocial interventions are encouraging and help to counter the stereotype often heard in clinical settings that it is impossible to treat children with CD. Clearly, a larger investment by our government in prevention programs with well-documented efficacy would help reduce crime rates in a fashion that is much more cost-effective than incarceration.

TOURETTE SYNDROME AND OBSESSIVE–COMPULSIVE DISORDER

> . . . he often had, seemingly, convulsive starts and odd gesticulations, which tended to excite at once surprise and ridicule.
> He had another particularity. . . . This was his anxious care to go out or in at a door or passage by a certain number of steps from a certain point. . . . I have, upon innumerable occasions, observed him suddenly stop, and then seem to count his steps with a deep earnestness, and when he had neglected or gone wrong in this sort of magical movement, I have seen him go back again, put himself in a proper posture to begin the ceremony, and, having gone through it, break from his abstraction, walk briskly on, and join his companion.
> —JAMES BOSWELL, *The Life of Johnson*

It is clear from Boswell's description that the famous English writer Samuel Johnson had tic-like symptoms and performed a compulsive ritual before crossing through a doorway. In addition to these symptoms, he also suffered from bouts of depression. Hence, Johnson may have had both a tic disorder and obsessive–compulsive disorder (OCD), as well as major depression. If so, Johnson illustrates both the frequent comorbidity between tic disorders and OCD, and that between OCD and depression. Obviously, despite these problems, we might say he had a productive life. Boswell's description of Johnson's symptoms captures some important aspects of both tics and compulsive rituals: their disruption of social interactions, the social disapproval they provoke, the anxiety that accompanies a compulsive ritual, and the need to perform it perfectly.

Although OCD is traditionally considered an anxiety disorder, it is included here with Tourette syndrome (TS) because the two disorders are related etiologically. There is also a subtype of OCD that is not related etiologically to TS. In what follows, the main focus is on TS, but I also review what is known about both subtypes of OCD.

In relation to the other action regulation disorders considered here, it is tempting to think of TS as somehow more "neurological," especially more than, say, CD. The symptoms in TS, motor and vocal tics, seem less voluntary than the symptoms in ADHD, which in turn seem less voluntary than those in CD. But as we will see, the expression of these symptoms in TS is very much influenced by psychosocial factors. In addition, even though tics are experienced as being involuntary, they can be temporarily suppressed. So TS lies on a boundary between voluntary and involuntary behavior, and challenges us to think about what we really mean by these terms. The terms "voluntary" and "involuntary," which are often accepted at face value in neuropsychology and psychiatry texts, are actually fairly blatant examples of how folk psychology gets smuggled into scientific terminology, since these terms take for granted the notion of free will. This is not to say that these terms have no value, only that they need to be defined in terms of brain function.

Like other disorders considered here, TS has served as a Rorschach blot for theorists. A late medieval account of a priest with both motor (periodically thrusting out his tongue) and vocal (yelling uncontrollably) tics is contained in the *Malleus Maleficarum* (Sprenger, 1489/1948), which is essentially a diagnostic manual to help the clergy identify witches. In this work, the priest in question is viewed as suffering from demonic possession. Gilles de la Tourette (1885) viewed TS as a hereditary disorder affecting the nervous system, which is closer to modern views than later views of psychoanalytic theorists, who viewed the symptoms in TS as a breakthrough of energy associated with unconscious conflicts (e.g., Fenichel, 1945).

Definition

Tics are sudden, nonrhythmic, repetitive, brief (< 1 second) stereotypical movements, gestures, or utterances of which the patient is initially unaware and which seem meaningless. Tics can be classified as motor or vocal and simple or complex (Evans, King, & Leckman, 1996). Examples of simple motor tics include eye blinking or other eye movements, grimacing, nose twitching, lip pouting, jaw snapping, tooth clicking, head jerks, arm jerks, shoulder shrugs, abdominal tensing, kicks, or finger movements. Simple vocal tics include throat clearing, coughing, sniffing, grunting, gurgling, hissing, and sucking, among others. Complex tics appear more purposeful and, at times, communicative. For example, complex motor tics include gestures of the face or hands, including obscene gestures, as well as sustained "looks," grooming behaviors, touching objects or self, or biting, throwing, or banging. Complex vocal tics involve speech—either syllables, words, or phrases—that can have unusual prosody and be obscene (e.g., the classic, but relatively uncommon, TS symptom of coprolalia) or inappropriate (e.g., "Shut up"). Tics occur in bouts, are partly suppressible, and wax and wane in severity. Patients with a tic disorder become aware of impending tics, which are experienced as an irresistible urge. Intriguingly, tics are also "infectious," in that a group of patients with tic disorders will unintentionally mirror each other's particular tics. So the mechanisms of tics may intersect with those involved in social mimicry and imitation. Tics are exacerbated by fatigue and stress, including the social stress of disapproval by teachers, parents, and peers. Obviously, tics are disruptive of normal social interactions and can be threatening or frightening to others, as well as a source of shame and embarrassment to the sufferer.

DSM-IV-TR (American Psychiatric Association, 2000) distinguishes three tic disorders—TS, chronic motor or vocal tic disorder, and transient tic disorder—which form a severity continuum, with TS being the most severe. If there is previous evidence of a more severe tic disorder, then the less severe diagnosis cannot be made. Thus, previous TS excludes both other diagnoses, and previous chronic tic disorder (CTD) excludes a diagnosis of transient tic disorder (TTD). The three diagnoses are distinguished by chronicity (in TS and CTD, the tics must be present for more than a year, whereas in TTD they can only have been present for a year at most) and by pervasiveness. (TS requires the presence of both motor and vocal tics, TTD permits the presence of both, but CTD is restricted to one or the other.) DSM-IV-TR also requires that the onset occur before 18 years, that the tics cause clinically significant distress or impairment, and that they not be caused by substance abuse or another neurological disease that produces involuntary movements (e.g., Huntington's disease, Sydenham's chorea, or Wilson's disease). Since TTD may develop into CTD, which may in turn develop into TS, these are not entirely distinct disorders. Indeed, as discussed later, all three are cofamilial, so it makes more sense to regard the three diagnoses as different regions of a continuum.

In addition, there is a phenotypic and etiological overlap with two other repetitive symptoms, obsessions and compulsions, which also overlap with tics in terms of brain mechanisms. Obsessions are repetitive and intrusive, inappropriate thoughts that cause marked anxiety or distress. They are distinct from both anxious thoughts about real-life problems and psychotic thoughts, which are experienced as being imposed from without. Common obsessions include fears of contamination, doubts about one's actions (e.g., "Did I lock the door?"), concerns about order, aggressive impulses (especially directed at family and friends), and sexual imagery. As will be discussed later, there is some value in thinking of obsessions as mental "tics." Compulsions are repetitive, seemingly purposive complex behaviors or rituals that are longer in duration than tics and performed to reduce the anxiety produced by an obsession or to ward off some dreaded outcome. Therefore, obsessions generate anxiety and compulsions relieve it. The proper execution of a compulsion can produce a "just right" feeling. Common compulsions include washing and cleaning, counting, checking, repeating actions, ordering, and seeking assurance. OCD is typically associated with even more distress and shame that is TS. Once again, obsessions and compulsions raise interesting questions about the boundary between voluntary and involuntary behavior, and provide interesting test cases for a neuropsychological theory of action selection.

Epidemiology

The prevalence of tic disorders, as defined here, is about 1–2% of the population (Popper & West, 1999). There is a much higher rate (as high as 18% of boys in a U.S. survey) of some tic-like behaviors as reported by parents, raising the possibility that tic disorders are the extreme tail of a normal distribution (Evans et al., 1996). TS, the most extreme disorder, is also the rarest, but hardly as rare as once thought. Prevalence estimates for TS range roughly between 0.1 and 30 per 10,000 (American Psychiatric Association, 2000; Evans et al., 1996; Tourette Syndrome Association International Consortium for Genetics, 1999), with a male predominance of about 2:1 (American Psychiatric Association, 2000). However, the prevalence may be as high as 1% in school-age males (Robertson & Stern, 1998).

The lifetime prevalence of OCD is 2.5%, with an equal gender ratio (American Psychiatric Association, 2000). Similar to tic disorders, OCD appears to lie on a continuum, since high rates of obsessional thoughts are reported by population samples of adolescents (46%) and adults (80–90%; see review in Carter, Pauls, & Leckman, 1995). As mentioned earlier, there appear to be at least two etiological subtypes of OCD, one cofamilial with TS and the other not. Among relatives of a TS proband, the gender ratio for OCD without tics shows a female predominance of about 3:1 (Pauls & Leckman, 1986). As will be discussed later, the expression of the TS genotype is thus pleiotropic and provides a good example of gender influence on genetic expression.

TS is comorbid with OCD (about 30–40% of patients also have OCD) and ADHD, with 40–50% of clinic samples of children with TS/CTD having histories of ADHD (Evans et al., 1996). Patterns of family transmission suggest different bases for these two comorbidities: a shared etiology for the comorbidity with OCD, and possibly a selection artifact (Berkson's bias) for the comorbidity with ADHD, although some evidence runs counter to this possibility.

OCD is comorbid with anxiety disorders (panic attacks, phobia, and separation anxiety) and depression (see review in Carter et al., 1995). OCD thus poses a challenge for how we think about diagnostic boundaries.

Etiology

TS provides a good example of some of the factors that complicate the search for specific genetic and environmental risk factors for complex behavioral disorders (see reviews in Alsobrook & Pauls, 1999; Evans et al., 1996; Tourette Syndrome Association International Consortium for Genetics, 1999). First, there are clearly etiological subtypes. One subtype consists of a familial and heritable phenotype that may manifest as either TS, chronic tics, OCD, or some combination of the three. There may be a second, familial and heritable subtype of OCD that is not cofamilial with tic disorders, and also sporadic (nonfamilial) cases of these disorders.

For example, up to one-third of children with TS appear to have an autoimmune disorder in which antibodies formed during a group A beta-hemolytic streptococcal infection then attack the basal ganglia (Swedo, 1994). Hence, TS provides one of the clearest examples we have of the contribution of an infection to the etiology of a psychiatric disorder. However, since streptococcal infections are a ubiquitous risk factor in children, it is quite possible that there might be genetic influences on the propensity for this adverse autoimmune reaction, as is true in other autoimmune disorders. Second, there is assortative mating for TS and related symptoms. Bilineal transmission of genetic risk factors, especially if a different genetic risk factor is transmitted from each side of the family, complicates traditional linkage analysis, which is attempting to find a single, major locus that contributes to the disorder. Third, despite fairly consistent evidence of major locus transmission in segregation analyses of TS (e.g., Pauls & Leckman, 1986), it is becoming increasingly clear that multiple genes are involved, so nonparametric sib-pair methods are more appropriate than traditional parametric linkage analysis (Tourette Syndrome Association International Consortium for Genetics, 1999).

Familiality

The rate of TS in siblings of a TS proband is about 11.5% for brothers and 4.8% for sisters, meaning that relative risk (λ) is greater than 10 (Tourette Syndrome Association International Consortium for Genetics, 1999). Hence, TS is one of the most familial of psychiatric disorders. Such siblings are also at increased risk for CTD or OCD, and the risk of any one of these three disorders in families of a TS proband is 42% (Pauls & Leckman, 1986), which is about seven to eight times the population risk.

Whether OCD apart from TS is familial is less clear. Existing studies do not separate TS families from non-TS families. Even so, not all of these studies find elevated rates of OCD in the relatives of OCD probands (see reviews in Carter et al., 1995, and Crowe, 1999). One of the largest family studies (Pauls, Alsobrook, Goodman, Rasmussen, & Leckman, 1995) found that the rates of both OCD (10.3% vs. 1.9%) and subsyndromal OCD (7.9% vs. 2.0%) were elevated in first-degree relatives of OCD probands versus those of controls. Hence, λ was 4.6 for the combined phenotype (OCD + subsyndromal OCD).

Heritability

MZ concordance rates are 50–60% for TS alone and increase to 77–90% if the phenotype is expanded to include CTD. Corresponding DZ concordance rates are 8% and 22%, respectively (Evans et al., 1996). If the phenotype is further expanded to include OCD, then both MZ and DZ concordance rates rise further, with the MZ concordance rate approaching 100% and a DZ rate of 30–35%. Across all three phenotypic definitions, the MZ concordance is substantially greater than the DZ concordance, providing evidence for substantial heritability and a common genetic etiology for the three cofamilial phenotypes (TS, CTD, and OCD).

There have been fewer twin studies of OCD than TS. Carey and Gottesman (1981) studied a small sample of MZ (N = 15) and DZ (N = 15) twin pairs in which the proband had OCD. Using a combined phenotype (OCD + subsyndromal OCD), they found an MZ concordance of 87% and a DZ concordance of 47%. In a large, unselected twin sample, Clifford, Murray, and Fulker (1984) found a heritability of 47% for obsessional symptoms. Taken together, these two twin studies indicate genetic influence on both OCD itself and OCD symptoms. These results are consistent with those of Pauls and colleagues (1995), which supported familiality for a quantitative trait of OCD symptoms; they extend that result by indicating that this familiality is partly genetic. In summary, while there is evidence for familiality and heritability for both OCD itself and OCD symptoms, suggesting that OCD is transmitted as a quantitative trait rather than a categorical one, we lack clear evidence on the transmission of OCD in non-TS families.

Mode of Transmission

Although segregation analyses support major locus transmission of TS, they vary in terms of whether the major locus is dominant (e.g., Pauls & Leckman, 1986) or additive, and whether there is a multifactorial background (Tourette Syndrome Association International Consortium for Genetics, 1999). As mentioned earlier, bilineal transmission is also a complication in these studies. Moreover, a major locus result does not necessarily mean that there is only one major locus.

Cosegregation analysis has been used to test the basis of the comorbidities observed in TS. As discussed earlier, if a common genetic etiology underlies the comorbidity, then relatives of probands with or without the comorbidity (e.g., TS only vs. TS + OCD) should exhibit equal elevations in risk for the comorbid condition, meaning that transmission of the two disorders is not independent. This is exactly what Pauls and colleagues (1986b) found for the relation between TS and OCD, consistent with the twin data reviewed earlier. In contrast, the rates of ADHD among relatives of TS + ADHD probands were significantly higher than those in relatives of TS-only probands, which were similar to population rates, consistent with independent transmission of the two disorders (Pauls et al., 1986a).

Hence, another explanation besides a shared genetic etiology is needed for the comorbidity between TS and ADHD. One possibility is a selection artifact (Berkson's bias). However, this comorbidity has been found in a population sample (Caine et al., 1988). Another possibility is a nonfamilial environmental risk factor that increases the risk for both disorders. For example, the autoimmune response, discussed earlier, that affects the basal ganglia could also increase the risk for ADHD, since basal ganglia alterations are also observed in ADHD. Such an environmental risk factor would produce a nonartifactual comorbidity. Consistent with this hypothesis, there is a 50% rate of ADHD among TS patients with this autoimmune syndrome, as well as an 80% rate of OCD (Swedo et al., 1998). However, susceptibility to this autoimmune response is probably genetically mediated, as discussed earlier, so the risk factor is not completely environmental. Also, for this explanation to work, the rates of ADHD in the autoimmune subtype of TS must be higher than in the rest of TS. It is not clear whether this is true. So both genes and environmental risk factors appear to contribute to the comorbidity between TS and OCD, whereas the comorbidity between TS and ADHD remains to be explained.

Gene Locations

Using a traditional parametric linkage approach, researchers have excluded about 80% of the genome as the location of the putative major locus for TS. This disappointing result has led to the hypothesis that multiple genetic risk factors may be involved (e.g., quantitative trait loci [QTLs]) and that nonparametric sib-pair approaches are more appropriate. A whole genome search using these methods (Tourette Syndrome Association International Consortium for Genetics, 1999) found two suggestive chromosomal locations, on 4q and 8p, as well as some support for a third region on 19p, for which a separate study of large families had also found suggestive results. Obviously, these three possible gene locations need to be replicated. Chromosomal anomalies (on 9, 18, and 22) have also been found associated with TS (Alsobrook & Pauls, 1999). One study (Grice et al., 1996) found a within-family association between TS and the 7-repeat allele of DRD4, which has been associated with ADHD in several studies reviewed earlier. If replicated, this finding would provide a genetic explanation for the comorbidity between TS and ADHD, but one that is inconsistent with the cosegregation results discussed earlier. In summary, more work is needed to test these various suggestive results.

For OCD, three candidate genes have been examined: those for the DRD3 receptor (Catalano et al., 1994), the serotonin transporter (Altemus, Murphy, Greenberg, & Lesch, 1996; Billet et al., 1997), and the enzyme catechol-O-methyltransferase (COMT; Karayioragou et al., 1997). DRD3 was a candidate because of the alterations in dopamine neurotransmission found in TS, which overlaps with OCD. The serotonin transporter (whose gene locus name is SLC6A4) was a candidate because of the efficacy of SSRIs in treating OCD. COMT was a candidate because it affects both dopamine and norepinephrine neurotransmission, also implicated In OCD.

The results for DRD3 were null, as were the results for the primary coding region of SLC6A4 (Altemus et al., 1996). However, a polymorphism in the regulatory region of SLC6A4 exhibited a marginally significant ($p = .06$) case–control association with OCD (Billet et al., 1997). As reviewed earlier, this same allele has been found to be associated with depression and anxiety in some, but not all, studies. Finally, a significant case–control association was found between an allele of the COMT gene and OCD in males (Karayiorgou et al., 1997). This allele causes a size reduction in COMT enzyme activity and would therefore be expected to affect neurotransmission. Since the two positive results did not use within-family association methods, they could be artifactual. In summary, while promising, these results need to be replicated in other labs using within-family association methods.

Environmental Risk Factors

Besides the autoimmune syndrome discussed earlier, other environmental risk factors for TS include perinatal risk factors (reviewed in Evans et al., 1996). Psychosocial stress clearly exacerbates the expression of tic disorders (Evans et al., 1996) and OCD (Carter et al., 1995).

Brain Mechanisms

Neurobiologically, tic disorders can be conceptualized roughly as being the opposite of Parkinson's disease. In Parkinson's, a reduction of dopamine in the basal ganglia leads to a slowing of movement. In contrast, in animal models of tics, application of dopamine agonists (e.g., Ritalin) to the basal ganglia produces tics. In this model, tics are conceptualized as arising from basic motor "programs," partly stored in the basal ganglia, that are released from inhibition because of a dopamine excess in the basal ganglia.

The fact that tics are preceded by premonitory urges and may be temporarily suppressed can be explained by the close reciprocal connections between the prefrontal cortex and the basal ganglia. The bottom-up activation of a candidate action would be registered in prefrontal cortex, and if strong enough, would reach consciousness. If the candidate action were inappropriate to the current representation of context maintained in active memory in prefrontal cortex, descending inhibitory connections to the basal ganglia would be activated in an attempt to stop the action from being launched. Hence, whether inhibition succeeded or not would depend on a dynamic interaction between bottom-up activation and top-down inhibition. This account of tics illustrates how top-down cognitive factors (voluntary or controlled processing) interact with bottom-up factors (involuntary or automatic processing) in the course of action selection. I hope this account also makes it clearer why the terms "voluntary" and "involuntary" are somewhat misleading.

Notice that the primary circuits implicated in tic generation, those between prefrontal cortex and basal ganglia, are nominally the same as those implicated in ADHD, and both disorders have been conceptualized as failures of inhibition. Nonetheless, the symptoms are different, and, most importantly, stimulant medication (a dopamine agonist) has *opposite* effects on the two disorders: It reduces symptoms in ADHD but increases them in tic disorders. Therefore, a satisfactory prefrontal–striatal model of both disorders will need to account for this apparent contradiction. It is very likely that different prefrontal–striatal circuits are involved in each disorder.

Indeed, as discussed earlier in the section on the action selection system in Chapter 2, recent work on the functional organization of the basal ganglia has revealed at least three distinct, feedforward circuits (Figure 13), which may be described as motor, cognitive, and limbic (Alexander, 1995; Mahurin, 1998). Topographically organized information from different parts of frontal cortex projects to different parts of the striatum (caudate, putamen, and ventral striatum), which in turn projects to different parts of the pallidum and then to distinct thalamic nuclei, which send projections back to the original part of frontal cortex. The motor circuit originates in premotor and supplementary motor cortex, the cognitive circuit in dorsolateral and lateral orbitoprefrontal cortex, and the limbic circuit in anterior cingulate and medial–orbitoprefrontal cortex. Each of these circuits receives somewhat different dopamine projections; for example, the motor circuit receives dopamine projections from the substantia nigra, whereas the limbic circuit receives them from the ventral tegmental area. There may also be different distributions of subtypes of dopamine receptors in the different circuits, so it is quite plausible that dopamine could have different effects in different circuits.

One can speculate that tic disorders (and Parkinson's disease) involve the motor circuit, ADHD involves the cognitive circuit, and OCD involves the limbic circuit. As we see later, neuroimaging data support this speculation about OCD. Such a speculation could also begin to help account for the different developmental trajectories of TS, ADHD, and OCD. The most common time of onset for ADHD is during the preschool years, and symptoms persist into adulthood. Time of onset for tics is early school age, with exacerbation in adolescence and a decrease in adulthood. For OCD, the most common time of onset is adolescence.

Structural Neuroimaging Studies

Predominantly left-sided volume reductions of the basal ganglia have been found in MRI studies of adults and children with TS, but not all studies have confirmed this result (see Lombroso & Leckman, 1999, for a review). In OCD, smaller caudate volumes have been found (see Carter et al., 1995, for a review).

Functional Neuroimaging Studies

Evidence for reduced cerebral metabolism in the basal ganglia in TS has been found across three neuroimaging studies, along with decreased activity in orbitofrontal, cingulate, and insular cortices (see Peterson, Leckman, & Cohen, 1995, for a review).

There have been many more functional neuroimaging studies of OCD. Baxter's (1999) review lists over 20 such studies and finds that the converging results across these studies include overactivity in orbitofrontal cortex and head of the caudate nucleus (part of the striatum). When OCD behaviors are provoked, these two structures are activated, along with the thalamus. When OCD is successfully treated, activity in these two structures declines and is no longer significantly correlated (as is the case in normal controls). These results support the view that overactivity of this particular basal ganglia circuit (the limbic circuit discussed earlier) has a causal relation to OCD symptoms. Another structure that is consistently overactive in OCD is the anterior cingulate, which is also part of the limbic circuit.

In summary, the neuroimaging studies of OCD tell a clearer story than those for TS. The involvement of a limbic basal ganglia circuit fits with the symptoms of OCD and its overlap with anxiety disorders. Obsessive thoughts generate anxiety, which compulsive rituals attempt to reduce. We can think of the orbitoprefrontal cortex as holding these anxious thoughts in active memory and activating compulsive actions whose implementation involves the basal ganglia. However, performance of the compulsion does not totally relieve the anxiety, so the sufferer of OCD is caught in a vicious circle of anxious arousal and stereotyped action selection. Treatment breaks up this vicious circle of tightly correlated brain activity.

With regard to TS, it is not clear why volume and metabolic reductions in the basal ganglia (presumably in the motor circuit) should lead to an *excess* of behavior, a failure of inhibition.

Neuropsychology

In the previous section, I have sketched a very preliminary neuropsychological model of tics, obsessions, and compulsions. There have been some initial attempts to develop computational models of basal ganglia functions (e.g., Mahurin, 1998), but more comprehensive models are needed that can accommodate the whole range of basal ganglia disorders (e.g., Parkinson's disease, ADHD, TS, and OCD).

Unfortunately, most existing neuropsychological studies of TS and OCD have not taken us very far toward the goal of a theoretical model. Many of these studies have used clinical neuropsychological batteries in an exploratory way in these groups. While there is evidence for neuropsychological dysfunction, the pattern of results is confusingly inconsistent (see Carter et al., 1995, and Pennington & Ozonoff, 1996, for reviews). In particular, there is not consistent evidence of executive dysfunction, at least on traditional measures. Obviously, this result does not fit with the view developed here: that these disorders arise from dysfunctions in the action selection system. Some of this inconsistency may arise from failure to control for conditions that are comorbid with TS and OCD (Ozonoff, Strayer, McMahon, & Filloux, 1998). In summary, there is a pressing need for better theoretical models of the functions of basal ganglia circuits and improved neuropsychological measures of these functions.

A recent study by Casey and colleagues (2001) differentiated TS from ADHD, OCD associated with Sydenham's chorea, and schizophrenia by using tasks based on the model of different frontal–basal ganglia circuits (Figure 13) presented earlier. Subjects with TS were selectively impaired on a response execution task; those with OCD, on a response selection task; those with schizophrenia, on a stimulus selection task; and those with ADHD, on both stimulus selection and response execution. Although these results need to be replicated in larger samples and tied more closely to the relevant circuits in the action selection system, this study clearly represents a step forward.

Treatment

For TS, the main treatment is pharmacological, usually with dopamine antagonists. There is also a need for supportive and educational psychotherapy for both individual patients and their families, to help them manage their own reactions and the often-stigmatizing reactions provoked by TS. In the past, neuroleptic drugs such as haloperidol (Haldol) were used effectively to treat TS, but these drugs have the disadvantage of producing motor side effects (e.g., tardive dyskinesia). Now there are atypical neuroleptics, such as risperidone (Risperdal) and olanzapine (Zyprexa), that have fewer motor side effects and effectively treat TS. Also effective in treating TS is clonidine (Catapres), which decreases norepinephrine neurotransmission and indirectly increases dopamine utilization. It is not known why these neurochemical changes reduce the symptoms of TS. In particular, the efficacy of increased dopamine utilization is puzzling given the efficacy of dopamine antagonists.

For OCD, the main pharmacological treatment is with selective serotonin reuptake inhibitors (SSRIs); the main psychotherapeutic treatment, a behavioral therapy, involves exposure with response prevention (see Hollander et al., 1999, and Holmes, 1997, for reviews). One such SSRI is clomipramine (Anafranil), but due to a high rate of side effects, it is used relatively rarely. Instead, other SSRIs are used in treating OCD.

Initially, the efficacy of these serotonin agonists in treating OCD was surprising (e.g., Kramer, 1993). How could the same drugs be effective treatments for both depression and OCD, when these two disorders were traditionally viewed as quite distinct from each other? But there is now fairly extensive evidence that serotonergic neurotransmission plays a causal role in OCD (reviewed in Hollander et al., 1999). As discussed earlier in the section on CD, there are serotonin receptors in parts of the limbic basal ganglia circuit (i.e., in orbitofrontal cortex) that, as discussed earlier, is important in OCD. Other limbic circuits are implicated in depression. So a resolution to the apparent paradox posed by the efficacy of SSRIs for the treatment of both OCD and depression is once again overlapping neural circuits in the two disorders and different subtypes of serotonin receptors, with different anatomical distributions. Of course, as with all the psychopharmacological treatments considered in this book, we do not have a complete understanding of why they work.

The behavior therapy proven to be effective in treating about half of adult patients with OCD, exposure with response prevention, involves presenting a stimulus to the patient that ordinarily triggers a compulsive ritual (for Samuel Johnson, this would be a doorway) and then preventing the ritual. So the link between stimulus and response is deconditioned. Finally, there appear to be few clinical trials of either psychopharmacological (see Walsh, 1998) or behavioral treatments of children with OCD.

SCHIZOPHRENIA

Schizophrenia, one of the most severe psychiatric illnesses, has been recognized as a distinct disorder for about 100 years. The term "schizophrenia," which means "splitting of the mind," was coined by Bleuler (1857–1939) to emphasize the disorganization in thinking that characterizes the disorder. So contrary to popular belief, the term schizophrenia does not mean "split personality," a term that might better describe multiple personality disorder, which is not related to schizophrenia. A term for a prominent characteristic of schizophrenic speech, "loose associations," also derives from Bleuler (1911/1950). Kraepelin (1856–1926), who laid the foundation for modern psychiatry by distinguishing psychoses according to their course, called schizophrenia *dementia praecox* ("precocious dementia"). Kraepelin (1919/1971) believed that, unlike the episodic psychoses sometimes associated with bipolar disorder or major depression, the psychosis in schizophrenia was chronic and reflective of a neurodegenerative process, similar to what is seen in Alzheimer's disease. As will become apparent in this discussion, current data are more consistent with the view that schizophrenia is a neurodevelopmental disorder rather than a neurodegenerative one, with about half of schizophrenics showing recovery in later adulthood.

Although schizophrenia was originally viewed as a brain disorder by Kraepelin and others, the advent of psychoanalysis led to psychosocial theories of its etiology. As recently as a few decades ago, future clinicians were taught about the role of "schizophrenogenic" mothers in producing this terrible disorder. It was hypothesized that such mothers were cold, distant, and rejecting; by exposing their offspring to "mixed messages," they helped produce schizophrenia. Just as is the case for autism, such psychosocial hypotheses regarding the etiology of schizophrenia have been thoroughly rejected. Once again, schizophrenia is viewed as a brain disorder, but now there is considerably more evidence for that view. Nonetheless, the outcome in schizophrenia, like autism, is affected by psychosocial influences. Several excellent reviews of schizophrenia research have appeared recently (Berman & Weinberger, 1999; Byne, Kemether, Jones, Haroutunian, & Davis, 1999; Cornblatt, Green, & Walker, 1999; Kendler, 1999; Marenco & Weinberger, 2000); this chapter attempts to synthesize those reviews.

Definition

DSM-IV-TR (American Psychiatric Association, 2000) defines schizophrenia as the presence (for 1 month) of two or more of the following five symptoms: (1) delusions, (2) hallucinations, (3) disorganized speech, (4) grossly disorganized or catatonic behavior, and (5) negative symptoms, including flat affect, poverty of speech (alogia), and diminished initiative (avolition). These symptoms must cause significant functional impairment, which must have lasted for at least 6 months. Exclusionary conditions include (1) schizoaffective disorder, (2) mood disorders with psychotic features, (3) substance use or a general medical condition, or (4) a pervasive developmental disorder, unless it is accompanied by delusions or hallucinations.

The first four types of symptoms are considered "positive" symptoms, meaning that they represent the appearance of new behaviors that are clearly abnormal. In contrast, "negative" symptoms refer to the loss of normal functions. This distinction between positive and negative symptoms derives from the great English neurologist John Hughlings-Jackson (1835–1911), who wanted to account for the different kinds of symptoms observed following acquired brain damage (Hughlings-Jackson, 1931). A negative symptom represented the loss of a normal function previously performed by a damaged brain region, whereas a positive symptom represented the failure of a region's inhibitory function after damage. Crow (1980) very productively applied this distinction to schizophrenia. He hypothesized that positive symptoms were caused by a reversible biochemical disorder; hence, patients with only positive symptoms (Type I schizophrenia) could be expected to return to normal functioning after successful medication treatment. In contrast, negative symptoms were caused by an irreversible structural brain disorder; hence, patients with negative symptoms (Type II schizophrenia) would be expected to exhibit neuropsychological dysfunction, a chronic course, and a poor outcome. As we see later, subsequent research has supported the view that positive and negative symptoms have different brain mechanisms.

Epidemiology

The lifetime prevalence of schizophrenia is about 1%, which varies little around the world (Cornblatt et al., 1999). However, culture does affect the manifestation and interpretation of symptoms (Satcher, 1999). The gender ratio is equal, but average age of onset is about 6 years earlier (around 21 years) in males than in females (Cornblatt et al., 1999). There are also gender differences in presentation, with more mood symptoms and better prognosis in females (Satcher, 1999). Rates of schizophrenia are higher in urban areas and in lower socioeconomic classes. Two competing hypotheses have been generated to account for this association with lower socioeconomic class. The *social stress hypothesis* posits that the adversity associated with lower socioeconomic status helps cause schizophrenia, whereas the *social drift hypothesis* posits an opposite relation, namely, that schizophrenia causes a decline in socioeconomic class. As reviewed in Seligman and colleagues (2001), studies that have examined this issue support the social drift hypothesis. For example, individuals with schizophrenia but not their (nonschizophrenic) fathers have a lower socioeconomic status than controls.

Schizophrenia is comorbid with substance abuse (particularly nicotine abuse), certain personality disorders (schizoid, schizotypal, and paranoid), and anxiety disorders (American Psychiatric Association, 2000). Some of these comorbidities could just mean that schizophrenia is a spectrum disorder, like autism. Schizophrenia, like mood disorders, is also associated with increased mortality, due in part to suicide (about a 10% risk) and in part to comorbid medical illnesses, which include vision and dental problems, hypertension, diabetes, and sexually transmitted diseases (Satcher, 1999). Although the reasons for these comorbid medical problems are not clearly understood, they may result in part from substance abuse, poor diet, and poor health care. For example, a significant proportion of the homeless population has schizophrenia (Cornblatt et al., 1999).

Schizophrenia is a particularly devastating illness because it effectively removes individuals from society during the most productive years of their life, thus lowering their social status. Besides this lost productivity, other societal costs include those of long-term medical and custodial care. The total costs to society have been estimated to be greater than those of all cancers combined (Kaplan & Sadock, 1988).

Developmental Continuity

Schizophrenia has a different developmental course than any of the other psychopathologies considered in this book. Prodromal symptoms may be detectable as early as infancy, suggesting congenital neurodevelopmental anomalies, including minor physical anomalies (pointing to an alteration in prenatal development), and motor, cognitive, and social anomalies observable in infancy and childhood (Marenco & Weinberger, 2000). After the onset of the full syndrome in young adulthood, there is a period of deterioration that lasts on average about 5 years, then gradual improvement, with a fairly full functional recovery in about half of schizophrenics (Marenco & Weinberger, 2000). Finally, it is worth noting that, much more rarely, the onset of schizophrenia occurs in childhood (hence, "childhood schizophrenia"). The factors that produce early onset are not well understood. (For a review of the clinical characteristics of childhood schizophrenia, see Russell, Bott, & Sammons, 1989.)

Most of the other disorders considered here are either chronic or episodic (i.e., mood disorders). Hence, the distinct developmental course in schizophrenia requires an explanation. In particular, two questions need to be answered:

1. If the neurodevelopmental anomaly is congenital, why is the onset of the disorder delayed until young adulthood?
2. Why does the disorder improve in later adulthood?

We still lack definitive answers. Neurodevelopmental hypotheses have been advanced to answer these questions, including late myelination of congenitally abnormal brain structures, producing a "sleeper" effect: The symptoms of the disorder emerge when the abnormal structures fail to come online (which only addresses the first question). Another hypothesis invokes documented lifespan developmental changes in dopamine levels, which peak in young adulthood and decline in later adulthood. If some of the symptoms of schizophrenia are caused by a dopamine imbalance, this imbalance could be worsened by a rise in dopamine levels. One could also pose a social–developmental hypothesis, namely, that something particularly demanding about the tasks of young adulthood magnifies an underlying weakness in individuals with schizophrenia. However, this hypothesis better explains negative than positive symptoms.

Etiology

Current thinking on the etiology of schizophrenia involves both a genetic diathesis and an early environmental insult, both of which change brain development. As we will see, some of the brain anomalies in schizophrenia are familial, whereas others appear to have a nonshared environmental cause.

Familiality

There have been over 40 family studies of schizophrenia (reviewed in Gottesman, 1991, and Plomin et al., 1997). These studies document that this disorder is clearly familial, with a relative risk (λ) of 9 for full siblings. Other first-degree relatives also exhibit elevated risk ($\lambda = 13$ for offspring and 6 for parents). The risk to parents is probably decreased because individuals with schizophrenia are less likely to marry; so parents may have risk alleles for schizophrenia without being schizophrenic themselves. In the rare event that both parents have schizophrenia, the risk to offspring rises considerably ($\lambda = 46$). Risk falls off systematically with decreasing genetic relation (e.g., $\lambda = 4$ for second-degree relatives).

The familial phenotype is broader than the diagnosis of schizophrenia and includes the comorbid disorders listed earlier (except, possibly, substance abuse) and endophenotypes found in about half the relatives of a schizophrenic proband, including relatives without a psychiatric diagnosis (Cornblatt et al., 1999; Kendler, 1999). Probably the two most studied endophenotypes are deficits in smooth pursuit eye movements (SPEM) and sensory gating, which is measured with an evoked response paradigm.

Heritability

The reviews referred to earlier also include twin and adoption studies of schizophrenia, which document that most of the increased familial risk (λ) is attributable to genetic influences. For example, adopted offspring of a biological parent with schizophrenia still have a relative risk (λ = 11), which is only slightly smaller than the risk (λ = 13) observed in nonadopted offspring. Moreover, the average concordance for schizophrenia in MZ pairs reared apart (64%) is not lower than the average concordance for MZ pairs reared together (48%); the latter figure is, of course, based on much larger samples than the former. In addition, the average MZ concordance of 48% is significantly larger than the average DZ concordance of 17% (Gottesman, 1991), which also documents schizophrenia's significant heritability. Because the MZ concordance is much less than 100%, there must be nonshared environmental risk factors for schizophrenia. Evidence for a different sort of environmental influence is provided by the discrepancy between the average sibling risk (λ = 9) and the DZ risk (λ = 17). Since siblings and DZ twins have the same degree of genetic relationship, this difference in risk must be environmental and may implicate a shared prenatal environment. If the liability for schizophrenia is considered to lie on a continuum, then the observed average MZ and DZ concordances cited earlier yield a liability heritability of about 60% (Plomin et al., 1997).

Mode of Transmission

As has been true for most of the disorders in this book, segregation analyses of schizophrenia generally support the conclusion that its transmission is complex rather than Mendelian (Cornblatt et al., 1999; Kendler, 1999).

Gene Locations

There have probably been more molecular genetic studies of schizophrenia than any other behaviorally defined disorder. Kendler (1999) recently reviewed research on this topic, and I summarize his main conclusions. Three linkage findings for schizophrenia have each been replicated in at least two samples other than the initial sample and one multigroup study; nonetheless, other studies have failed to replicate all three linkages. This overall pattern is similar to results found for several other disorders discussed in this book and would be consistent with multiple risk alleles, each with a small effect. There may also be genetic heterogeneity across samples. Such a pattern of results is not consistent with a single major locus hypothesis.

These three best replicated linkages for schizophrenia are on 6p 24–22, 8p 22–21, and 22q 12–13. The region on 22 is of interest because microdeletions here cause velocardiofacial syndrome (VCFS), which has been associated with schizophrenia and schizotypal disorder in some studies. More preliminary linkage results have been found on 5p 21–23 and 15q 14 (Freedman et al., 1997; Leonard et al., 1998). The 15q 14 site is close to the gene for the alpha 7-nicotinic acetylcholine receptor gene; a defect in this gene could provide an explanation for the nicotine addiction that is so common in schizophrenia. Interestingly, evidence for linkage increased considerably in the Freedman and colleagues (1997) study when the endophenotype of a deficit in sensory gating was used instead of a diagnostic phenotype. The work by Freedman's group illustrates what an integrated neuroscientific account of at least one aspect of schizophrenia might look like: A risk allele alters an aspect of neurotransmission, which in turn affects an aspect of information processing (sensory gating) and explains a behavioral symptom (increased smoking). Obviously, this finding and the other linkages reviewed here need more replication; this field is changing so rapidly that aspects of this review will undoubtedly be out of date by the time this book is published.

In contrast to these promising linkage findings, numerous association studies of schizophrenia, each targeting alleles of genes for neurotransmitter (i.e., dopamine, GABA, glutamate, serotonin, and N-methyl-D-aspartate [NMDA]) receptors and transporters have all found null results.

Environmental Risk Factors

As discussed earlier, twin studies implicate nonshared environmental and prenatal influences (which may be shared or not shared by twins) in the etiology of schizophrenia. Other studies, reviewed in Marenco and Weinberger (2000), have begun to identify what these environmental influences might be. Both place (urban) and time of birth (late winter) increase risk for schizophrenia. Such associations are very unlikely to be genetically mediated and instead implicate environmental risk factors (such as exposure to viruses). Several, but not all, studies of the association between viral epidemics (e.g., influenza) during pregnancy and rates of later schizophrenia have found positive results, but the effect is small and not specific to schizophrenia. Across studies, obstetrical complications (such as maternal preeclampsia, which consists of hypertension and edema, and can compromise blood flow to the fetus) increase the risk for schizophrenia about twofold. Again, the effect is small and nonspecific. It is also not clear whether this effect is entirely environmental, since a genetically abnormal fetus can produce an increased rate of obstetrical complications.

Although there is very little evidence that psychosocial factors influence the onset of schizophrenia, similar to the case with bipolar illness, there is good evidence that such factors influence its course (see Hooley & Candela, 1999, for a review). Much of the research on this topic has focused on the construct of "expressed emotion" (EE), which means the extent to which family members communicate with a patient in a critical, hostile, or emotionally overinvolved way. Across numerous studies, high EE in relatives more than doubles the relapse rate found in patients with relatives low in EE. However, the relation between EE and severity of schizophrenia is a two-way street. As the illness returns and becomes more severe, relatives' critical and hostile reactions increase (Scazufca & Kuipers, 1998).

Brain Mechanisms

Brain mechanisms include studies of neurotransmission, brain structure, and neuroimaging, all of which reveal differences in individuals with schizophrenia, supporting the general hypothesis that schizophrenia is a brain disorder. At the same time, the exact nature of the neuropathology remains elusive.

Neurotransmission

This summary is based on the reviews of Cornblatt and colleagues (1999) and Byne and colleagues (1999). Similar to what has occurred in research on mood and anxiety disorders, a single neurotransmitter hypothesis of schizophrenia has been rejected as evidence has accumulated for the involvement of multiple neurotransmitters. The single neurotransmitter hypothesis of schizophrenia postulated an excess of dopamine, especially in the limbic system.

This hypothesis was supported by the fact that high doses of amphetamines (which are dopamine agonists) induce a psychosis that is clinically indistinguishable from schizophrenia, and that neuroleptics (such as Thorazine and Haldol), which are dopamine antagonists, are effective treatments. However, other predictions of this hypothesis were not supported by dopamine metabolite and receptor studies. If there is an excess of dopamine, there ought to be higher levels of the dopamine metabolite, homovanillic acid (HVA), in individuals with schizophrenia. An excess of dopamine should also downregulate the number of dopamine receptors. But across studies, these predicted results were generally not found. In addition, a substantial proportion of individuals with schizophrenia are not helped by neuroleptics. Moreover, negative symptoms are neither aided by neuroleptics nor exacerbated by dopamine agonists. Finally, there is also evidence of alterations in other neurotransmitters in schizophrenia, such as glutamate, GABA, and, in the Freedman and colleagues (1997) work, acetylcholine.

A new dopamine hypothesis has been formulated (Byne, Kemether, Jones, Haroutunian, & Davis, 1999), in which negative symptoms are associated with decreased cortical (mainly prefrontal) dopamine activity, and positive symptoms are associated with increased subcortical dopamine activity. There is also some evidence that decreased cortical dopamine activity may lead to a subcortical increase in dopamine activity, which would come close to Hughlings-Jackson's (1931) view of how a positive symptom arises (failure of a cortical structure to regulate the activity of a subcortical one). This new dopamine hypothesis also includes changes in other aspects of neurotransmission.

Drugs of abuse besides amphetamines have also produced models of schizophrenia. Phencyclidine (PCP) blocks the ion channel of the NMDA receptor and produces a psychotic syndrome with both positive and negative symptoms, but so far there is not direct evidence of NMDA hypofunction in schizophrenia, although it is known that NMDA hypofunction can result from dopamine overactivity. Lysergic acid (LSD) increases serotonin activity and leads to perceptual distortions that are similar to the hallucinations seen in schizophrenia. Moreover, there is evidence for alterations in the ratio of different serotonin receptors in schizophrenia.

In summary, the symptoms of schizophrenia are likely to be associated with alterations in multiple neurotransmitter systems. Which, if any, of these neurotransmitter alterations are primary is unknown, as is how they relate to changes in brain structure that have also been documented in schizophrenia. The neurotransmitter alterations could cause the structural changes or vice versa, or the two could be separate but interacting causes.

Structural Neuroimaging Studies

These studies are reviewed in Cornblatt and colleagues (1999), Fannon and colleagues (2000), and Marenco and Weinberger (2000). The best replicated structural difference in schizophrenia is ventricular enlargement, which could result either from failure of development or later atrophy of adjacent brain tissue (average effect size across studies = .7). Consistent with the neurodevelopmental hypothesis, ventricular enlargement is present at the first episode (Fannon et al., 2000) and does not change over time in longitudinal studies. MZ twins discordant for schizophrenia are also discordant for ventricular enlargement, which indicates that the etiology of this structural difference must be due to a nonshared environmental influence, such as a prenatal insult of some kind. Obviously, ventricular enlargement is not specific to schizophrenia, since it is found in a number of other disorders. Other structural differences that have been observed include a smaller brain size (with sulcal enlargement); a smaller cerebellum; smaller temporal lobe structures, including the superior temporal gyrus and the hippocampus; and a smaller thalamus. There are also reports of alterations in the symmetry of temporal lobe structures, such as the planum temporale.

Postmortem studies are also consistent with the neurodevelopmental hypothesis (Marenco & Weinberger, 2000) and do not find markers of neurodegeneration, such as gliosis (an accumulation of glial cells around injured neural tissue) or plaques and neurofibrillary tangles (which are observed in neurodegenerative diseases such as Alzheimer's). In contrast, these studies do find some positive evidence consistent with alterations in early brain development, including mediotemporal decreases in neuron size and neuropil (the dense "feltwork" of axons and dendrites that connect neurons and are formed mainly in early brain development), as well as reductions of proteins (e.g., neuronal cell adhesion molecules [NCAMs]), involved in neuronal migration. Some studies, but not others, have found ectopias (neurons that have failed to migrate properly), something that would have to occur early in brain development.

Functional Neuroimaging Studies

Research on this topic is reviewed in Berman and Weinberger (1999). There have been many functional neuroimaging studies of schizophrenia; inevitably, the small sample sizes and methodological variations across studies have led to some conflicting results, as is true in the functional neuroimaging literature generally. However, there is some convergence on a few broad conclusions. Unlike findings observed in neurodegenerative disorders, there is not a global decrease in cerebral metabolism in schizophrenia, which, again, is consistent with the neurodevelopmental hypothesis. Initially, functional neuroimaging studies of patients with schizophrenia at rest produced a pattern of reduced blood flow to the frontal lobes (called "hypofrontality"). This finding is consistent with the negative symptoms found in the disorder, since the frontal lobes are crucial for the initiation of complex behaviors. However, later studies did not replicate this finding. Hypofrontality during activation studies, in which the subject performs a cognitive task known to be mediated by the frontal lobes, such as the Wisconsin Card Sorting Test (WCST), is a more consistent result. Moreover, various control studies have shown that this finding is not an artifact of either neuroleptic medication, poor performance on the activation task (normal controls with similar poor performance on the WCST do not exhibit similar hypofrontality), or performance of a difficult task per se (schizophrenics do not exhibit hypofrontality on difficult nonfrontal tasks). Although reduced frontal blood flow is also found in major depression, it resolves with medication treatment, unlike the finding in schizophrenia. So hypofrontality during tasks that require prefrontal mediation appear to be a trait rather than a state marker in schizophrenia, one that may help explain the negative symptoms of the disorder.

Less consistently, studies have found temporal–limbic overactivity in schizophrenia. A theory has been advanced positing a disconnection between prefrontal and temporal–limbic regions in schizophrenia (Friston & Frith, 1995). A few studies have examined the neuroimaging correlates of symptoms in schizophrenia, such as auditory hallucinations (differences are found in left-hemisphere language areas) and psychomotor poverty (decreased dorsolateral prefrontal activity).

A general view that emerges from all this work is that negative symptoms in schizophrenia are associated with prefrontal underactivity, and that positive symptoms are associated with temporal–limbic overactivity.

Neuropsychology

Studies of this topic are reviewed in Cohen and Servan-Schreiber (1992), Cornblatt and colleagues (1999), and Pennington and Welsh

(1995). Earlier applications of neuropsychology were focused on the diagnostic question of whether a clinical neuropsychological evaluation could distinguish patients with chronic schizophrenia from those with acquired brain damage (e.g., Heaton, Baade, & Johnson, 1978). Although this question sounds unusual today, because schizophrenia is now viewed as a brain disorder, at the time it was posed, it was still common to assume a psychosocial etiology for schizophrenia. The general conclusion from this work, which was surprising at the time, was that persons with chronic schizophrenia had brain dysfunction that could not be distinguished from that found in patients with known neurological insults. Although this work failed to find a specific neuropsychological phenotype in schizophrenia, it did contribute to the growing recognition that schizophrenia is a brain disorder.

This and other research has documented that groups with schizophrenia have (1) lower IQs; (2) deficits in sustained attention (such as on the Contingent-Ax version of the Continuous Performance Test [CPT-AX]); (3) deficits on executive function measures (such as the WCST, the Tower of Hanoi, and the Stroop); (4) deficits on measures of working memory, both verbal (Fleming, Gold, Goldberg, & Weinberger, 1995) and spatial (Park & Holzman, 1992); and (5) deficits on measures of long-term memory (e.g., Saykin et al., 1991). This pattern of deficits would be consistent with a combination of prefrontal and temporal lobe dysfunction, which is also suggested by the functional neuroimaging results.

While this summary suggests some specificity in the neuropsychological profile of schizophrenia, demonstrating this specificity in a rigorous way has been difficult. Generalized impairment in schizophrenia make specific deficits more difficult to detect. Measures of attention, executive function, working memory, and long-term memory are all particularly sensitive to generalized impairment, so the impression of specificity might just represent a resource artifact: Tasks that are more demanding of cognitive resources in general are more likely to be impaired. This problem was discussed some time ago by Chapman and Chapman (1973) in a review article that clarified the psychometric and statistical requirements for a true finding of differential deficit.

Neurocomputational Modeling

Cohen and Servan-Schreiber (1992) developed connectionist models of the working memory deficit in schizophrenia. Using a three-layered architecture, they modeled three tasks on which groups with schizophrenia show deficits. Each model contained an input layer, a hidden layer, and an output layer. The three tasks were the Stroop, the contingent CPT-AX, and a lexical disambiguation task (choose the meaning of an ambiguous word, such as "pen," that fits a sentence context). In each task, correct performance depended on maintaining context information in working memory. Each model contained context units that interacted with other processing units. To simulate the performance of individuals with schizophrenia, a particular parameter of the performance of these context units was manipulated—their gain parameter, which affects the shape of the unit's threshold function. This parameter was selected based on neurophysiological research on the effects of dopamine on target cells; instead of simply being inhibitory or excitatory, dopamine modulates or "sharpens" the response of target neurons. So in these models, a decrease in the gain parameter simulated the effects of reduced dopaminergic input to the prefrontal cortex, which other evidence suggests is the case in schizophrenia. A reduction in the gain parameter thus flattened the threshold function of the context units. This manipulation had the effect of weakening the influence of context on performance, resulting in increased errors on the three tasks, similar to previous results seen in groups with schizophrenia.

What is exciting about this work is that it provides the kind of integrated neuroscientific explanation of an aspect of a psychopathology that is generally needed in this field. This work starts with neuropsychological results (deficits on tasks that require working memory), which are also relevant for understanding negative symptoms in schizophrenia, and then explains these deficits using two other levels of analysis, neurochemistry and neurocomputation. Hence, Cohen and Servan-Schreiber (1992) have made the kind of "round-trip" that, as I argued earlier, is necessary for understanding psychopathology. They start with a behavioral deficit, reduce it to a molecular one, and then reconstruct how this molecular deficit alters neurocomputation to produce the behavioral deficit. Although these are "demonstration" rather than fully realistic models and only simulate one aspect of the disorder, they nonetheless represent an important advance.

Treatment

As is true for many of the disorders already considered in this book, both pharmacological and psychosocial treatments have proven useful in treating schizophrenia (see Satcher, 1999, and Hooley & Candela, 1999, for reviews). Different treatments are needed at different phases of the illness, and optimal treatment requires the coordination of a variety of services provided by different disciplines. During the acute phase, the first-line intervention is pharmacotherapy with antipsychotic medication (neuroleptics); stabilizing a patient in the acute phase may often require a psychiatric hospitalization. After the acute phase, neuroleptic medication must be continued to prevent relapse, along with psychosocial interventions, which include social skills training for the patient, family interventions (such as those based on research on EE, discussed earlier), and vocational and daily living skills rehabilitation. Individuals with schizophrenia, because of their negative symptoms, need help meeting other basic needs, such as housing (sometimes a sheltered living situation is needed), transportation, and medical care. Given all this, it is easy to see why the care of schizophrenia is expensive, and, why, in a country that lacks universal health care, such as the United States, care for individuals with schizophrenia may frequently be suboptimal. Therefore, it is not too surprising that individuals with schizophrenia face an increased risk of medical illness and mortality, as discussed earlier.

Neuroleptic medications fall into two broad categories: conventional and atypical. Conventional neuroleptics include chlorpromazine (Thorazine) and haloperidol (Haldol); these and other conventional neuroleptics work by blocking the dopamine 2 (D2) receptor, so they are dopamine antagonists. The presumed site of action is D2 receptors in the limbic system. As discussed earlier, positive symptoms are thought to arise from excessive dopamine activity in the limbic system, so blocking dopamine receptors there should reduce this activity. Conventional neuroleptics are highly effective in both relieving positive symptoms in an acute episode and preventing relapses. Positive symptoms are relieved by treatment with conventional neuroleptics in about 70% of patients, which is significantly greater than the proportion (25%) exhibiting symptom relief after placebo treatment. However, there are two main drawbacks to conventional neuroleptics: (1) They do not improve negative symptoms, and (2) they produce parkinsonian side effects, because they also block dopamine receptors in the basal ganglia.

Atypical neuroleptics include clozapine (Clozaril), risperidone (Risperdal), olanzapine (Zyprexa), and quetiapine (Seroquel). These antipsychotics are called "atypical" because they have a broader mode of action than the conventional medications just discussed; they are antagonists to a much wider range of receptors (dopamine, serotonin, norepinephrine, and acetylcholine). Because they do not bind as strongly and selectively to D2 receptors, they are much less likely to produce parkinsonian side effects. Additional benefits of these atypical antipsychotics are that they work with more patients and improve negative symptoms. Unfortunately, clozapine (Clozaril) has a rare but potentially fatal side effect, loss of white blood cells (agranulocytosis), necessary for a normal immune response. As a result, the use of clozapine is generally restricted to patients who cannot tolerate other neuroleptics. In such patients, weekly monitoring of white blood cell levels can detect signs of agranulocytosis, which is reversible if detected early.

Chapter 5

Disorders of Language and Cognitive Development

Three disorders are included in this chapter: (1) autism, (2) mental retardation, and (3) dyslexia and other language disorders. Autism provides the worst fit to this overall category. Although its symptoms certainly include deviations in language and cognitive development, there are also problems in action selection and emotion regulation. Hence, of the disorders considered in this book, autism is the most pervasive.

AUTISM

One could argue that autism is the most severe psychopathology, since it disrupts very basic aspects of personhood and does so very early in development. Autism is also the most recently recognized psychopathology (at least, of those considered in this book). The first descriptions of this syndrome (Asperger, 1944/1991; Kanner, 1943) were published less than 60 years ago, whereas some of the other disorders considered here have been recognized since antiquity. Even other childhood disorders, such as dyslexia and ADHD, have been in the scientific literature for over a century. Considered together, these two facts about autism, its severity and its late recognition, present us with a puzzle. How did earlier generations regard people with autism? What treatments did such people receive, and what became of them? Perhaps part of the answer to this puzzle lies in a very recent change in social attitudes toward persons with severe developmental disabilities such as autism and mental retardation. Not very long ago, such individuals were considered essentially untreatable and were institutionalized very early in life.

Public awareness of autism has increased recently because of movies (e.g., *Rain Man*) and books about high-functioning people with autism, such as the autobiographical book by Professor Temple Grandin at Colorado State University, *Thinking in Pictures: And Other Reports from My Life with Autism* (1995). While these portrayals are quite useful introductions to this disorder, it is important to remember that most people with autism are not high functioning. Three-fourths of such individuals are mentally retarded and about half of them lack speech.

Autism, like many of the disorders considered here, has been a projective test for theorists; changes in conceptions of autism have reflected changes in more general notions about the nature of psychopathology. As we will see later, autism is one of the least understood psychopathologies; thus, it still has a lot to teach us about errors in our conceptual frameworks. The term "autism" (from the Greek word *autos*, meaning "self") was introduced by Bleuler (1911/1950) to describe a symptom of schizophrenia, namely, extreme self-absorption leading to a loss of contact with external reality. (This is a somewhat ironic term to describe the syndrome that is autism, since many theorists agree that developing a self depends on relations with others, such that extreme early social isolation would lead to *less* rather than more of a self. I return to the topic of the early development of the self in the review of competing neuropsychological theories of the development of autism.) Partly because Bleuler's term, "autism," for a symptom of schizophrenia was chosen as the name for this new syndrome, the two disorders were confused (a good example of Piaget's concept of assimilation). Autism was originally considered just another form of childhood schizophrenia, but it is now clear that these disorders are etiologically distinct, with different developmental courses, despite some superficial symptom overlap.

Both Kanner (1943) and Asperger (1944/1991) selected Bleuler's term, "autism," to characterize the extreme lack of social awareness in the children they were describing, whether extreme social isolation without speech (the "lives in a shell" quality) or didactic and tangential speech about obscure subjects (such as vacuum cleaners or parking garages) of little interest to the listener. For instance, in Kanner's paper, "Autistic Disturbances of Affective Contact," he spoke of "extreme autistic aloneness" (p. 242). Other features of the syndrome noted by Kanner included (1) an "obsessive desire for the maintenance of sameness" (p. 245); (2) a fascination with objects; (3) mutism and other language abnormalities, such as echolalia; (4) a normal physical appearance; and (5) evidence of preserved intellectual skill, such as a good rote memory or good performance on spatial tasks. Finally, Kanner, good clinician that he was, noted a high frequency of large head circumferences among his 11 patients. As I discuss later, one of the most consistent brain structure correlates of autism is macrocephaly, so Kanner was prescient in this regard.

The title of Asperger's paper was " 'Autistic Psychopathy' in Childhood" (1944/1991). His independent description of a different sample of cases strikingly noted many of the same characteristics, the main differences being the better language skills, unusual specialized interests, and somewhat greater social awareness in Asperger's sample (Wing, 1991). Indeed, many authors regard the syndromes described by Kanner and Asperger as two points on the same continuum or spectrum, with one sample just happening to be higher functioning than the other. Indeed, Miller and Ozonoff (1997) found that all four of Asperger's (1944/1991) original cases met DSM-IV criteria for autism and *not* Asperger syndrome. But other experts believe these are two distinct syndromes. I review data bearing on this controversy in different sections of this chapter. As we will see, the data from family members of probands with autism strongly support such a continuum, since subclinical variants of autism are found in these family members. So research on autism provides an example of both splitting (autism from schizophrenia) and, potentially, lumping (autism with Asperger syndrome).

Although both Kanner (1943) and Asperger (1944/1991) believed their syndromes were of constitutional origin (and Asperger explicitly hypothesized genetic transmission), psychoanalytic theorists (e.g., Bettelheim, 1967; Mahler, 1952) postulated a psychosocial etiology for autism. Even Kanner himself later adopted this view. Mahler postulated that there was a normal developmental stage of "autism," and that children with autism, partly for environmental reasons, became stuck in this stage. Stern (1985) and others later argued that actual studies of normal, early social development did not support the hypothesis of "autism" as a normal developmental stage. In fact, normal infants are remarkable in their social orientation; something about this normal social orientation is disrupted in autism. Another psychoanalytic view held that rejecting "refrigerator" mothers caused these children to withdraw from social interaction, and treatment focused on changes in parenting. Although, as we will see later, it is possible for very extreme environmental deprivation to produce at least some of the symptoms of autism, it is much less plausible that parental coldness could produce such a devastating developmental outcome. Indeed, these psychosocial theories of autism were based only on clinical observations, not on systematic research. Subsequent research has shown that, on average, mothers of children with autism interact *more* than mothers of typically developing children, rather than less, most likely because they are trying to engage their children. Since parents of a child with atypical development almost inevitably blame themselves for the problem, these erroneous theories undoubtedly increased parents' guilt and suffering—a fairly striking example of how clinical ignorance can lead to a violation of the Hippocratic maxim: "First, do no harm."

Rimland (1964), a scientist and also a parent of a child with autism, was among the first to argue that this disorder is neurological rather than psychosocial in origin. A neurological etiology was supported by the association of autism with maternal rubella (Chess, 1977), late-onset seizures (Schain & Yannett, 1960), and certain genetic conditions, such as untreated phenylketonuria. The contemporary view of autism emphasizes its biological origin; as we will see, autism is probably the most heritable of the psychopathologies considered here. Current research is focused on identifying the genetic risk factors, the neurological phenotypes, and the resulting changes in neuropsychological development. At the same time, the psychosocial environment remains very important in the development of individuals with autism. Early interventions have shown that the behavioral deficits found in young children with autism are much more malleable than was previously thought, although there is as yet no cure.

Definition

In DSM-IV-TR (American Psychiatric Association, 2000), the diagnoses of autism and Asperger syndrome fall under the broader category of pervasive developmental disorders (PDDs). The other three members of this category are Rett's disorder, childhood disintegrative disorder (CDD), and PDD not otherwise specified (PDD-NOS). All five PDDs share symptoms of autism, which is defined by a triad of qualitative impairments in (1) social interaction, (2) communication, and (3) range of behavior, interests, and activities. The five PDDs differ in the extent of these symptoms and in developmental course. Both Rett's disorder and CDD require regression after a period of normal development (from 5 to 30 months in Rett's and from 2 to 10 years in CDD). So, in both these disorders, an apparently normal child loses developmental gains in motor, language, and social skills, and develops at least some of the symptoms of autism. Rett's disorder is a rare, progressive neurological disease (in which there is a deceleration in brain growth and, as a result, head circumference) that occurs only in girls. CDD is assumed to be due to an acquired neurological insult, but in many cases the etiology is unknown. Asperger syndrome is distinguished from autism by a normal early language development. Thus, for an individual to meet diagnostic criteria for Asperger syndrome, there can be no significant delay in language or cognitive development. So, by definition, Asperger syndrome in DSM-IV-TR is a less severe form of autism, without language impairment and mental retardation. Finally, PDD-NOS is reserved for cases where symptoms of autism are present but criteria for one of the other four PDDs are not met, either because of subthreshold levels of symptoms or even later onset. In summary, the definition of these five PDDs implies an autistic spectrum that runs from autism proper to Asperger syndrome to PDD-NOS and includes two autism-like syndromes that have a deteriorating course.

I now describe the autistic triad in more detail. A qualitative impairment in social interaction requires at least two of four symptoms: (1) marked impairment in the use of multiple nonverbal behaviors (such as eye contact, facial expression, body postures, and gestures) to regulate social interaction; (2) failure to develop age-appropriate peer relations; (3) lack of spontaneous sharing of enjoyment, interests, or achievements with other people; and (4) lack of social or emotional reciprocity. A marked impairment in communication requires one of four symptoms: (1) delay or lack of spoken language development, without an attempt to compensate through gesture or mime; (2) if speech is present, marked impairment in initiating or sustaining conversation; (3) stereotyped and repetitive, or idiosyncratic, use of language; and (4) lack of spontaneous, varied pretend play. The last part of the triad—restricted, repetitive, and stereotyped patterns of behavior—requires at least one of four symptoms: (1) an encompassing preoccupation, with a narrow interest; (2) inflexible adherence to specific, nonfunctional routines or rituals; (3) motor stereotypies (e.g., hand flapping); and (4) persistent preoccupation with parts of objects. In addition, the total number of symptoms must be six or more. For the diagnosis of autism, the onset must occur before age 3.

These diagnostic criteria for autism have been operationalized by a standardized, semistructured parent interview, the Autism Diagnostic Interview—Revised (ADI-R; Lord, Rutter, & LeCouteur, 1994). The ADI-R has an interrater reliability of at least 90%, and both its sensitivity and specificity also exceed 90% (Lord et al., 1994). Therefore, it is the current "gold standard" for diagnosing autism and is the phenotype being used in current, large, collaborative molecular genetic studies of this disorder. However, just as is true for the other behaviorally defined disorders considered in this book, the question of which phenotypes to use with which boundaries in such studies is a difficult issue. Perhaps a dimensional phenotype is more appropriate than a categorical one, or perhaps some other phenotype better captures what is transmitted in families, even though it is not part of the diagnostic definition. In other words, genetic studies will help refine the phenotype, and refinements in phenotype definition will inform genetic studies. As with other disorders, we should be careful to not reify current phenotype definitions.

Epidemiology

The median lifetime prevalence of autism is about 5 per 10,000 (American Psychiatric Association, 2000), although more recent studies with broader diagnostic criteria have found a higher prevalence, about 10–12 per 10,000 (Bryson & Smith, 1998). There has been some recent concern that the true rates of autism have actually increased due to greater exposure to some environmental risk factor (e.g., vaccinations). However, there is little evidence for a true increase in rate (Frombonne, 2001). Thus, autism is roughly 8–20 times more rare than schizophrenia, and rarer still than other developmental disabilities, such as ADHD, dyslexia, other developmental language disorders, or mental retardation. Apparently, the developmental processes that are disrupted in autism are more difficult to perturb than those that characterize these other disorders.

The male:female ratio in autism is 3–4:1. Females with autism have lower average IQs and hence a higher rate of mental retardation (reviewed in Klinger & Dawson, 1996). The reasons for these gender differences are unknown. The prevalence of autism has not been found to vary across cultures or as a function of social class (Klinger & Dawson, 1996).

Developmental Continuity

For the vast majority of individuals with this diagnosis, autism is a life-long developmental disability that limits independent living, but early intervention can make a difference, as will be discussed later. In a large Japanese outcome study of 197 young adults with autism, only 1% were living independently, only 27% were either employed or pursuing postsecondary education, and only 50% had enough language to permit verbal communication (Kobayashi, Murata, & Yoshinaga, 1992). Across a number of studies, both IQ and the presence of some communicative speech before age 5 are the best early predictors of a more favorable out-come (reviewed in Klinger & Dawson, 1996). As would be expected, romantic relationships are rare, and among individuals with autism, only a very few manage to marry and have children.

Etiology

The presentation here summarizes excellent, recent reviews of the etiol-ogy of autism (Bailey, Phillips, & Rutter, 1996; Rutter, 2000). Genetic influences on autism were long doubted by both psychodynamic theo-rists and geneticists, who noted the apparent lack of both vertical transmission and associated chromosomal anomalies (Rutter, 2000). Ironically, more recent research has documented that autism is both the most familial and possibly the most heritable of all psychiatric diagno-ses, with a significant minority of cases associated with chromosome anomalies or known genetic syndromes. In what follows, we see how research results changed the view that autism is not genetic.

Familiality

Because individuals with autism very rarely marry and have children, vertical transmission of the diagnosis of autism from parent to child is rarely observed. But this fact does not exclude genetic transmission, since parents could transmit genetic risk factors without having the di-agnosis themselves. Although the rate of autism in siblings (2% in ear-lier studies, 3% in later ones) appeared low, it was considerably higher than the population rates cited earlier. Dividing the sibling rates by the appropriate population rates, one obtains a sibling relative risk (λ) of 30 to 100, which is considerably higher than that of other psychiatric disorders.

Recent studies have also made it clear that the behavioral phenotype transmitted in families of individuals with autism is broader than the diagnosis itself. Hence, the familial phenotype may be dimensional rather than categorical. First-degree relatives of probands with autism have increased rates of symptoms of autism, shyness and aloofness, and pragmatic language problems compared to control relatives (Rutter, 2000). In the Maudsley study (Bolton et al., 1994), if the phenotype was broadened to any PDD, the rate in siblings was 6% versus 0% in controls. Broader phenotypes, defined by symptoms of autism and cognitive deficits, were found in 12% of relatives versus 2% of control relatives, and 20% versus 3%, respectively, depending on the stringency of the cutoff. With continuous measures of these phenotypic features and large samples, one could test whether the familial phenotype is dimensional rather than categorical. If dimensional, powerful genetic methods for identifying quantitative trait loci (discussed earlier in Genetic Methods) could be employed. Several studies have also found higher rates of anxiety and depressive disorders among relatives of probands with autism. However, these disorders did not cosegregate with the broader autism phenotype (the BAP, which is defined by social and cognitive deficits), and unlike the BAP, their rate did not increase with the severity of autism in the proband (Rutter, 2000). Although individuals with the BAP had higher rates of reading and spelling problems, perhaps because of other cognitive and language problems, a specific reading and spelling problem (i.e., dyslexia) was not more common in such families, nor were mental retardation or seizure disorders, which are increased in probands. Although more work is needed to define the BAP, especially work using neuropsychological markers, these studies are exciting and clearly have implications for what phenotypes are used in molecular studies.

Heritability

This question has necessarily been pursued through twin studies, because adoption studies of autism are not feasible. In the first, now classic, twin study of autism conducted by Folstein and Rutter (1977), the concordance rate in MZ pairs (36%) was significantly greater than that found in DZ pairs (0%). If the phenotype was broadened to include a cognitive or language disorder, these concordance rates became 82% and 10%, respectively. So this study provided evidence that autism is significantly heritable and that the heritable phenotype is broader than the diagnosis of autism itself, consistent with the family studies just discussed. Two subsequent studies (Bailey et al., 1995; Steffenburg et al., 1989) also found significant heritability for autism. In the Steffenburg and colleagues (1989) study, the MZ and DZ concordance rates were 91% and 0%, respectively. The Bailey and colleagues (1995) study is the most sophisticated of the three studies methodologically because it (1) used a total population ascertainment; (2) based diagnoses on both parent interviews and observations of the child, using standardized diagnostic instruments, the ADI, and the Autism Diagnostic Observatory Schedule (ADOS); (3) excluded nonidiopathic cases (those with medical conditions and chromosomal abnormalities); and (4) tested zygosity with blood groups. In this study, the MZ concordance rate for autism was 60% versus 5% in DZ pairs, whereas these rates rose to 90% versus 10%, respectively, when a broader phenotype of social or cognitive deficits was used. These two results confirm the two key results of the earlier Folstein and Rutter (1977) study, although the definition of the broader phenotype shifted in the later study to focus more on social abnormality. Interestingly, a similar social deficit was found in subjects with the broader phenotype in a follow-up of the earlier sample (Rutter, 2000). Finally, within the 16 MZ pairs concordant for autism or atypical autism, there were wide differences in IQ and clinical symptomatology, such that similarity within these MZ pairs for these features was no greater than that between individuals picked at random from different pairs. This finding argues that although the diagnosis of autism is highly heritable, there is hardly rigid genetic determinism for an exact phenotype. Instead, even with an identical genotype, epigenetic interactions and nonshared environmental influences must produce divergence in phenotypes.

Across these three twin studies of autism, we can see that the disparity between MZ and DZ concordance rates is quite large, with the MZ:DZ ratio averaging around 10. For other psychiatric disorders, such as schizophrenia, depression, and bipolar disorder, this ratio is considerably lower, about 2 to 4. Such a marked discrepancy in MZ versus DZ concordance rates indicates that nonadditive genetic effects are operating. In the case of autism, these nonadditive effects most likely represent interactions among several different genes, called "epistasis," rather than nonadditive effects (dominance) of a single major locus (Rutter, 2000). The large disparity between MZ and DZ concordance rates, as well as the very high MZ concordance rate for the broader phenotype, indicate a high heritability for autism. Quantitative analysis of the Bailey and colleagues (1995) data indicate a heritability greater than 90%, making autism one of the most heritable of psychiatric disorders. So the diathesis–stress model seems to fit autism less well than it does many of the other disorders we have considered; there are interactions in the development of autism, but they appear to be mainly among genes. There are also unknown epigenetic interactions that produce wide phenotypic variability found within concordant MZ pairs.

Mode of Transmission

These results indicate that the mode of transmission is complex, as is the case for virtually all the behaviorally defined disorders considered in this book. Earlier segregation analyses of autism, like those for other disorders considered here, have not converged on a simple Mendelian model of transmission (reviewed in Bailey et al., 1996).

Gene Locations

Several large, multisite molecular studies are in progress, with some results emerging, although none are definitive as yet (see review by Lamb, Moore, Bailey, & Monaco, 2000). The strongest linkage finding so far is for a locus on chromosome 7q (International Molecular Genetic Study of Autism Consortium [IMGSAC], 1998), which has been replicated by this group and three other independent studies (Lamb et al., 2000). Although the location of the 7q locus varies somewhat across studies, the confidence interval for a quantitative trait locus (QTL) affecting a complex trait is large (as great as 25cM) given sample sizes similar to those in these studies (Lamb et al., 2000). More preliminary linkage results have been reported for loci on chromosomes 1p, 2q, 6q, 13q, 16p, 18q, and 19p (Lamb et al., 2000). All of these linkages except the ones on 1p and 6q have been found in two separate samples, but more replication is needed. Another promising locus on 15q 11–13 was originally suggested in single cases by the association between autism and chromosome anomalies in this region (Rutter, 2000), although this location has not been identified in whole genome searches (Lamb et al., 2000). This consortium (IMGSAC, 2001) recently reported a whole genome search in an expanded sample. The 2q, 7q, and 16p linkages continued to receive support, with the 2q result providing the strongest evidence for linkage, whereas the evidence for other, previously identified locations diminished.

Association studies with candidate genes have also been attempted. Some of these investigated a GABA receptor gene located in the 15q region, implicated by cytogenetic abnormalities, and other studies pursued serotonin receptor genes, based on the well-replicated finding of peripheral serotonin elevations in autism (discussed below). The majority of results in both cases are negative (Lamb et al., 2000), although it is possible that these candidates may be important for a subtype of autism. There are also recent reports of associations with an allele of a homeobox gene, HOXA1 (Ingram et al., 2000; Rodier, 2000), and the reelin gene (Persico et al., 2001). The existence of several large family samples will speed the verification of these linkage and association results.

Associations with Genetic Disorders

The two strongest associations are with tuberous sclerosis and fragile X syndrome (Bailey et al., 1996). In tuberous sclerosis, an autosomal dominant neurocutaneous (affecting both brain and skin) disorder, with a prevalence rate of about 1 in 10,000, there is abnormal tissue growth in the skin, brain, and other organs. Both physical and behavioral phenotypes are quite variable. Behaviorally, the phenotype can range from normal functioning to severe problems, with the latter including severe mental retardation, seizure disorder, and symptoms of autism. Less severe behavioral problems associated with tuberous sclerosis include learning disabilities, hyperactivity–impulsivity, aggression, and uncooperative behavior (see review in Patzer & Volkmar, 1999). Across studies, there is evidence for a significant, two-way association between tuberous sclerosis and autism. Rates of autism in individuals with tuberous sclerosis range between 17% and 61%, and rates of tuberous sclerosis in individuals with autism range between 0.4% and 9.0% (reviewed in Bailey et al., 1996, and Patzer & Volkmar, 1999). All of these results are well beyond the chance rate of roughly 1 in 10 million. Since the association is strongest in individuals with tuberous sclerosis and both mental retardation and seizure disorder, it seems unlikely that a direct or specific effect of the genes for tuberous sclerosis causes the symptoms of autism. Instead, it seems much more likely that the abnormal tissue growth (nonmalignant tumors) in tuberous sclerosis sometimes occurs in particular parts of the brain, damage to which is important for the development of autism (see Bailey et al., 1996). Nonetheless, localizing these nonmalignant brain tumors in individuals with retardation and tuberous sclerosis, both with and without autism, could shed light on which brain structures, when damaged, are important in the development of autism. Indeed, a recent study did just that, finding that tumors in the medial–temporal lobe are associated with autism (Bolton & Griffiths, 1997).

The association between fragile X syndrome (FXS) and autism in earlier studies appeared much stronger than in later studies, likely because of earlier studies' small samples and use of cytogenetic rather than DNA measures of the fragile X mutation, and clinical rather than standardized assessments of autism (Bailey et al., 1996). In recent, methodologically adequate studies, rates of autism in fragile X syndrome range from about 3% to 5% and of fragile X syndrome in autism, about 2.5% to 4.0% (Bailey et al., 1996; Patzer & Volkmar, 1999). These rates still support a significant two-way association, at least if chance is determined simply by multiplying the prevalence of autism by the prevalence of fragile X syndrome (which yields a liberal chance value of 1 in 1 million). While there is a robust, two-way association relative to population base rates, it can be argued that the appropriate base rates need to be derived from populations with intellectual levels similar to those found in males with fragile X syndrome and males with autism, both of which fall in the mental retardation range. For example, the rate of fragile X syndrome in unselected males with retardation is about 1.9% (Sherman, 1996), which is still clearly less than the rate of fragile X syndrome in males with autism, although it could still be argued that the intellectual levels might differ across the two sets of studies.

A better study would compare the rates of autism in fragile X syndrome-negative and -positive males matched on IQ and drawn from the same population with mental retardation. To my knowledge, only two such studies exist (Einfeld, Maloney, & Hall, 1989; Maes, Fryns, Van Walleghem, & Van den Berghe, 1993). Both studies found *no* differences in the rates of autism in FXS-positive versus FSX-negative males with similar levels of mental retardation. However, both did find higher rates of certain autistic symptoms in the FSX-positive group, specifically, gaze avoidance and hand flapping in the Einfeld and colleagues study, and stereotypical movements (including hand flapping; rocking; and hitting, scratching, or rubbing their own bodies), echolalia, gaze avoidance, and ritualistic behaviors in the Maes and colleagues study.

Further evidence has been found for an association between fragile X syndrome and certain autistic features, such as stereotypies, perseveration, and avoidance of eye contact, which are found in over 80% of males with fragile X syndrome (Hagerman, 1996). Moreover, fragile X syndrome is distinctive among mental retardation syndromes in exhibiting this association with autistic features, which, for example, are not found in either Down or Williams syndromes. Lachiewicz, Spiridigliozzi, Gullion, and Ransford (1994) studied 55 boys with fragile X syndrome and 57 IQ-matched controls with several behavioral questionnaires, and found that boys with fragile X syndrome were four times more likely to have both tactile defensiveness and abnormal speech (perseveration and rapid speech) compared to controls. A controlled study by Reiss and Freund (1992) demonstrated a unique profile of behavior within the DSM-III-R criteria for autism in males with fragile X syndrome, including more difficulty with peer interactions compared to adult interactions, more stereotypes, and unusual nonverbal interactions compared to IQ-matched controls. Closer analysis of these autistic features in males with fragile X syndrome has yielded some interesting contrasts with idiopathic autism. Cohen, Vietze, Sudhalter, Jenkins, and Brown (1989) showed that males with fragile X syndrome are more sensitive to an adult's initiation of social gaze and subsequently demonstrate a greater aversion to mutual gaze than do individuals with autism without fragile X syndrome. Other studies have found that the eye contact disturbance in autism is not so much a decrease or avoidance of eye contact as it is inappropriate use of eye contact, which is likely due to deficits in joint attention. Sudhalter, Cohen, Silverman, and Wolf-Schein (1990) found that the speech of patients with fragile X syndrome exhibited more perseveration of words and phrases and less echolalia than that of autistic patients without fragile X syndrome and controls with mental retardation.

In summary, since not all forms of mental retardation (e.g., Down or Williams syndromes) are associated with increased risk for autism, it appears there is something more specific to the association between fragile X syndrome and at least certain symptoms of autism. One intriguing possibility is that since both disorders are characterized by increases in brain size, unlike the microcephaly that is characteristic of Down syndrome and many other forms of mental retardation, such increases (perhaps reflecting too many connections due to a lack of pruning) somehow lead to these shared symptoms.

Finally, about 5% of cases with behaviorally defined autism have chromosomal anomalies detectable with standard cytogenetic methods (Bailey et al., 1996). Summing across the three genetic associations reviewed here (tuberous sclerosis, fragile X syndrome, and various chromosomal anomalies), it is clear that a sizable minority (up to about 18%) of cases of individuals diagnosed with autism will have identifiable genetic anomalies. Hence, a genetic evaluation should be a standard part of the clinical workup. It is also clear that the majority of such individuals will not have an identifiable etiology (they will fall in the idiopathic category). As progress is made in understanding the molecular genetics of idiopathic autism, this proportion will drop.

Environmental Risk Factors

Although earlier reports implicated prenatal infections (i.e., maternal rubella; see Chess, 1977) and obstetrical complications in the etiology of autism, neither of these environmental influences have proven to be very important. On follow-up, children with congenital rubella no longer appeared autistic (Chess, 1977), and other studies of possible infectious influences have been mostly negative (see Bailey et al., 1996). The weight of evidence indicates that obstetrical complications are caused by a genetically abnormal fetus (e.g., with congenital malformations, or with a greater familial loading for autism), rather than themselves being etiological (see discussion in Bailey et al., 1996). Incidentally, it appears that this explanation of associated obstetrical complications has not been adequately explored in some psychopathologies (e.g., schizophrenia).

It is worth noting that extreme environmental deprivation, including decreased social stimulation, can produce a rough phenocopy of autism, such as that found in congenital blindness (Brown, Hobson, & Lee, 1997; Rogers & Pennington, 1991) and in some orphans placed in minimally stimulating institutions as infants (e.g., in Romania; see Rutter et al., 1999). The existence of these phenocopies is very important theoretically, because it reminds us that social relatedness is not innate, but rather depends on interactions with a caregiver. Factors that strongly limit these interactions, whether environmental or genetic, can lead to the development of the symptoms of autism. In inherited autism, one key theoretical puzzle in infants who will develop autism is to identify which early psychological deficits strongly limit the ability to participate in socializing interactions with a caregiver (see discussion in Rogers & Pennington, 1991). I consider possible answers to this puzzle in the section on Neuropsychology.

Brain Mechanisms

This section includes studies of brain structure, neuroimaging, and neurotransmission. Although differences in each type of brain study have been found in individuals with autism, the list of well-replicated findings is very short, and the neurological cause of autism remains unknown.

Structural Neuroimaging Studies

The best-replicated structural finding is macrocephaly in about one-fourth of cases. As mentioned earlier, Kanner's (1943) original case report noted the children's enlarged head circumferences. More recently, macrocephaly has been found in structural MRI studies (Filipek et al., 1992; Piven et al., 1995) and in autopsy samples (reviewed in Bailey et al., 1996). The change in brain development that produces this macrocephaly and how it relates to brain function are currently unknown. Can we exclude the experience of growing up with autism as the cause of this brain phenotype? Other examples of macrocephaly are due to changes in prenatal processes of brain development, mainly in the cortex (see Bailey et al., 1996), such as an excess of neuronal proliferation or a failure of early neuronal elimination (apoptosis, or programmed cell death). However, a reduction in the synaptic pruning that occurs in later childhood and adolescence could produce a larger brain relative to age norms. This hypothesis is supported by the lack of macrocephaly at birth in autism (Lainhart et al., 1997). A reduction in synaptic pruning could be due to altered environmental experience secondary to autism. Clearly, more work is needed to understand the role of macrocephaly in autism. Interestingly, macrocephaly is also found in both fragile X syndrome and tuberous sclerosis.

Other candidate structural differences in autism have not been consistently replicated, such as the hypoplasia in the cerebellar vermis, first reported by Courchesne, Yeung-Courchesne, Press, Hesselink, and Jernigan (1988), or lateral ventricular enlargement (see review in Bailey et al., 1996). Such ventricular enlargement would be suggestive of volume reductions in medial–temporal lobe structures, such as the hippocampus and amygdala, whose role in memory and emotion could be theoretically important for autism. Consistent with this possibility, in their autopsy studies, Bauman and Kemper (1994) found abnormally small, densely packed neurons in these and other limbic structures, although this finding is not consistent across other autopsy studies (reviewed in Bailey et al., 1996). In addition, recent structural MRI studies have found alterations in amygdala volumes in autism (Abell et al., 1999; Aylward et al., 1999). Unfortunately, the first study found an *enlarged* volume, whereas the second found a reduced volume.

Functional Neuroimaging Studies

The main findings in this domain consist of a (1) reduced P300 response to novel stimuli in event-related potential studies (reviewed in Klinger & Dawson, 1996); (2) more variability in regional metabolic rates in PET studies, suggesting less coordinated processing across brain regions (reviewed in Bailey et al., 1996); and (3) recent fMRI findings of differences in the brain substrates used to process social stimuli, such as faces (Baron-Cohen et al., 1999; Bookheimer, 2000; Shultz et al, 2000). Some earlier PET studies found global hypermetabolism in groups with autism, but this result has not been replicated in other studies (reviewed in Bailey et al., 1996).

Recent fMRI studies indicate brain activation differences in processing social stimuli. Shultz and colleagues (2000) contrasted brain activation for face versus object processing in subjects with autism and controls. Subjects looked at pairs of faces and objects to determine whether they were same or different. In controls, the face task produced focal activation in the classical face area (bilateral fusiform gyrus [FG], which is on the ventral surface of the occipital and adjacent temporal lobes), whereas the object task produced focal activation in the inferior temporal gyrus (ITG). In contrast, in subjects with autism, the face task did not activate the FG, but instead activated the adjacent ITG. These results suggest that subjects with autism have not developed the typical specialized cortical area for face recognition and instead process faces and other objects in the same manner. Although such a difference could be innate, these authors speculate that this difference is due to reduced social experience in autism. Bookheimer (2000) examined processing of facial emotion in an fMRI study in which subjects had to either match or label angry or fearful facial expressions. In controls, both tasks activated the face area (FG), and the matching task also activated the amygdala bilaterally. In contrast, in subjects with autism, neither FG nor amygdala activation was observed; instead, Broca's area was activated.

A third group (Baron-Cohen et al., 1999, 2000) examined brain activation on the Eyes task, in which a subject sees a photograph of the eyes portion of a face and decides which of two descriptors (e.g., concerned vs. unconcerned) best describes the mental state of the individual in the picture. The control task was to identify the gender of the individual in the same photographs. Unlike the group with autism, controls specifically activated the amygdala in the mental state task. They also exhibited more activation of the inferior frontal gyrus and the insula, whereas the group with autism had greater activation in the superior temporal gyrus. In summary, across these studies of processing different aspects of faces (identity, emotion, and mental state), there are converging differences in the group with autism in the FG and the amygdala. The amygdala differences are consistent with some of the structural differences discussed earlier and suggest problems that individuals with autism have with basic aspects of processing emotion, a topic I also consider in the Neuropsychology section.

Neurotransmission

This topic is reviewed in Bailey and colleagues (1996) and Patzer and Volkmar (1999); their main conclusions are summarized here. The search for neurotransmitter abnormalities in autism has gone on for about 40 years but with very few consistent results. Unlike many of the disorders considered in this book, there is much less evidence of an abnormality in neurotransmission in the central nervous system, and there is currently no effective neurochemical treatment for the main symptoms of autism. Investigations of the dopaminergic, noradrenergic, and opiate neuropeptide systems have not produced evidence of consistent abnormalities (Bailey et al., 1996).

The sole consistent result is elevated serotonin levels in peripheral blood (hyperserotonemia) in about one-fourth of individuals with autism, which is caused by increased amounts of serotonin in blood platelets. However, there are no elevations of the serotonin metabolite 5-HIAA in the cerebrospinal fluid of individuals with autism, suggesting that the serotonin elevation does not extend to the central nervous system. Hyperserotonemia is also found in severe mental retardation, raising the possibility that this neurochemical abnormality is related to mental retardation rather than to autism. However, reports of hyperserotonemia in the nonretarded relatives of individuals with autism (Bailey et al., 1996) suggest some specificity. The finding of hyperserotonemia prompted an attempt to treat autism neurochemically with a serotonin antagonist, fenfluramine, which lowers platelet levels of serotonin. However, a multicenter treatment study of fenfluramine did not produce clear, positive results, so fenfluramine is not an empirically validated treatment for autism. In summary, we still do not understand the etiological significance, if any, of hyperserotonemia—the one replicated neurochemical correlate of autism.

Neuropsychology

Recent research on the neuropsychology of autism provides an excellent example of the power of the developmental psychopathology approach. This interdisciplinary work illustrates the reciprocal relation between studies of normal and abnormal development. Not only has autism research drawn on the latest theories and paradigms from studies of normal early development but also it has become an important stimulus for these studies, as evidenced by the numerous articles on normal development of a theory of mind in the recent literature. Autism research has brought the early social and cognitive accomplishments of normal human infants into sharper relief, making clearer what needs to be explained in early development and which early skills may be useful to examine in both within- and cross-species comparisons. These research accomplishments have relevance for deep and fundamental questions in psychology and philosophy. For example, how do we become aware of other minds? What is a person, and how do infants form a concept of persons? How does the self develop? What are the cognitive requirements for intersubjectivity and later human relatedness? How are early social and cognitive development intertwined? I touch on the relevance of autism research for these issues in the review that follows.

Theorizing about the nature of the primary psychological deficit in autism has come full circle. As discussed earlier, Kanner (1943), in his original description of the autism syndrome, suggested the possibility that such children were born with an innate inability to form emotional contacts with other people. But a psychogenic hypothesis prevailed for the next two decades in psychoanalytic accounts of autism (e.g.,

Mahler, 1952). As evidence for an organic etiology of autism accumulated, researchers concerned with the underlying processing deficit shifted their focus to various cognitive possibilities, neglecting Kanner's original insight that the disorder might represent a primary *social* deficit of constitutional origin. Various possible, primary cognitive deficits were investigated, including deficits in arousal, language, symbolic thought, memory, and cross-modal processing. However, when children with autism were compared to nonautistic children with retardation, of similar mental age, few reliable differences were found in these various cognitive processes. Even when reliable differences were found, there were other reasons why the apparent deficit in these areas was unlikely to be primary (Fein, Pennington, Markowitz, Braverman, & Waterhouse, 1986). Specifically, most of these cognitive processes develop after the onset of autistic symptoms and are theoretically inadequate to explain autistic aloofness; they cannot be found in all children with autism and may be the very cognitive abilities that depend most heavily on normal social functioning. Other reasons for regarding the social symptoms as primary in autism include (1) the dissociability of social and cognitive impairments both within and across developmentally disabled populations, (2) the special difficulty that children with autism have with social stimuli, and (3) the rarity of social relatedness deficits in even severely damaged babies and their resistance to change in autism.

Research published subsequent to the Fein and colleagues (1986) review has refined our understanding of impaired and intact social processes in autism. Somewhat surprisingly, some early social behaviors in children with autism have proved *not* to be specifically impaired compared to mental age-matched controls, including attachment behaviors, self-recognition, person recognition, and differential social responsivity (reviewed in Ozonoff, Pennington, & Rogers, 1990; Rogers & Pennington, 1991).

Clearly impaired social processes in autism include social orientation, joint attention, imitation, theory of mind, empathy, and aspects of emotional expression (reviewed in Klinger & Dawson, 1996). Some of these deficits, for example, those in social orientation and joint attention, are present early in the development of the disorder (Osterling & Dawson, 1994), whereas others (i.e., theory of mind) cannot be measured until later in development. It is currently unclear when deficits in imitation, empathy, and emotional expression appear in the development of autism. All of these social processes contribute to the typical protracted development of intersubjectivity (see, e.g., Stern, 1985;

Trevarthen, 1979), which is the awareness of mental states (i.e., emotions, other motivations, attention, intentions, and beliefs) in both self and others, and the use of this awareness in social interactions. Almost by definition, individuals with autism are deficient in intersubjectivity. The key questions are which aspects of intersubjectivity are deficient, and what underlying neuropsychological deficit or deficits disrupt the development of these aspects of intersubjectivity? For example, very young infants share emotions with caregivers through imitative exchanges (Stern, 1985). An infant with deficits in either imitation or emotion would have trouble participating in these exchanges and would thus miss some of the experiences necessary for the development of very early aspects of intersubjectivity. Around the end of the first year, infants share attention with caregivers (joint attention) and give evidence of some understanding of intentions (see, e.g., Csibra, Gergely, Biro, Koos, & Brockbank, 1999). An infant could have difficulty with this part of the development of intersubjectivity because of a general or specific processing deficit, and this in turn would be expected to undermine later, developing aspects of intersubjectivity. Or selective difficulties could arise at later points in the development of intersubjectivity. The developmental dependencies among these different aspects of intersubjectivity are not completely understood, which makes it difficult to evaluate competing neuropsycholgical theories of autism.

Because a great deal of human development depends on social transmission, a child deficient in intersubjectivity would miss much of the input necessary for typical development. Since brain development depends on environmental input, as discussed earlier, this lack of input would change brain development in autism (Mundy & Neal, 2000). Some of the deficits in autism (e.g., language and IQ) might be seen as secondary to this missing input. Consistent with this hypothesis, one robust cognitive correlate of intelligence, speed of information processing (measured by an inspection time paradigm), has been found to be normal in individuals with autism despite their low IQs (Anderson, O'Connor, & Hermelin, 1998; Scheuffgen, Happé, Anderson, & Frith, 2000). While missing this typical input, some individuals with autism may "specialize" in learning other things about the environment; such "specialization" could explain the savant skills that characterize this disorder. This hypothesis would also explain why intensive early intervention can succeed in children with autism, because such intervention reduces this secondary deprivation (Mundy & Neal, 2000).

A successful neuropsychological theory of autism must account for not only these impaired social processes but also the triad of symptoms and other features that define the disorder, such as the high rate of mental retardation and the uneven profile of cognitive abilities. The hypothesized primary psychological deficit must also (1) be present before the onset of the disorder (i.e., very early in development), (2) be pervasive among individuals with the disorder, and (3) be specific to autism. This is a tall order, and there is fairly good agreement among autism researchers that no current psychological theory of autism meets all these criteria (see discussion in Bailey et al., 1996). Some of these current theories are (1) the theory of mind theory (Baron-Cohen, Leslie, & Frith, 1985, 1986), (2) the executive theory (Ozonoff, Pennington, & Rogers, 1991; Russell, 1996, 1997), (3) the praxis/imitation theory (Meltzoff & Gopnik, 1993; Rogers & Pennington, 1991), and (4) the emotion theory (Hobson, 1989, 1993). These major, contending theories of the development of autism all agree that intersubjectivity is disrupted in some way in this disorder but disagree about why it is disrupted. An initial deficit in any one of these areas could conceivably derail the development of intersubjectivity and lead to deficits in the other areas. The praxis/imitation theory (Rogers & Pennington, 1991) holds that the initial deficit is in imitation. In emotion theory (Hobson, 1993), the initial deficit is in affective contact. The theory of mind theory holds that the initial deficit is a cognitive inability to compute second-order representations, or metarepresentations, which are necessary for pretense and understanding others' intentions and beliefs. The executive theory (Russell, 1996) posits that a deficit in action monitoring leads to a deficit in understanding others' intentions and beliefs.

Although cross-sectional studies have consistently found deficits in each of these four areas in groups with autism, we do not know which, if any, of these deficits have causal priority in the development of the intersubjectivity deficit in autism.

Each theory has significant shortcomings. Theory of mind per se does not develop until a considerable time after the onset of autism. In addition, deficits on theory of mind tasks are not found in some individuals with autism (lack of universality), but they are found in other populations (e.g., children with deafness, blindness, mental retardation, and specific language impairment), indicating a lack of specificity (see Tager-Flusberg, in press, for a review). Theory of mind theorists also freely admit that this theory does not account for the repetitive, stereotypical symptoms. The executive theory readily explains these repetitive symptoms but does not as straightforwardly explain the social and communicative symptoms that the theory of mind explains so well. In addition, executive problems are not specific to autism (see discussion in Pennington & Ozonoff, 1996), and a recent study has failed to find early executive deficits in the development of autism (Griffith, Pennington, Wehner, & Rogers, 1999). The praxis/imitation theory must explain why children with worse praxis deficits than those found in autism (such as children with cerebral palsy) do not develop autism. Deficits in praxis may nonetheless contribute to the failure of speech development in this disorder and help define a subtype of autism (Gernsbacher & Goldsmith, in press). Finally, the emotion theory has not been sufficiently explored; recent theoretical analyses of emotion processing have identified components that have not been evaluated in autism.

Notice that one aspect of developing intersubjectivity, the understanding of others' intentions, is crucial to at least two of these theories: the theory of mind and the executive theory. Both theories assume that the robust, early deficit in joint attention behaviors (see, e.g., Mundy, Sigman, Ungerer, & Sherman, 1986) found even in very young children with autism is an early marker of a failure to understand another's mental states, attention, and intentions (see discussions in Russell, 1996, and Tager-Flusberg, in press). But this is an inference, since measures of joint attention do not directly test understanding of others' intentions. Conceivably, other underlying deficits could disrupt joint attention behaviors, such as a deficit in aspects of emotion (Mundy & Sigman, 1989). Hence, it is logically possible that a young child with autism could understand another's intentions but still not exhibit joint attention behaviors. If this were the case, it would seriously challenge both the theory of mind and the executive theory of autism, and perhaps the praxis/imitation theory as well.

Thus, the question of whether young children with autism understand others' intentions is crucial for testing competing theories of this disorder. Yet this particular aspect of early social cognition has not been as intensively studied in autism. A recent study by Carpenter, Pennington, and Rogers (2001) used Meltzoff's Unfulfilled Intentions Task to examine this issue in a group of preschool children with autism compared to a control group of similar chronological and mental age with developmental disabilities. Meltzoff's (1995) task assesses understanding of another's intentions in an imitation context with novel objects. In his study, typically developing 18-month-old infants were as likely to produce a target action on an object (e.g., pulling two halves of a dumbbell apart) regardless of whether they saw the experimenter perform this action successfully ("target" condition) or attempt this action but fail ("intention" condition). Moreover, these infants performed the target action significantly more often in these two conditions than in either of two control conditions, a "baseline" condition, with no demonstration, or a "manipulation" condition, in which the experimenter performed an unrelated action on the object. The fact that infants in the "intention" condition produced the target action instead of what the experimenter actually did indicates that they understood his intention. Carpenter and colleagues used this paradigm but added an "end-state" condition (in which subjects saw the transformed object, without any actions being performed on it). Both groups (the autism group and the group with other developmental disabilities) gave evidence of understanding intentions, because there were no significant differences between the "target" and "intention" conditions in either group, whereas there were significant differences between the "intention" and "baseline" conditions in both groups. There were also no between-group differences. Although the pattern of results suggested a slightly less mature understanding of intention, the group with autism nonetheless had a much more marked deficit in joint attention.

These results suggest that the early, robust joint attention deficit in children with autism may *not* reflect a deficit in one aspect of intersubjectivity: understanding others' intentions. Moreover, a similar null result on this Meltzoff task has been found in two other studies of young children with autism (Aldridge, Stone, Sweeney, & Bower, 2000; Rogers, Wehner, & Pennington, 2002). In addition, null results on a different measure of understanding intentions were found in an older sample of children by Russell and Hill (2001). In a similar vein, Hobson and colleagues (Hobson & Lee, 1999; Moore, Hobson, & Lee, 1997) found that individuals with autism were able to recognize and imitate human actions, but they had difficulty recognizing or imitating the "style" or attitude those actions convey.

If children with autism understand others' intentions (at least their intentions toward objects), then both the executive theory and the theory of mind can be rejected. This means some other deficit, possibly in some aspect of emotion, must underlie their earlier and later social deficits. In summary, although we now have a much better understanding of what is impaired and what is intact in the development of social cognition in people with autism, much more remains to be done to determine (1) why the development of intersubjectivity is disrupted in this disorder, (2) what secondary effects this lack of intersubjectivity produces, and (3) what interventions may compensate for these problems.

Treatment

Autism changes development more pervasively than any disorder considered in this book, even mental retardation. Language, cognitive, and social development all depend on many thousands of hours of learning that strengthen connections in the relevant neural networks. Because a child with autism has missed much of this natural learning, it would be very surprising if a neurochemical intervention could abruptly reverse the symptoms of autism. However, intensive early interventions targeting these areas of development have been more successful in reversing some of the symptoms of autism.

As mentioned earlier, there are no proven pharmacological treatments for the main symptoms of autism, although medications can be helpful with associated symptoms, such as attention problems, aggressive or self-injurious behavior, and seizures. For example, Ritalin can help improve attention problems, and standard anticonvulsants are used to control seizures.

The most efficacious current treatments are psychosocial, involving intensive early intervention, although more research is needed to evaluate rigorously what aspects of these psychosocial treatments are helpful. The short-term goals of these intensive early interventions are to improve social and language skills, and to reduce behaviors that interfere with learning. The long-term goals are to promote adaptive and vocational skills. As reviewed earlier, a wide range of adult outcomes are found among individuals with autism, from a need for complete, custodial care to independent living. It is currently unknown to what extent intensive early interventions improve adult outcome.

One of the first evaluations of an intensive, early intervention program was the report by Lovaas (1987) on a 2-year, 40-hours-per-week program of behavior modification that actively included parents. This intervention appeared to produce dramatic improvement, in that nearly half of the children in the treatment program had a normal IQ and successfully completed first grade in a standard classroom, whereas none of the control children had either outcome. In later follow-up of these samples, McEachin, Smith, and Lovaas (1993) found that about half of the treated children compared to almost none of the controls continued to succeed in a normal classroom. However, this study has been criticized for lack of random assignment of cases to the treatment and control conditions, and lack of data on behavior, including symptoms of autism. Nonetheless, at least some aspects of this approach appear to be useful and have influenced other early intervention programs. Some of these (e.g., Ozonoff & Cathcart, 1998; Rogers, 1998) have focused more explicitly on teaching the deficient social skills, such as imitation, which were reviewed earlier.

Dawson and Osterling (1997) reviewed eight different, university-based, early intervention programs for children with autism. Upon entry into these programs, all children were mentally retarded, with a mean IQ below 55. After treatment, there was an average IQ gain of 23 points, and half the children were successfully placed in regular elementary school classrooms. These authors identified several common elements across these different programs, including (1) a curriculum focused on attention, imitation, communication, social, and play skills; (2) a highly structured teaching environment, with a low student:staff ratio; (3) strategies for generalizing skills to a wide range of contexts; (4) a predictable and routine daily schedule; (5) a functional rather than aversive approach to problem behaviors; (6) emphasis on skills needed for the transition to a regular classroom; and (7) a high level of family involvement. There have also been recent advances in the early identification of autism (e.g., A. Cox et al., 1999), making even earlier interventions feasible.

Despite considerable progress in developing early treatments for autism, we still lack a rigorous treatment study with random assignment of individuals to treatment conditions. The work of Lovaas and colleagues suggests that the gains from early intervention are maintained years later, but more rigorous evidence is needed on that point as well.

MENTAL RETARDATION

Mental retardation (MR) has been recognized since antiquity, as witnessed by the distinction (expressed in pejorative terms) between those who had lost their reasoning ("lunatics") and those who had never developed it ("idiots"). However, in earlier times, persons with MR were either neglected or placed in asylums. Efforts to train individuals with MR, to treat them humanely, and to understand their problems scientifically are much more recent and began with the Enlightenment, although much remains to be done to attain all three goals. Despite these efforts, stigma and abuse of persons with MR (as well as those with other psychopathologies) remain contemporary problems.

In France, in 1799, Jean Itard found an abandoned boy with MR and possibly autism in the forest (the Wild Boy of Averyon, also named Victor) and attempted to train him using instructional methods already in use with the deaf (Achenbach, 1982). His work with Victor is dramatized in François Truffaut's movie *l'Enfant Sauvage* ("the wild child"). Itard's efforts succeeded to some extent, showing that training could help those with MR, but he eventually abandoned Victor, who lived out his days in lonely custodial care. Edward Seguin (1812–1880) attempted systematically to train individuals with MR, both in France and the United States (Achenbach, 1982). By the middle of the 19th century, several training schools for individuals with MR were established, and in 1876, the directors of these schools in the United States formed a society that later became the American Association on Mental Retardation (AAMR) (Hodapp & Dykens, 1996). The AAMR, the main professional organization in the field of MR, publishes two journals and promotes research, intervention, and social policy efforts.

Despite the good intentions of the founders of the AAMR, the training schools often devolved into custodial "warehouses." In addition, at the end of the 19th century, widespread acceptance of the "science" of eugenics led to much more hostile attitudes toward those with MR. Eugenics conceived of familial MR as a threat to the gene pool; such a threat was dramatized by supposedly scientific accounts of extended families with limited intellectual functioning, such as *The Jukes* (Dugdale, 1877) and *The Kallikak Family* (Goddard, 1912). These concerns led to the reprehensible practice of enforced sterilization of those with MR. Since very little was actually known about the etiology of MR at the time, such a practice was not only ethically but also scientifically questionable.

The contemporary view of the treatment of persons with MR is partly a humane reaction against this history of past abuses and emphasizes the rights of those with disabilities. An important emphasis is on the concepts of "normalization" and "inclusion," or "mainstreaming." The basic idea behind these concepts is that, given appropriate accommodations, those with MR can and should be integrated as much as possible into normal life—in families, schools, and communities. I return to the topic of treatment later in this chapter.

Scientific understanding of some of the causes of MR is actually quite recent; such causes include genetic syndromes, early neurological insults, polygenic inheritance, and environmental deprivation. Although Down's (1866) description of the syndrome that bears his name is well over 100 years old, the genetic basis of Down syndrome was only discovered about 40 years ago (LeJeune, Gautier, & Turpin, 1959). Our understanding of the molecular basis of fragile X syndrome, another common genetic cause of mental retardation, is much more recent. There are now more than 100 known genetic causes of MR (Plomin et al., 1997), with more yet to be discovered. Other known genetic causes of MR include phenylketonuria, Lesch–Nyhan syndrome, neurofibromatosis, tuberous sclerosis, and Prader–Willi syndrome, to name a few.

   This chapter reviews general issues pertaining to MR and focuses on three MR syndromes—Down syndrome, fragile X syndrome, and Williams syndrome—that exemplify the progress made toward a neuroscientific understanding of MR. As we will see, each of these syndromes has a distinctive cognitive *and* social phenotype. The contrasting social phenotypes in these three disorders involve dimensions, such as gregariousness, empathy, and social anxiety, that are highly relevant for understanding other psychopathologies. By tracing the complex developmental pathways that run from genetic alterations through brain development to these distinctive behavioral phenotypes, we will very likely learn not only about mechanisms that operate in other psychopathologies but also how domains traditionally viewed as disparate— namely, cognition, language, and temperament—may share partly common developmental roots. These domains interact in important ways to produce the behavioral phenotypes characteristic of different disorders. Whereas other approaches to understanding psychopathology have often left MR off the list of phenomena to be considered, recent neuroscientific research on MR syndromes has shown them to be of central importance for understanding other psychopathologies. MR syndromes present in a more extreme form the dissociations that are also found in these other disorders. As I discuss in more detail later, MR syndromes provide a very important universality test for developmental theory.

Definition

The definition of MR provides a good example of the issues involved in both dimensional versus categorical conceptions of psychopathology and etiological versus behavioral definitions. Part of what we call MR (especially mild MR) lies on a continuum—in this case, a continuum of intelligence and adaptive functioning, the two constructs used in definitions of MR. On the one hand, the IQ and adaptive behavior cutoffs for MR, as well as subtypes of MR, are inevitably somewhat arbitrary and have changed over the years. On the other hand, there is clear bimodality in the lower tail of the IQ distribution, and many cases of moderate or more severe MR are part of a distinct distribution, with distinct etiologies, as is discussed later. Moreover, even with mild MR, it is obvious that a categorical diagnosis is needed to determine who qualifies for publicly funded services.

At first glance, it might appear that we should prefer etiological definitions of MR whenever they are available. More than is the case for any other disorder considered in this book, it is possible to define many forms of MR etiologically. But since persons who share an etiology (e.g., trisomy 21, the cause of Down syndrome) nonetheless vary in their level of cognitive and adaptive functioning, it is not all clear that etiological definitions should replace behavioral ones, especially for most treatment purposes. Obviously, an individual with Down syndrome and mild MR needs different services than another individual with Down syndrome and moderate or severe MR. For any psychopathology, there is no doubt that etiological definitions will help focus medical interventions, but short of a medical cure, we will also need behavioral definitions to guide treatments.

Most current definitions of MR (such as the one found in DSM-IV-TR) have three requirements: an IQ deficit, an adaptive behavior deficit, and onset before age 18 years. More specifically, IQ must be at least 2 standard deviations below the mean on an individually administered IQ test (e.g., an IQ of 70 or lower on the Wechsler). Earlier definitions had a higher IQ cutoff (1 standard deviation below the mean) and did not require an adaptive behavior deficit. As a result, about 16% of the population met criteria for MR. Since many such individuals did not have significant social and occupational problems as adults, the validity of this diagnostic definition was questionable. The lower IQ cutoff of 2 standard deviations below the mean only identifies about 3% of the general population. Individuals with IQs that low are much more likely to have problems meeting the demands of everyday life, but even with a lower IQ cutoff, there will inevitably be some false-positive diagnoses. This possibility is especially troublesome in ethnic and socioeconomic groups whose average IQ is below the population mean of 100.

To illustrate this problem, let us consider a hypothetical ethnic group with a mean IQ of 85, a normal distribution of IQ, and a standard deviation similar in magnitude to that found in the general population (i.e., 15). In this particular case, about 16% of the subpopulation would fall below an IQ cutoff of 70, again raising questions about the validity of the definition. To eliminate the false-positive problem in some ethnic and socioeconomic groups, the adaptive behavior deficit criterion was added to the definition of MR in the 1970s. The combination of the two criteria, an IQ 2 standard deviations below the mean and an adaptive behavior deficit, is much more likely to identify individuals who have significant problems in everyday life because of low intelligence.

The AAMR's controversial 1992 definition of MR essentially raised the IQ cutoff to 75. By changing the cutoff by just one-third of a standard deviation, this definition *doubled* the number of persons potentially eligible for the diagnosis. This change in cutoff has been controversial, and more recent definitions, such as the 1994 DSM-IV definition, have retained the lower cutoff (−2 standard deviations, or an IQ of 70).

In summary, the shifting IQ cutoffs in definitions of MR illustrate that imposing a cutoff on a continuum is somewhat arbitrary. Any cutoff will have a mix of costs and benefits in terms of research, external validity, clinical benefits to individuals, and societal needs. Moreover, these different uses of the diagnosis will be unlikely to agree on the best cutoff. One can imagine that as the global economy increasingly demands technological sophistication from workers, arguments for raising the IQ cutoff for MR could again become more common.

Of the three diagnostic criteria for MR, the least well-defined criterion is the adaptive behavior deficit. DSM-IV-TR requires that there must be a significant deficit in at least two (of 11) areas of adaptive functioning, such as self-care, communication, social skills, or occupational skills. Definitions of MR vary in the number of areas of adaptive functioning they consider, and there is some controversy about which areas should count and how they are measured. For example, should a deficit in "leisure" (many academics unfortunately have leisure impairments!) count the same as a deficit in self-care? Some definitions distinguish as many as 10 or 11 areas of adaptive functioning, but factor-analytic studies of adaptive behavior inventories find a smaller number of underlying factors, with a single general factor accounting for most of the variance (reviewed in Hodapp & Dykens, 1996).

To illustrate some of these points, let us consider a commonly used measure of adaptive functioning, the Vineland Adaptive Behavior Scales

(Sparrow, Balla, & Cicchetti, 1984), which have excellent psychometric characteristics in terms of reliability, construct validity, and discriminant validity, and clearly measure something besides IQ, because in normal children the correlation with IQ measures is about .30. The Vineland has three main scales, Communication, Daily Living Skills, and Socialization, whose internal validity is generally supported by factor analysis. Nonetheless, principal components analyses of domain standard scores across eight age groups in the standardization sample all found substantial general factors that accounted for between 55% and 70% of the total variance. The Vineland is very likely superior psychometrically to clinical impressions of multiple domains of adaptive functioning. Moreover, these two measures of adaptive functioning could produce conflicting and counterintuitive results with regard to whether a given child with an IQ under 70 has MR. A child might have a significant deficit on the Vineland Adaptive Behavior Composite, which best measures the general factor, but not meet the diagnostic criterion because only one of the three Vineland scales was below the cutoff. A second child, who, if assessed on the Vineland, would not be impaired on either the overall Composite or any one of its three scales, might meet this criterion for an adaptive behavior deficit based on a clinical interview covering 11 areas of adaptive functioning. Obviously, the first child would have a more significant overall adaptive behavior deficit than the second child, but only the second child would receive the diagnosis of MR.

In summary, diagnostic decisions about MR vary as a function of which measure of adaptive behavior is used. This diagnostic uncertainty is greater for individuals with milder deficits in IQ and adaptive behavior (i.e., those with IQs close to 70). Despite this uncertainty, the reliability of the diagnosis of MR is higher than that of many disorders considered in this book, because it requires the convergence of two separate behavioral criteria, IQ and adaptive behavior, each of which can be highly reliable.

The other continuum versus category issue in the definition of MR concerns severity subtypes, which are important clinically because they help predict both service needs and prognosis, yet are also somewhat arbitrary divisions of a continuum. Four subtypes recognized in the DSM-IV and ICD-10 taxonomies were defined by IQ ranges: mild (IQ = 55–70), moderate (IQ = 40–54), severe (IQ = 25–39), and profound (IQ < 25). In contrast, the 1992 AAMR definition eliminated these subtypes and replaced them with four levels of services required by an individual with MR: intermittent, limited, extensive, and pervasive. This change was motivated by the understanding that the kind of services needed represent an interaction between characteristics of an individual and his or her particular social context. This aspect of the 1992 AAMR definition has also been controversial, partly because the measurement of service needs is less precise and objective than the measurement of IQ. For example, levels of funding available to service providers (such as schools, health maintenance organizations, and the Social Security Administration) could easily bias assessments of what services are needed.

Epidemiology

As the foregoing discussion makes clear, the prevalence of MR depends on which cutoffs are used. Using the definition described here (an IQ 2 standard deviations below the mean, an adaptive behavior deficit, and onset before age 18), the prevalence is between 1% and 3% (Hodapp & Dykens, 1996), with the majority of that 1–3% having mild MR. The prevalence of the other three subtypes (moderate, severe, and profound) combined is 0.4%, or 4 per 1,000 (Hodapp & Dykens, 1996). Thus, depending on which overall prevalence estimate is used, between 60% and 87% of the total MR population have mild MR.

MR is more common in males than females (1.5:1; American Psychiatric Association, 2000). This male predominance is partly due to the large number of X-linked MR syndromes, the most common of which is fragile X syndrome, which is discussed in more detail later. Comorbidity with other psychiatric diagnoses is a common aspect of MR; hence, many individuals with MR have "dual diagnoses," and it is important that they receive appropriate treatment of both MR and the comorbid disorder. Symptoms of ADHD are very common across most forms of MR.

Known genetic syndromes, such as Down syndrome or fragile X syndrome, account for many of the cases of moderate or more severe MR. In what follows, I discuss the epidemiology of three of the best-known genetic MR syndromes: Down syndrome, fragile X syndrome, and Williams syndrome. Each represents a different type of genetic mechanism.

The most prevalent form of MR with a known genetic etiology is Down syndrome, which is found in 1 in 600 live births (a population prevalence of 0.17%), and affects males and females equally. Although

Down syndrome is genetic, most cases are not familial, as will be discussed later. Therefore, Down syndrome is not the most common *familial* form of MR with a known genetic etiology. Instead, fragile X syndrome fits that description.

Although fragile X syndrome is familial, its transmission is not simply Mendelian, as will be discussed later. The prevalence of fragile X syndrome varies somewhat across countries, probably because of founder effects; overall, it is found in about 1 in 4,000 males and about half as many females, so the population prevalence is about 0.019% (Sherman, 1996).

Finally, Williams syndrome is caused by a usually spontaneous, contiguous microdeletion of genes on chromosome 7. It affects both genders equally and occurs in about 1 in 25,000 births (0.004%). About one-fourth of individuals with Williams syndrome have moderate or worse MR.

Since the majority of individuals with Down syndrome and males with fragile X syndrome have moderate or worse MR, these two disorders together come close to accounting for half of individuals with moderate or worse MR, who represent 0.4% of the general population. Williams syndrome accounts for less than 1% (roughly 0.25%) of this total. While genetic, only one of these syndromes—fragile X syndrome—is familial, and the complexities of its transmission reduce familial risk. In addition, although males with fragile X syndrome are technically fertile, they rarely reproduce because of their cognitive and behavioral problems. If most of the remaining causes of moderate or worse MR are likewise nonfamilial, we should expect little risk for MR in the relatives of probands with moderate or worse MR.

Etiology

Both genes and environment contribute to the etiology of MR. One of the most frequent environmental causes is fetal alcohol syndrome. I first review evidence that supports a difference in the etiology of mild versus moderate or worse MR and then consider the etiology of three MR syndromes—Down syndrome, fragile X syndrome, and Williams syndrome.

Both direct and indirect evidence support the conclusion that the etiology of moderate or worse MR is substantially distinct from the etiology of mild MR. We have already seen that some of these etiologies of moderate or worse MR are nonfamilial (e.g., Down syndrome). Other nonfamilial organic etiologies, such as teratogens, perinatal complications, and postnatal neurological insults (e.g., meningitis and head injuries), are also much more common in moderate or worse MR (Hodapp & Dykens, 1996).

Moreover, as I mentioned earlier, the lower tail of the IQ distribution is bimodal (Dingman & Tarjan, 1960), which also suggests distinct etiologies of MR for individuals in the second, smaller distribution. Therefore, we might predict that siblings drawn from probands in this second, smaller distribution should not be at risk for MR. Consistent with this prediction, the siblings of probands with moderate and worse MR have a mean IQ of 103 (Nichols, 1984); that is, they have regressed all the way back to the population mean, indicating that the etiology of the probands' extreme low IQ scores is nonfamilial and cannot be due either to genes or environments shared by family members.

In contrast, mild MR, part of the lower tail of the IQ distribution, is clearly familial. In a classic family study of MR, Reed and Reed (1965) examined 289 probands with mild MR and their relatives. If mild MR is familial, the mean IQ of siblings of probands with mild MR should not regress all the way back to the population mean, unlike the case in moderate or worse MR. In the study by Reed and Reed, the mean sibling IQ was about 1 standard deviation below the population mean (i.e., about 85), thus supporting familiality. A second test of familiality involved transmission from parents to offspring. In this study, if one parent had mild MR, the risk for MR in the children was 20%, whereas if both parents had mild MR, offspring risk rose to 50%, again supporting familiality.

The distributional and etiological differences between mild and more severe MR have led to a distinction between "organic" and "cultural–familial" MR, which is called the "two-group" approach (Hodapp & Dykens, 1996). Earlier in this book, I discussed the implicit dualism involved in labeling some disorders "organic" and others not. Another problem with this distinction in the current context is that it might lead to the assumption that the familial influences on mild MR are all environmental. Although we do not have a twin or adoption study of probands with mild MR per se, we do know that the overall heritability of IQ is about 50%, and that twin studies of individuals with below average IQs find a similar value (Plomin et al., 1997). In a recent study of over 3,000 infant twin pairs, Eley and colleagues (1999a) found that the heritability of IQ in the lowest 5% was similar to that in the rest of the sample. So the most parsimonious hypothesis is that IQ is similarly heritable across the whole distribution, which would mean that mild MR is about 50% heritable. However, it is always possible that environmental influences could be stronger at the low end of the IQ distribution, because children of parents with low IQs would be exposed to a greater range of environmental adversities, including poorer health care, nutrition, and schools. These possibilities become even more salient when we consider minority groups that are at greater risk for such adversities. We next consider the specific genetic mechanisms that operate in Down syndrome, fragile X syndrome, and Williams syndrome.

As I discussed earlier, most (about 94%) cases of Down syndrome are not familial. Instead, a parent with a normal chromosome number produces an offspring with an extra copy of chromosome 21 (trisomy 21) through a process called "nondisjunction," which is failure of one of the paired chromosomes to separate in meiosis. Nondisjunction is more likely in mothers, especially older ones, than in fathers, because all of a mother's eggs are present in an immature form before her birth. In contrast, new sperm are continually being produced by fathers across their reproductive lifespan. Each month, one of these immature eggs goes through the final, reductive division in meiosis and becomes available for fertilization. Hence, the older the mother, the older the egg, and for reasons that are not completely understood, the older the egg, the greater risk for nondisjunction. So the risk for Down syndrome is only 1 in 2,400 in mothers 15–19 years old, but it rises to 1 in 40 in mothers who are 45–49 years old. The small remainder of Down syndrome cases are familial and reflect either translocation of an extra piece of the long arm of 21 to another chromosome or mosaicism, in which both parent and offspring have trisomy 21 in some but not all of their cells. In both translocation and mosaic Down syndrome, the parents can be apparently unaffected carriers, because they either have a balanced translocation or most of their mosaic cells are normal. These protective factors are not necessarily transmitted to the offspring.

Incidentally, nondisjunction is quite common across all the chromosomes, but most trisomies or monosomies are not viable and lead to early, spontaneous abortions. More than half of all conceptions end early, the majority of these affected by nondisjunction. Thus, viable aneuploidies (individuals with an abnormal chromosome number) can only involve a small number of extra or missing genes. This is the case if the aneuploid chromosome is small. Chromosome 21 actually has the fewest genes of any autosomal chromosome. The Y chromosome, which contributes to viable aneuploidies (e.g., 47, XYY), has the fewest genes of any chromosome. The one exception is the X chromosome, which is large and gene-rich but contributes to viable aneuploidies. However, all but one copy of the X chromosome are largely inactivated early in development. Nonetheless, there is some cost to having the wrong number of inactive X chromosomes, since females without an inactive X (45 X) have Turner's syndrome, and individuals with extra inactivated X's (such as 47, XXY males or 47, XXX females) have developmental disabilities.

So the genetic etiology of Down syndrome is due to an extra dose of the products of normal genes. Understanding this genetic etiology at the molecular level is a difficult task, because it requires that we (1) have identified all the genes on chromosome 21, (2) know which of these are overexpressed (other genes or epigenetic interactions may produce dosage compensation for some of the genes on 21), and (3) know which of the overexpressed genes are expressed early enough in development to cause a congenital disorder. To understand the etiology of the neurobehavioral phenotype in Down syndrome, we need to add a fourth constraint, namely, that the gene is expressed in the brain, or at least affects brain development.

Earlier work with partial trisomies had established that only part of chromosome 21, on the long arm, is involved in the etiology of Down syndrome. But there are still many genes in that region. Recently, the physical map of chromosome 21 was completed (Hattori et al., 2000), and it appears that the number of genes is only about 225, which is less than the size of the chromosome would predict (smaller chromosome 22 has about twice as many genes). A majority subset of these genes are in the Down syndrome region on 21q.

Work is now under way to determine which genes in this subset meet the other criteria listed earlier to qualify as a potential etiology of the neurobehavioral phenotype. Mouse models with trisomies of either single candidate genes or segments of the Down syndrome region have been constructed and are being tested for their neurological and neurobehavioral phenotype. In a review, Crnic and Pennington (2000) discussed some of the promising candidate genes that have already been identified, including the amyloid precursor protein gene (APP), which is also implicated in Alzheimer's disease; a glutamate receptor subunit gene (CRIK1); the human minibrain homologue (MNB); and the neuronal intracellular adhesion molecule (DSCAM).

In summary, the genetic etiology of Down syndrome is the most complicated of the three syndromes considered here because it involves many more genes. Indeed, it is always possible that trisomy induces developmental instability in a general way and that we will not be able to map specific phenotypic features of Down syndrome to extra doses of specific genes (Reeves, Baxter, & Richtsmeir, 2001). Nonetheless, recent advances in mapping the human genome and constructing mouse models have accelerated progress toward understanding the genetic basis of the neurobehavioral phenotype in Down syndrome.

Fragile X syndrome is a single-gene disorder in which the fragile X mental retardation 1 (FMR1) gene becomes inactivated (methylated) because it contains a large number (> 200) of trinucleotide (i.e., CGG) repeats (Verkerk et al., 1991). Normal individuals have a small number (< 50) of repeats, but sometimes the number of repeats increases when gametes are produced, so that an FMR1 gene with a larger number (50–200) of repeats is transmitted to the offspring. A gene with this many repeats is called a "premutation," because it functions normally but increases the risk of an even larger number of repeats in the next (third) generation. If that number exceeds 200, the grandchild is considered to have the fragile X syndrome mutation, because the FMR1 gene is very likely to be inactivated and will not produce the protein it codes for (FMR protein, or FMRP). The absence of this gene product in development causes fragile X syndrome. A male grandchild with this mutation will very likely have the full syndrome, including MR, because males have only one X chromosome. On the other hand, a female grandchild with this mutation on one of her X chromosomes will nevertheless have a normal FMR1 gene on her second X chromosome, so she can still produce some FMRP. How much FMRP she can produce partly depends on what proportion of her cells have this second X chromosome active, since the normal process of X inactivation (also called "Lyonization," after the person who discovered it) leaves only one X chromosome active in each cell. This proportion, called the X activation ratio, predicts the degree of phenotypic involvement in females with the fragile X mutation. So because the FMR1 gene is on the X chromosome, fragile X syndrome acts like a more typical X-linked disorder and produces an excess of males with this syndrome. But unlike a typical, Mendelian, X-linked disorder (e.g., hemophilia), fragile X syndrome also exhibits what is called "anticipation," which means that severity increases and age of onset decreases across generations. In contrast, in a Mendelian disorder, the phenotype stays the same across generations. Anticipation in fragile X syndrome is explained by the expansion of repetitive sequences across generations; a similar phenomenon is found in Huntington's disease, which also exhibits anticipation.

The degree of expansion across generations, and hence the degree of anticipation in both fragile X syndrome and Huntington's disease, depends on the gender of the transmitting parent, which is the second non-Mendelian aspect of these two disorders. In fragile X syndrome, expansion is greater in a transmitting mother, whereas in Huntington's disease, it is greater in a transmitting father. These are examples of a phenomenon called "imprinting," which is non-Mendelian because of the classic assumption that gene expression does not vary as a function of the parent from which the gene came.

In summary, the genetic transmission of fragile X syndrome is complicated. In extended families with fragile X syndrome, there will be (1) a greater number of cases in more recent generations (anticipation), (2) more males with fragile X syndrome than females (X-linkage), (3) more children with fragile X syndrome born to mothers than to fathers with a premutation (imprinting), and (4) a wider range of phenotypic severity in females than in males with the mutation (partly because of variation in the X activation ratio in females). But understanding fragile X syndrome at the gene level is a much simpler task than is the case for Down or Williams syndromes, because only a single gene—FMR1—is involved. The role of FMR1 in brain development is now being elucidated (Witt et al., 1995); it appears that it plays a widespread role in postsynaptic pruning of neuronal connections. Absence of this gene product (FMRP) could therefore interfere with an important mechanism in brain development—elimination of excess synapses—that is necessary for efficient neural networks. A reduction in synaptic pruning would therefore help to explain both an important aspect of the neurological phenotype (macrocephaly) and the MR in this syndrome.

As mentioned earlier, Williams syndrome is caused by a usually sporadic, contiguous deletion of genes on chromosome 7q11.23. This deletion is 1.5 megabases in length, hemizygous (i.e., only on one of the two copies of chromosome 7), and involves at least 16 genes, two of which have been characterized (Mervis & Klein-Tasman, 2000). Recent molecular work has identified these two genes and has begun to determine how they influence the physical and cognitive phenotype. The physical phenotype includes characteristic facial, cardiac (particularly supravalvular aortic stenosis [SVAS]), and connective tissue features (see Mervis, Morris, Bertrand, & Robinson, 1999). Because there is an autosomal dominant form of SVAS, with some family members exhibiting other physical features of Williams syndrome, it appeared there might be a shared genetic etiology for Williams syndrome and SVAS. Linkage studies of kindreds with familial SVAS eventually identified mutations in the elastin gene (ELN) on chromosome 7q as the cause of this familial disorder (Ewart et al., 1993b, 1994). Some of these families had microdeletions of portions of the ELN gene, raising the possibility that an even larger deletion on 7q was the cause of Williams syndrome. This hypothesis was confirmed by Ewart and colleagues (1993a) and by subsequent studies. ELN produces elastin protein, which is important for the heart and connective tissues; hence, deletion of ELN could explain much of the physical phenotype in Williams syndrome (see Mervis et al., 1999).

But since ELN is minimally expressed in brain and familial SVAS due to ELN deletions does not involve cognitive changes, other genes must be involved in the cognitive and behavioral phenotype of Williams syndrome. Subsequent studies identified a second gene in the Williams syndrome deletion region on 7q11.23, LIM-kinase 1 (LIMK1), which was found to influence the deficit in spatial cognition found in the syndrome (Frangiskakis et al., 1996). This deficit is not found in most individuals with familial SVAS.

In summary, research on the etiology of Williams syndrome provides an example of a third genetic mechanism in the etiology of MR, namely, microdeletions. As in Down syndrome, the genes involved are normal but with abnormal expression. Whereas Down syndrome involves overexpression of some genes, Williams syndrome involves underexpression. Theoretically, 50% of the gene product is available in development because one of the two normal genes is missing. Work is currently proceeding to identify the remaining genes in the Williams syndrome deletion region and to trace their phenotypic effects. Because the size of the microdeletion in the Williams syndrome region on 7q varies across individuals, it will be possible to evaluate how these new genes relate to different aspects of the Williams syndrome phenotype.

In sum, there has been rapid progress in identifying genes involved in these three MR syndromes and in relating them to aspects of their phenotypes. This progress illustrates well the potential power of collaborations between molecular geneticists and cognitive neuroscientists for understanding the other psychopathologies considered in this book.

Brain Mechanisms

In this section, I focus on what is known about brain mechanisms in Down syndrome, fragile X syndrome, and Williams syndrome. Nadel (1999) recently reviewed what is known about brain development in

Down syndrome. Broadly speaking, development appears normal at birth and is invariably abnormal by adulthood, since virtually all adults with Down syndrome have developed some of the neuropathological features of Alzheimer's disease by around age 35. In addition, by adulthood, the brain is clearly microcephalic; differentially greater volume reductions occur in the hippocampus, prefrontal cortex, and cerebellum (Kesslak, Nagata, Lott, & Nalciouglu, 1994; Lögdberg & Brun, 1993; Raz et al., 1995; Weiss, 1991). Much less clear from the existing data is when these aspects of abnormal brain development first appear in individuals with Down syndrome.

A wide range of studies has found no differences at birth between brains of normals and individuals with Down syndrome (e.g., Schmidt-Sidor, Wisniewski, Shepard, & Sersen, 1990). Differences that appear in the first few months of life include delayed myelination, reduced growth of the frontal lobes, a narrowing of the superior temporal gyrus, diminished size of the brainstem and cerebellum, and a major reduction (20–50%) in the number of cortical granular neurons (Nadel, 1999). However, these differences in brain development are not invariant across all cases. So several features of the adult brain phenotype begin to emerge in the first years of life, including microcephaly and reduced volumes of the cerebellum and frontal lobes. However, evidence for hippocampal volume reduction in the first years of life has not been reported.

Less is known about brain development in children and adolescents with Down syndrome. One structural MRI study of adolescents (Jernigan, Bellugi, Sowell, Doherty, & Hesselink, 1993) found a pattern of results similar to that found in adults, that is, microcephaly and relatively smaller volumes of frontal cortex, hippocampus, and cerebellum. These investigators compared a small sample ($N = 6$) with Down syndrome to both normal chronological-age-matched controls ($N = 21$) and adolescents with Williams syndrome ($N = 9$). Both of the MR groups had overall microcephaly, but only the group with Down syndrome had cerebellar volume reduction relative to age controls. In Williams syndrome, despite microcephaly, the cerebellar volume was similar to that of age-matched controls. There were also contrasts between the groups with Down and Williams syndromes in the proportions of grey matter for several other structures. The group with Down syndrome had a smaller proportion of anterior cortex and temporal limbic cortex, including the hippocampus (compared to both Williams syndrome and the chronological-age-matched control group). In contrast, the posterior cortex, the lenticular nucleus, and the diencephalon were all proportionally larger in the group with Down syndrome compared to the other two groups.

In summary, the adult brain phenotype in Down syndrome is characterized by both general (microcephaly) and specific (frontal lobes, hippocampus, and cerebellum) volume reductions, some of which may emerge earlier in development than others.

Neuroanatomical abnormalities in fragile X syndrome have included decreased size of the posterior cerebellar vermis (Reiss, Aylward, Freund, Joshi, & Bryan, 1991), which may be related to abnormalities in sensory motor integration, activity level, and social interactions. Mild ventricular enlargements have been demonstrated, which would be consistent with mild frontal or parietal atrophy, or hypersecretion of cerebrospinal fluid (Wisniewski, Segan, Miezejeski, Sersen, & Rudelli, 1991). Finally, there appears to be brain enlargement in fragile X syndrome, since their head circumferences are large (Prouty et al., 1988). These findings contrast the microcephaly found in Down syndrome and many other MR syndromes, and suggest a failure of neuronal pruning mechanisms in early brain development. As we have seen, there is also evidence for macrocephaly in autism.

In summary, we do not yet know how the mutation causes brain changes or which brain changes cause the MR associated with fragile X syndrome. However, the fact that this is a single-gene disorder, in which the gene has been identified, makes the elucidation of this causal pathway much easier than it will be for Down syndrome.

In Williams syndrome, structural studies have found a neurological phenotype that contrasts sharply with that found in Down syndrome (see Bellugi, Mills, Jernigan, Hickok, & Galaburda, 1999). Although there is microcephaly in both Williams and Down syndromes, unlike both fragile X syndrome and autism, not all structures are equally reduced in size, nor are the same structures reduced in each syndrome. In Williams syndrome, there is relative sparing of frontal, limbic, and cerebellar volumes, whereas these volumes are reduced in Down syndrome (Bellugi et al., 1999). Limbic structures include the hippocampus, providing further evidence for a hippocampal deficit in Down syndrome. In contrast, there is sparing of the lenticular nuclei (part of the basal ganglia) in Down syndrome but not in Williams syndrome. Posterior temporal cortex, including primary auditory cortex (Heschel's gyrus), is of normal size in Williams syndrome in contrast to Down syndrome (Bellugi et al., 1999). This difference could help explain both hyperacusis (lower hearing thresholds) and relatively preserved language development in Williams syndrome. The neuroanatomical contrasts across these three MR syndromes are beginning to help us understand their contrasting neuropsychological phenotypes, which I discuss next.

Neuropsychology

The neuropsychology of MR has been reviewed in Pennington and Bennetto (1998) and Crnic and Pennington (2000). The following discussion updates those reviews. Ironically, we mostly lack a neuropsychology of MR, just as we lack a neuropsychology of intelligence. Neuropsychologists have focused more on specific, acquired disorders of cognition than on general, developmental ones. The study of intelligence has been pursued mainly by psychometricians; its brain correlates have only recently been studied. Nonetheless, the study of MR is relevant for fundamental issues concerning the nature of cognitive development (see, e.g., Anderson, 2001). There are two fundamental facts about human cognitive development: (1) There are wide differences in diverse cognitive abilities both across age and between individuals at a given age, and (2) because differences are moderately correlated across wide content domains, there must be some *general* cognitive factors that partly explain individual and developmental differences in intelligence. The study of MR can help answer the following questions:

1. What are these general factors?
2. How do general factors underlying individual differences relate to those underlying developmental differences?
3. How do both relate to brain development?
4. How, despite these general influences, are there also differences in *specific* aspects of cognitive development?
5. How do these specific differences relate to brain development?
6. How universal are the hypothesized sequences of brain and behavioral development?

Some recent efforts to use a neuropsychological approach to study various MR syndromes have been much more concerned with which specific functions are relatively impaired or spared, than with why there is an impairment in general intelligence. This approach tends to assume that the cognitive architecture consists of a set of relatively independent and isolable modules, and that the only difference between MR and other examples of brain damage or dysfunction is that more modules are dysfunctional in MR. In this view, we would study MR in much the same way we study specific learning disorders such as developmental dyslexia, by looking for the profile of specific strengths and weaknesses that characterize a particular MR syndrome. However, as discussed earlier, this approach to understanding developmental disorders has significant limitations (Oliver et al., 2000).

In what follows, I place the above six questions in a historical context and then consider what we have learned about them from the study of specific MR syndromes.

It is useful to view current work on the neuropsychology of MR in the context of issues that have been important in the history of psychological approaches to understanding MR (Hodapp et al., 1998). One key debate has been between those who espouse either a developmental approach (Zigler, 1969) or specific deficit approach, whether in verbal mediation (Luria, 1961), stimulus traces (Ellis, 1963), attention (Zeaman & House, 1963), executive processes (Belmont & Butterfield, 1971), or some other cognitive process. The latter approach has attempted to account for all of MR, regardless of etiology, with a single cognitive deficit. In contrast, the developmental approach has divided MR into organic and nonorganic types and has argued that for the nonorganic or cultural–familial type, there has been a general slowing of development across all domains. Consequently, both the sequence of developmental acquisitions ("similar sequence hypothesis") and the profile across domains ("similar structure hypothesis") would be similar to what is found in typically developing children at the same mental age level. So the debate has centered on the relevance of specific versus general cognitive processes for understanding MR, as well as the relevance of etiology and, of course, development. These two positions highlight significant aspects of MR that any comprehensive neuroscientific account will have to explain, yet each has committed significant errors.

In terms of aspects to explain, there is the fact that individuals with MR do develop, that they follow a normal sequence of developmental acquisitions much more often than not, and that their performance on most, but not all, tasks is well predicted by mental age. In fact development is even more robust in MR than expected by the developmental position, since these generalizations also apply to "organic" MR syndromes with known genetic causes, such as trisomy 21 or the fragile X mutation. So the similar sequence and structure hypotheses have largely been supported. Both point to the potential importance of general cognitive processes in understanding MR, although a modularity theorist could conceivably argue that similarity in sequence and structure derives from independent modules, each slowed to a similar extent in development. An important goal for the neuropsychological approach is to identify parameters of brain development that, when altered, would affect general cognitive processes and lead to this general slowing of development. Possible candidates include number of neurons, synaptic connections (either too few or too many), or neurotransmitter systems.

However, the specific deficit approach is partly correct as well. There is now accumulating evidence of some degree of specificity in both developmental sequence and cognitive profile across MR syndromes. For instance, language development in Williams syndrome contradicts an assumed universal sequence in two respects: Pointing does not precede referential labeling, and exhaustive sorting of objects does not co-occur with the vocabulary spurt (Mervis & Bertrand, 1997). In terms of profile, verbal short-term memory is above mental age level in Williams syndrome and below it in Down syndrome, whereas the reverse is the case for visuospatial skills (Mervis, 1999; Wang & Bellugi, 1994). At the same time, this double dissociation across the two syndromes does not indicate independence of the two cognitive domains in MR, since there are moderate partial correlations (controlling for age) among these and other cognitive measures in Williams syndrome (Mervis et al., 1999). In fact, greater correlations among various domains of cognition may be a general characteristic of MR (Detterman & Daniel, 1989). Moreover, even though below mental age level, development in the weak area can follow a normal developmental sequence, as has been shown in studies of the development of drawing skills in Williams syndrome (Bertrand & Mervis, 1996; Bertrand, Mervis, & Eisenberg, 1997).

In summary, general developmental processes are robust in MR, even in "organic syndromes," but there is evidence of specificity as well. Both the general slowing of development and the different specific deficits that characterize different syndromes require a neuroscientific explanation. At the cognitive level, explanations have attempted to identify some fundamental process(es) that explain the general aspect of both developmental and individual differences in intelligence. One probably too simplistic position is that both developmental and individual differences can largely be reduced to differences in a single cognitive process, such as working memory (see, e.g., Pennington, 1994). Another position, also probably too simplistic, is that a different fundamental cognitive process underlies each kind of difference. Hence, Anderson's (2001) two-factor theory proposes that differences in speed of processing account for individual differences in intelligence, whereas working memory and inhibition account for developmental differences in intelligence. Research on MR syndromes allows us to test such theories.

The findings just reviewed also highlight how the developmental approach to understanding MR is a two-way street; not only does what we have learned about normal development help us to understand MR but also MR syndrome research provides an important test of the generality of developmental theories. In fact, MR syndromes provide a particularly powerful test of putative developmental universals because (1) development proceeds more slowly in MR, allowing a more sensitive test of developmental sequences; (2) more dissociations are found between (and within) cognitive and language development in MR; and (3) contrasting profiles of dissociations exist across MR syndromes.

In terms of errors, both approaches to MR were wrong about etiology in somewhat different ways: The specific deficit approach ignored etiology, and the developmental approach drew too sharp a distinction between organic and nonorganic etiologies. All forms of MR must affect brain development in some way or another, and both genetic and environmental factors (and their interaction) are important in both syndromal and (currently) idiopathic, mild MR (i.e., the cultural–familial subgroup discussed earlier). Recent research has found that mild MR has a pathological etiology in as many as 30–50% of children (Simonoff, Bolton, & Rutter, 1998). A medical geneticist would argue that some of the remaining cases are due to syndromes not yet recognized. But many cases of mild MR are due to an accumulation of unfavorable alleles of quantitative trait loci (QTLs) and environmental risk factors. No one of these etiological factors is pathological by itself.

Even when the etiology of mild MR is thus multifactorial, how those multifactors act on brain and cognitive development is important to understand and will likely reveal commonalities with mechanisms operating in so-called "pathological" cases. For instance, we have already explained that in Down and Williams syndromes there are no pathological alleles, but rather extra or reduced doses of the products of normal alleles. Therefore, too sharp a line has been drawn between organic and nonorganic, and pathological and nonpathological; instead of a categorical distinction, we really have a continuum. From the perspective of developmental neuroscience, both normal and abnormal development require an explanation in terms of genetic and environmental influences on brain development. Studying MR syndromes such as Down syndrome will identify some of these influences. I now turn to the neuropsychology of the three specific MR syndromes considered here: Down syndrome, fragile X syndrome, and Williams syndrome.

Down Syndrome

What is known about the brain phenotype in Down syndrome leads us to predict both overall neuropsychological dysfunction and somewhat more specific deficits on measures of prefrontal, hippocampal, and cerebellar functions. Because different aspects of the brain phenotype appear to emerge at different points in development, we would also predict different developmental trajectories for different domains of dysfunction. Specifically, we would predict that hippocampal dysfunction may appear later in development than dysfunction in the other domains (Nadel, 1986). I next examine whether existing data support these hypotheses.

I begin with areas of cognitive development that have been thoroughly studied, including the level and trajectory of IQ, speech–language functions, short-term memory, and visuoconstructive functions, and conclude with the few studies of hippocampal functions (i.e., allocentric spatial cognition and explicit long-term memory) in Down syndrome. To my knowledge, there are no previous studies of prefrontal functions in Down syndrome.

LEVEL AND TRAJECTORY OF IQ

Down syndrome does not specify a particular IQ but instead exerts on it a powerful, downward main effect. Just as in normally developing children, IQ in Down syndrome is also influenced by other genetic and environmental factors. For example, a positive relation exists between parental IQ and the IQ of individuals with Down syndrome, and part of this relation is very likely genetic, just as in nonretarded children.

In contrast to IQ in normally developing children, a progressive IQ decline in Down syndrome begins in the first year of life. In other words, the mental age: chronological age ratio is not constant (Hodapp & Zigler, 1990). By adulthood, IQ is usually in the moderately to severely retarded range (IQ = 25–55), with an upper mental age limit of approximately 7–8 years (Gibson, 1978), though a few individuals with Down syndrome have IQs in the normal range (Epstein, 1989). The trajectory of IQ in adulthood is also different in Down syndrome because of the increased risk of early-onset Alzheimer's disease; consequently, IQ declines much sooner in adulthood than it does in normal aging (Epstein, 1989).

Little is known about the etiology of this virtually linear decline in IQ in the early development of individuals with Down syndrome. Determining the brain bases of the IQ trajectory in Down syndrome could illuminate the relations between normal brain and cognitive development. More specifically, either microcephaly or dysfunction in specific structures (i.e., prefrontal cortices, hippocampus, or cerebellum) could conceivably reduce IQ in Down syndrome and affect its trajectory, but in different ways in each structure. Each specific structure helps to mediate general cognitive processes that operate across content domains. Hence, dysfunction in each structure could be expected to have a general effect on cognitive development.

SPEECH, LANGUAGE, AND VERBAL SHORT-TERM MEMORY

These functions have been studied extensively in Down syndrome and other than IQ, are probably the most well-documented aspect of its cognitive phenotype. They also decline early, thus contributing to the IQ decline, since IQ tests partly measure language development. This speech and language profile contrasts markedly with what is observed in autism, fragile X syndrome, and Williams syndrome, a finding that potentially limits the causal role for some speech and language processes in explaining MR across syndromes.

Several areas of speech and language development are delayed below mental age expectations in Down syndrome. Specifically, articulation (Fowler, Gelman, & Gleitman, 1994; Hulme & Mackenzie, 1992), phonology (Rondal, 1993), vocal imitation (Dunst, 1990), mean length of utterance, and expressive syntax (Fowler et al., 1994) are all below the expected mental age level.

The development of verbal short-term memory lags behind mental age in Down syndrome (Hulme & Mackenzie, 1992). This well-replicated deficit may help explain some of the speech and language difficulties found in Down syndrome, as a number of researchers have suggested for the syntactic deficit (Chapman, 1999; Fowler, 1998; Marcell & Weeks, 1988). This relation makes sense both theoretically and empirically. Theoretically, comprehending syntactic relations requires temporary memory storage of parts of a phrase. There are in consistent moderate correlations between measures of verbal short-term memory and language in groups with developmental disabilities and those with typical development. Verbal short-term memory is a relative strength in Williams syndrome, as is language, and the two are moderately correlated (r's = .47–.69 with chronological age partialed; Mervis et al., 1999).

Hulme and Mackenzie (1992) demonstrated that slower articulation is not responsible for the verbal short-term memory deficit in Down syndrome. They proposed that children with Down syndrome were not rehearsing the to-be-remembered information in the articulatory loop. Consistent with the position I take here, they also suggested that deficits in verbal short-term memory may play an important causal role in MR.

Hence, the verbal short-term memory deficit in Down syndrome likely helps explain the language deficit, which in turn contributes to the IQ deficit. But we do not know the brain basis of the verbal short-term memory deficits in Down syndrome.

VISUOCONSTRUCTIVE FUNCTIONS

Certain spatial abilities are a strength relative to mental age in Down syndrome. For instance, Silverstein, Legutski, Friedman, and Tayakama (1982) found that a group with Down syndrome outperformed a group with non-Down-syndrome MR individually matched on chronological and mental age on several drawing and other visuoconstructive tasks from the Stanford–Binet test. This relative strength in Down syndrome contrasts with a relative weakness on similar tasks in Williams syndrome (Wang & Bellugi, 1994; Wang, Doherty, Rourke, & Bellugi, 1995).

HIPPOCAMPAL FUNCTIONS

There are a few studies of hippocampal functions in individuals with Down syndrome across the lifespan, but most of this work is on adults. Mangan (1992) studied preschool (16–30 months old) children with Down syndrome and chronological-age-matched controls on three spatial tasks, one of which (place learning and recall) tapped hippocampal functions. The group with Down syndrome performed worse than chronological-age-matched controls on the learning portion of all three tasks but was severely and selectively impaired on only the delayed recall probes for the place learning tasks. However, there was not a mental-age-matched control group in this study.

Carlesimo, Marrotta, and Vicar (1997) tested implicit (stem completion) and explicit verbal memory (word list learning and prose recall), as well as explicit nonverbal memory (Rey's Figure Form B) in adolescents with Down syndrome (N = 15), non-DS MR (N = 15), and mental-age-matched controls (N = 30). They found similar verbal priming in all three groups for the stem completion tasks. For the two explicit tasks, the group with Down syndrome performed significantly worse than the other two groups in learning but was not differentially impaired in delayed recall or recognition. In fact, the Down syndrome group improved on recognition trials relative to its recall performance. These authors interpret their results as supporting a hippocampally mediated deficit in episodic memory in Down syndrome, one that particularly affects encoding and retrieval. However, verbal memory tests are somewhat problematic in individuals with Down syndrome because of their well-documented language and verbal short-term memory deficits. Therefore, it would be valuable to see a test of nonverbal long-term memory in Down syndrome, using a task that does not depend on visuomotor skills.

Three studies of adults with Down syndrome have found particularly marked long-term memory deficits (Caltagirone, Nocentini, & Vicari, 1990; Devenny, Hill, Patxot, Silverman, & Wisniewski, 1992; Ellis, Woodley-Zanthos, & Dulaney, 1989). For example, Ellis and colleagues (1989) examined nonverbal long-term memory using pictures in a book. Their group with Down syndrome was impaired at both recognizing pictures and remembering their locations—a result that is consistent with hippocampal dysfunction. However, a subset of this group with Down syndrome performed very well on this task.

In summary, previous long-term memory research supports hippocampal dysfunction in Down syndrome. However, the only two studies in nonadult samples both have methodological shortcomings. So more work is needed to determine whether hippocampal dysfunction in Down syndrome occurs before adulthood, and if so, how early it occurs.

We (Pennington, Moon, Edgin, Stedron, & Nadel, 2001) recently conducted a study of prefrontal and hippocampal functions in a sample of 28 school-age (mean = 14.7 years, standard deviation = 2.7) individuals with Down syndrome compared to 28 (mean = 4.9 years, standard deviation = 0.75) typically developing children individually matched on mental age. Both neuropsychological domains were tested with multiple behavioral measures. "Benchmark" measures of verbal and spatial function demonstrated that this sample with Down syndrome was similar to others in the literature.

The main finding was a significant group-by-domain interaction effect indicating differential hippocampal dysfunction in the group with Down syndrome. However, there was a moderate partial correlation ($r = .54$), controlling for chronological age, between hippocampal and prefrontal composite scores in the group with Down syndrome, and both composites contributed unique variance to the prediction of mental age and adaptive behavior in that group.

In summary, these results indicate a particular weakness in hippocampal functions in Down syndrome in the context of overall cognitive dysfunction. Interestingly, these results are similar to those found in a mouse model of Down syndrome. Such a model will make it easier to understand the neurobiological mechanisms that produce hippocampal dysfunction in Down syndrome.

This study provides evidence relevant to the theoretical issues discussed earlier. We found at least three different developmental trajectories in Down syndrome. One domain of development—adaptive behavior—was *above* mental age level. So one determinant of adaptive behavior is chronological age, or time in the world. Nonetheless, adaptive behavior in Down syndrome is well below chronological age level and is correlated with IQ and mental age.

Another domain of development—prefrontally mediated executive functions—was at mental age level. It may be that key aspects of psychometric intelligence (e.g., fluid intelligence) are closely related to executive functions (Pennington, 1994). Consequently, we would hypothesize that executive dysfunction is an important contributor to low IQ in all MR syndromes. Nonetheless, MR syndromes may vary in whether executive functions are at or below mental age level (as they are in fragile X syndrome). No MR syndrome has yet been described in which executive functions are above mental age level.

Three other domains of development—verbal short-term memory, structural language (such as lexical and syntactic skills), and hippocampal functions—are *below* mental age level in Down syndrome. As argued earlier, the verbal short-term memory deficit may help explain the structural language deficit. However, it seems very unlikely that the verbal short-term memory deficit can be explained by hippocampal dysfunction. In classical hippocampal amnesia, verbal short-term memory is spared (Shallice, 1988), as it is in children with early selective hippocampal damage (Varga-Khadem et al., 1997), whose structural language development also appeared to be basically intact. Moreover, verbal short-term memory and hippocampally mediated long-term memory are doubly dissociable, since there are adults with a profound deficit in verbal short-term memory (Shallice, 1988) but intact, explicit long-term memory.

Hippocampal dysfunction, by itself, is also unlikely as a sufficient explanation for the MR in Down syndrome, because the children with early selective hippocampal damage described by Varga-Khadem and colleagues (1997) did not have MR.

So returning to the key issue of explaining the causes of both developmental and individual cognitive differences, the evidence from Down syndrome argues that *both* one- and two-factor theories are too simple. To explain the developmental profile in Down syndrome, we need at least four cognitive constructs: explicit memory, executive functions, verbal short-term memory, and another construct to explain the acquisition of adaptive behavioral skills that are above mental age level.

Fragile X Syndrome

LEVEL AND TRAJECTORY OF IQ

The average IQ of males with fragile X syndrome is in the moderate range of MR; the median average IQ for older males is 41–47 in the studies reviewed in Bennetto and Pennington (in press). In that review, the median value for younger males is 54, illustrating the decline of IQ with age found in males with fragile X syndrome. In females with the fragile X mutation, the average IQ is higher, with a median value of 83 (Bennetto & Pennington, in press), and there is not a decline with age. As explained earlier, this gender difference in IQ is explained by X-linked transmission. Approximately one-fourth of females with the full mutation have MR; most of the remainder exhibit learning problems (Hagerman et al., 1992; Staley et al., 1993).

Longitudinal analyses of IQ in males with fragile X syndrome have now shown that the IQ decline is a real phenomenon and not an artifact of comparing different samples or using different IQ tests at different ages (see Bennetto & Pennington, 1996, in press, for reviews).

SPEECH AND LANGUAGE SKILLS

Abnormalities in both speech production and language competence have consistently been noted in males with fragile X syndrome, who often demonstrate delays in articulation and syntactic ability that are typically no different than those produced by normally developing children as they acquire language competence (Sudhalter, Scarborough, & Cohen, 1991). Males with fragile X syndrome tend to show deviance in several areas of speech and language beyond that expected for their level of cognitive impairment. Their speech is often described as dysrhythmic, litany-like, and "cluttered." This latter term refers to a fast or fluctuating rate of talking in which sounds or words are occasionally repeated or garbled (Hanson, Jackson, & Hagerman, 1986).

Males with fragile X syndrome also show deviance in pragmatics and conversational skills. Their language is often described as perseverative and inappropriate or tangential in conversation style. Furthermore, language is often marked by palilalia (direct self-repetition), echolalia (repetition of others), or frequent use of stereotypical statements. The deviant language pattern does not appear to be due to overall lower IQ: Males with fragile X syndrome are more likely, for example, to perseverate on a topic, produce stereotyped vocalizations, and fail to read referential gestures in others than are males with Down syndrome (Sudhalter et al., 1990). Finally, women with fragile X syndrome have also been shown to have less goal direction and organization in their thinking and speech than comparison women (Sobesky, Hull, & Hagerman, 1994).

In contrast to their poor pragmatic skills, males with fragile X syndrome tend to show strengths in expressive and receptive vocabulary (Sudhalter, 1987). Cognitive profiles of males and females with fragile X syndrome on the Stanford–Binet Intelligence Scale (4th ed.) indicated strengths in vocabulary, verbal labeling, and verbal comprehension (Freund & Reiss, 1991). On achievement tests, the males have shown relative strengths in early reading skills and spelling ability (Hagerman, Kemper, & Hudson, 1985; Kemper, Hagerman, Altshul-Stark, 1988).

MEMORY

On the memory subtests of the Stanford–Binet, males with fragile X syndrome showed consistent weaknesses on short-term memory for sentences and bead memory (a visual memory task) but did relatively well on object memory (Freund & Reiss, 1991). The authors interpreted these results as suggesting that the memory deficit in fragile X syndrome is dependent on the type of information to be remembered. Abstract visual information that is not easily labeled (e.g., bead memory), or information that requires sequencing or syntactic ability (e.g., sentence memory) may be difficult for males, because these tasks require organizational or analytic skill. Freund and Reiss found the same dissociation between abstract and meaningful visual memory in the females. Other studies of females with fragile X syndrome have found a consistent pattern of relative weakness on subtests that require visual–spatial, quantitative, and auditory short-term memory skills (e.g., Brainard, Schreiner, & Hagerman, 1991; Kemper, Hagerman, Ahmad, & Mariner, 1986; Miezejeski et al., 1986). However, long-term memory for meaningful verbal information is a significant strength for females with fragile X syndrome, and they often perform above mental age level in this area (Bennetto & Pennington, in press).

SPATIAL ABILITIES

Both males and females with fragile X syndrome have demonstrated an apparent deficit in spatial ability. Visual–spatial tasks, such as Block Design on Wechsler tests, are typically among the lowest IQ subtests in profiles of individuals with fragile X syndrome (see, e.g., Kemper et al., 1986; Theobold, Hay, & Judge, 1987). Kemper and colleagues (1986) found a deficit in spatial short-term memory in a group of males, and Mazzocco, Hagerman, Cronister-Silverman, and Pennington (1992) found a pattern of weaker figural than verbal memory in a sample of expressing females. Individuals with fragile X syndrome also typically show deficits in arithmetic (Dykens, Hodapp, & Leckman, 1987; Kemper et al., 1986).

EXECUTIVE FUNCTIONS

There is clear evidence of a specific deficit in executive functions in women with fragile X syndrome (Bennetto, Pennington, Porter, Taylor, & Hagerman, 2001; Mazzocco et al., 1992; Mazzocco, Pennington, & Hagerman, 1993). Moreover, X activation ratio in such women predicts executive function (Bennetto et al., 2001). Furthermore, in these studies, the deficits in executive function remained after the authors covaried out the effects of IQ. There is preliminary evidence of executive deficits in males with fragile X syndrome (Bennetto & Pennington, in press).

In addition to impairment on standard executive function tasks, individuals with fragile X syndrome tend to show a pattern of deficits on other tasks that is consistent with impaired executive functioning.

Boys with fragile X syndrome perform worse on the sequential processing score than the simultaneous processing score of the Kaufman Assessment Battery for Children (Dykens, Hodapp, & Leckman, 1987; Kemper et al., 1988). Tasks of sequential processing, such as imitating sequential hand movements, often rely on an individual's ability to hold a sequence of actions online in working memory and formulate a motor plan to execute a response. Other tasks of motor sequencing have been shown to be sensitive to frontal lobe deficits (Kolb & Whishaw, 1990). This dissociation between performance on sequential and simultaneous tasks provides further neurocognitive differentiation between individuals with fragile X syndrome and Down syndrome. In contrast to boys with fragile X syndrome, individuals with Down syndrome showed no differences between levels of simultaneous and sequential processing (Pueschel, Gallagher, Zartler, & Pezzullo, 1987; Hodapp et al., 1992).

SOCIAL AND BEHAVIORAL PHENOTYPE

The social and behavioral phenotype in fragile X syndrome has also been studied. This has already been described in the previous section on autism, since males with fragile X syndrome have some of the symptoms of autism. One striking symptom is their marked avoidance of eye contact, as well as social anxiety and shyness. Nonetheless, they have more interest in social interactions than individuals with autism. Females with fragile X syndrome exhibit shyness, social anxiety, and problems with mood (Hagerman, 1999).

The constellation of behavioral problems often observed in individuals with fragile X syndrome is also consistent with a deficit in executive function, including distractibility, impulsivity, and difficulty with attentional control and with transitions or shifting from one cognitive set to another (Hagerman, 1987). A deficit in executive function would also help to explain a number of the deviant speech and language areas. For example, perseverative thinking, difficulty with topic maintenance, and tangential conversational style are all consistent with an executive function deficit. Evidence consistent with this hypothesis was found in a recent experimental study of discourse processing in females with fragile X syndrome (Simon, Keenan, Pennington, Taylor, & Hagerman, 2001). The discourse deficit in this sample correlated with both X activation ratio and a measure of verbal working memory.

Williams Syndrome

The neuropsychology of Williams syndrome provides an interesting contrast to what is found in both Down and fragile X syndromes. The following summary of the neuropsychological phenotype in Williams syndrome is based on three recent reviews (Bellugi et al., 1999; Mervis & Klein-Tasman, 2000; Mervis, Morris, Bertrand, & Robinson, 1999).

LEVEL AND TRAJECTORY OF IQ

The average IQ in Williams syndrome is somewhat higher than that found in Down and fragile X syndromes, and falls in the mild range of MR, with a mean IQ of about 60. For example, in a sample of 100 individuals with Williams syndrome, the mean IQ was 60, with a range from 40 to 100 (Bellugi et al., 1999). In another sample of 38 children and adolescents with Williams syndrome, the mean IQ was 59.3 (standard deviation = 10.7), with a range from 38 to 84 (Mervis et al., 1999). Roughly 25% of individuals with Williams syndrome will have IQs and adaptive behavior scores above the cutoff for MR, roughly 50% will fall in the mild range of MR, and the remaining 25% will have moderate or worse MR (Mervis & Klein-Tasman, 2000). Also in contrast to both Down and fragile X syndromes, there is no evidence for a decline in IQ in Williams syndrome. Raw scores on both language and spatial IQ measures show a moderate positive correlation with age ($r = .55–.59$) across childhood, whereas standard scores are not significantly correlated with age (Mervis et al., 1999). If there were an IQ decline, the correlation of raw scores with age would be smaller, and there would be a significant *negative* correlation between standard scores and age.

SPEECH AND LANGUAGE SKILLS

Another notable contrast is in terms of *speech and language* skills. Unlike results in Down syndrome, both verbal short-term memory (i.e., digit span) and receptive vocabulary (Peabody Picture Vocabulary Test—Revised) are above mental age level, and grammatical understanding is at mental age level, in groups with Williams syndrome (Bellugi et al., 1999; Mervis et al., 1999). Groups with Down syndrome are *below* mental age level on these aspects of language development. In both Down syndrome and Williams syndrome, moderate correlations between verbal short-term memory and language skills suggest that verbal short-term memory plays an important role in language development, whether below or above MA level.

In the other two MR syndromes considered here, Down and fragile X syndromes, and in autism, we have seen dissociations between structural language competence (phonological, lexical, and syntactic development) and pragmatic competence. Pragmatic language is a relative strength in groups with Down syndrome, despite their deficit in structural language, whereas it is a deficit in both autism and fragile X syndrome despite relatively preserved structural language. In Williams syndrome, we can say that at least some aspects of pragmatic language are a "super" strength. Such individuals are chatty and seek social contact; their narratives exhibit hyperaffectivity and a greater than normal use of affective prosody to convey meaning (Bellugi et al., 1999).

SPATIAL ABILITIES

Williams syndrome is also distinct from these other syndromes in terms of spatial cognition, which is consistently *below* mental age expectation in this disorder, whereas it is a relative strength in autism and Down syndrome. For example, subjects with Williams syndrome do very poorly on drawing and block design tasks, as well as on spatial tasks that do not require production of a spatial pattern (i.e., judgment of line orientation; see Bellugi et al., 1999). Their performance on block design is consistently poor, both in absolute terms and relative to their other abilities. Thus, an operational definition of this profile across Differential Ability Scales subtests showed excellent sensitivity and specificity (both above .90) in discriminating individuals with Williams syndrome from those with other developmental disabilities (Mervis et al., 1999). The sensitivity and specificity of this profile is holding up in new samples (Mervis & Klein-Tasman, 2000). Despite this pronounced deficit in spatial cognition, individuals with Williams syndrome are relatively unimpaired in recognizing faces (Bellugi et al., 1999) and perform similarly to other groups in processing global aspects of spatial stimuli (Mervis et al., 1999). In fact, reducing the salience of the global pattern on the block design model by leaving spaces between blocks improved the performance of individuals with Williams syndrome, just as it did for individuals with other developmental disabilities or younger, typically developing children (Mervis et al., 1999).

EXECUTIVE FUNCTIONS

In terms of executive functions, there is less research on Williams syndrome than on the other groups considered here. One study found that children with Williams syndrome performed similarly on two executive tasks to a group of children with Prader–Willi syndrome; the two groups were also similar in both mental age and chronological age (Tager-Flusberg, Sullivan, & Boshart, 1997). This one result suggests that executive functions are not spared in Williams syndrome. Other comparisons are needed to determine whether executive functions in Williams syndrome are below mental age level, as they are in fragile X syndrome and in older individuals with autism.

Although in Williams syndrome there is a marked dissociation between verbal and spatial cognition in the cognitive profile, these dissociated domains nonetheless tap some common processes. For example, the partial (controlling for age) correlations between a block design measure and three verbal measures—backwards digit span (arguably a measure of verbal working memory), receptive vocabulary, and receptive syntax—ranged from .50 to .52 (Mervis et al., 1999). This result argues for the importance of considering both general and specific cognitive processes in this MR syndrome, as discussed earlier.

SOCIAL AND BEHAVIORAL PHENOTYPE

In terms of social and behavioral phenotype, Williams syndrome also has a distinctive profile that contrasts with some of the other MR syndromes considered here. Both clinical observations and formal temperament and personality measures document "high gregariousness, strong orientation toward other people, high empathy, high sensitivity to criticism, and high anxiety" (Mervis & Klein-Tasman, 2000, p. 157). Strong social drive appears soon in the development of children with Williams syndrome; at early ages, they stare very intently at a new person (Mervis & Klein-Tasman, 2000). This intensity of eye contact is the direct opposite of what is observed in fragile X syndrome. Theory of mind performance in Williams syndrome sheds light on potential dissociations within the domain of social cognition. Despite their empathy and hyperaffectivity (and better than mental age level performance on the Eyes task, discussed earlier), individuals with Williams syndrome consistently perform at or below mental age level on false-belief tasks (Tager-Flusberg et al., 1997; Tager-Flusberg, Boshart, & Baron-Cohen,

1998; Tager-Flusberg & Sullivan, 2000). Since the social behavior of these children is in many ways the *opposite* of that found in autism, it is striking that there is nonetheless a deficit on theory of mind tasks in Williams syndrome. This result further questions whether a deficit in representational or cognitive theory of mind could be the primary deficit in autism. How could such a primary deficit be associated with opposite profiles of social behavior? Instead, other aspects of intersubjectivity, perhaps those related to social orientation, emotion, and empathy, may be more important in accounting for the opposite social phenotypes found in Williams syndrome and autism. Tager-Flusberg and Sullivan (2000) have distinguished social-cognitive (i.e., representational theory of mind) and social-perceptual (e.g., emotion perception and empathy) aspects of social knowledge. They argue that children with Williams syndrome are impaired in the former but not the latter. Deficits in social-cognitive knowledge could interfere with maintaining friendships, which is a problem for individuals with Williams syndrome despite their high social drive (Mervis & Klein-Tasman, 2000). Friendships usually require communication skills that depend on taking another's knowledge into account. Being chatty and empathetic but nonetheless talking about topics irrelevant to the listener could alienate potential friends.

In summary, across these three MR syndromes and autism, we have evidence for associations and dissociations that have important implications for developmental theory. In terms of associations, problems with executive functions and attention are found in all four syndromes; problems with false-belief tasks are widespread as well. We also have evidence for three double dissociations: (1) spatial cognition versus structural language (Down syndrome vs. Williams syndrome), (2) structural language versus pragmatic language (Down syndrome vs. autism and fragile X syndrome), and (3) pragmatic language versus spatial cognition (autism vs. Williams syndrome). These double dissociations provide evidence that these different cognitive domains can develop somewhat independently of each other.

One interesting possibility is a competitive relation between language and spatial development, especially in a brain with diminished processing capacity (as is the case in MR). If language development is compromised (either by a social deficit, as in autism, or by a deficit specific to language, such as a deficit in verbal short-term memory, as in Down syndrome), then there is overdevelopment of spatial cognition. If language development is not compromised, than there is underdevelopment of spatial cognition (as is the case in Williams syndrome). So initial deficits in one area may set off a cascade of secondary effects.

But I do not want to argue for total independence across different developmental domains in MR. Even the areas of strength in each MR syndrome are still below age level, and dissociated domains are nonetheless correlated, as illustrated earlier. So various MR syndromes appear to share a general cognitive deficit that affects all domains of cognitive development to some extent, whereas they may differ in their profiles of strengths and weaknesses in specific cognitive domains. The challenge for a neuroscientific account of MR is to specify which aspects of altered brain development produce the general cognitive deficit, and which lead to the specific cognitive profile.

This chapter also illustrates the considerable progress toward an integrated, neuroscientific understanding of these three MR syndromes, indeed *more* progress than for many of the psychopathologies considered in this book. What we learn about pathways running from genes to brain to behavior in these MR syndromes will likely provide useful hypotheses for studying other disorders.

Treatment

The main treatments for MR are behavioral and involve intensive early intervention and special education. Individuals with more severe levels of MR nonetheless need lifelong sheltered living situations. Behavior modification (applied behavioral analysis) can be useful in reducing troublesome behaviors and increasing appropriate ones, just as is true for autism.

Medications are used to treat problematic symptoms, including symptoms of comorbid disorders. For example, Ritalin effectively reduces symptoms of ADHD in persons with MR. Naltrexone, an opioid antagonist, effectively reduces self-injurious behavior. With more severe forms of MR, antipsychotic medications are used to control difficult behaviors, although there are concerns about overuse.

In terms of *prevention*, improved prenatal care, including reduced exposure to teratogens such as alcohol, would lower MR rates. Improved postnatal health care and nutrition would likely also make a contribution. An intensive early educational intervention program, the Abecedarian project (Ramey & Campbell, 1984), reduced the rates of MR among children at high risk because of prematurity and low birth weight.

Prenatal genetic testing followed by termination of abnormal pregnancies has reduced the rates of some genetic MR syndromes, although not every family would find this means of prevention ethically acceptable.

DYSLEXIA AND OTHER LANGUAGE DISORDERS

The three main types of abnormal language development are discussed in this section: (1) developmental dyslexia, or reading disability (RD), in which the defining problems are with written rather than spoken language; (2) phonological disorder (PD), in which the defining problem lies in the development of speech production; and (3) specific language impairment (SLI), in which the defining problem involves the development of expression or comprehension of spoken language. There are proposed subtypes of each, but the external validity of these subtypes is still an open issue, as we will see. At the same time, these three disorders are comorbid and share etiological risk factors, which suggests that we may be able to consolidate them to some extent. For example, many children with PD also have SLI and later develop RD. Do such children have three distinct disorders, or are all three disorders different manifestations of the same neuropsychological deficit and underlying etiology? In other words, is there a severity continuum, such that the most severe cases have all three disorders, the moderately severe cases have PD and RD, and the mildest cases have only RD? Although we do not yet have complete answers to these questions, relevant evidence is reviewed here. I next consider the history of these disorders.

Dyslexia, or RD, was first described over a century ago by Pringle-Morgan (1896) and Kerr (1897), but real advances in our understanding of its cognitive phenotype have only come about in the last 20 years. These advances have made it much clearer that dyslexia is a type of language disorder whose underlying deficit involves the development of phonological representations. Earlier theories of dyslexia that postulated a basic deficit in visual processing focused on the reversal errors made by individuals with dyslexia, such as writing *b* for *d* or "was" for "saw." Orton (1925, 1937) termed this deficit "strephosymbolia"—"twisted symbols"—and hypothesized that this visual problem arose because of a failure of hemispheric dominance, in which mirror images of visual stimuli were not inhibited, thus leading to reversal errors. Vellutino (1979) demonstrated that such reversal errors in dyslexia, restricted to processing print in one's own language, were thus really linguistic rather than visual in nature. However, it is still possible that other sorts of visual processing problems correlate with dyslexia.

Leonard's (2000) history of SLI and PD is briefly summarized here. The first case report of a child with limited speech was published by Gall in 1822, and many case reports followed, spurred in part by advances in understanding acquired aphasia (hence, the term "congenital aphasia" for such cases). The children in these case reports had extremely limited speech output despite apparently normal language comprehension and nonverbal intelligence. Later labels included "developmental aphasia" and "developmental dysphasia." Eventually, this neurological terminology was dropped in favor of terms such as "developmental language disorder" or "specific language impairment." The definitions of these latter categories excluded children who had an acquired aphasia or other identifiable cause for their language problem. Thus, these definitions focused on children with an *idiopathic* problem in language development. Other changes in 20th-century conceptions of SLI and PD have included (1) increasing awareness that such children have language problems other than limited speech output, such as grammatical deficits; and (2) increasing emphasis on subtypes, such as receptive and expressive SLI.

Definition

All current definitions of RD, PD, and SLI have two parts: (1) a diagnostic threshold and (2) a list of exclusionary conditions, which usually include a peripheral sensory impairment (e.g., deafness), a peripheral deficit in the vocal apparatus, acquired neurological insults, environmental deprivation, and other, more severe developmental disorders (e.g., MR and autism). Setting a diagnostic threshold for these disorders on what are essentially continua is inevitably somewhat arbitrary, as has been discussed repeatedly in other chapters. For these three disorders, a further issue is whether the diagnostic threshold should be relative to age or IQ expectations for the particular ability involved.

Traditional definitions of RD and SLI have required that the reading or language deficit be significantly below the child's IQ level (nonverbal IQ in the cases of PD and SLI), which means that many children with reading or language problems will not fit the definition, even though their reading or language is significantly below age expectations and interferes with everyday functioning. Besides excluding some children from services, IQ discrepancy definitions face a fundamental logical problem. Measures of IQ, even nonverbal IQ, are moderately correlated with measures of both reading and language, but we do not fully understand the causal basis of this correlation. IQ could influence reading and language development, reading and language development could influence IQ, or all three could be related to a third variable. As an example of a potential third variable, certain cognitive skills that are important for reading and language development, such as verbal short-term memory, are also part of what is measured by an IQ test. IQ discrepancy definitions assume that the causal basis of this correlation is that IQ influences reading and language development, the first possibility listed earlier. According to this logic, children with lower IQs inevitably have poor reading and language skills, and for a *different* reason (low IQ) than children with higher IQs. But it is very likely that the other two possibilities are also involved in these correlations. Reading and language skills very likely affect IQ scores, even nonverbal IQ scores, and these measures also share cognitive components. Therefore, children who are age, but not IQ, discrepant may have the most severe cases of RD or SLI, and they likely have the *same* underlying cognitive deficit as children who meet the IQ discrepancy definition. It seems ironic that the definition of a disorder should systematically exclude individuals with the most severe form of the disorder!

There is now an emerging research literature on the external validity of the distinction between age and IQ discrepancy definitions of RD and SLI (see reviews in Bishop, 1997, and Fletcher, Foorman, Shaywitz, & Shaywitz, 1999). In the case of RD, there is no evidence for external validity in terms of either the underlying deficit (i.e., in phonological processing) or the kind of treatment that is helpful. Although there is less research on this issue with regard to SLI, what research there is does not support the validity of this distinction (Bishop, 1997). Researchers may still want to use an IQ discrepancy to identify the "purest" cases, but retaining this distinction for clinical purposes seems difficult to justify if the same treatments are efficacious for children with and without an IQ discrepancy.

Epidemiology

Prevalence estimates, of course, depend on definition. For RD, typical estimates using an IQ discrepancy definition range from 5 to 10% (Benton & Pearl, 1978). In an epidemiological sample of second and third graders, a regression-based, IQ discrepancy definition of RD (i.e., 1.5 standard deviations or more below the reading score predicted by

IQ) identified 8.7–9.8% of boys and 6.0–6.9% of girls as having RD (Shaywitz, Shaywitz, Fletcher, & Escobar, 1990). If a similar age discrepancy definition is used (1.5 standard deviations or more below the mean for age), about the same proportion (7%) of the population will meet this definition. Of course, less extreme cutoffs will identify a larger proportion of children. However, some children will only meet the first definition (high ability, poor readers) and others will only meet the second (low ability, poor readers), so researchers and clinicians need to decide which groups to diagnose with RD. Ideally, researchers should include all these groups and test how their results vary as a function of which definition of RD is utilized.

The gender ratio in epidemiological RD samples generally shows a slight but sometimes nonsignificant male predominance, from about 1.3 to 1.7:1 (Smith, Gilger, & Pennington, 2001). For example, in the Shaywitz and colleagues (1990) study just discussed, the gender ratios were 1.26:1 in second grade and 1.50:1 in third grade. In contrast, there is a greater male predominance in referred samples, from about threefold to sixfold (Smith et al., in press). The difference in gender ratios between epidemiological and referred samples means that girls with RD are *less* likely to be referred for services!

The reason for this differential rate of referral appears to be higher rates of comorbid externalizing disorders (ADHD, ODD, and CD) in boys with RD; girls with RD are more likely to have comorbid internalizing disorders, such as dysthymia (Willcutt & Pennington, 2000). In this population-based sample, the overall male:female gender ratio was 1.3:1, similar to other epidemiological samples. However, among subjects with RD and a comorbid externalizing disorder, the male predominance was twice as great, 2.6:1, and in the range found in referred samples.

In this study and others in our lab, we have tested the basis of the comorbidities of RD. Once we have controlled for comorbidity with ADHD, the association between RD and either ODD or CD becomes nonsignificant (Willcutt & Pennington, 2000). A longitudinal study in our lab (Boetsch, 1996) found that children with future dyslexia did not differ from controls on measures of dysthymia before kindergarten, indicating that dysthymia is secondary to dyslexia. In contrast, in that same study, the children with future dyslexia did have higher rates of ADHD symptoms before kindergarten, consistent with our other results indicating a shared genetic etiology between RD and ADHD (Willcutt, Pennington, & DeFries, 2000a; Willcutt et al., in press). So some of the comorbidities of RD (i.e., dysthymia, ODD, and CD) are secondary to RD or comorbid ADHD. The remaining ones—PD, SLI, and ADHD—all appear to be due to a shared genetic etiology, as I discuss later.

The prevalence of PD in a recent epidemiological sample was 3.8%, with a male:female gender ratio of 1.5:1 (Shriberg, Tomblin, & McSweeny, 1999). In five earlier epidemiological samples reviewed by Shriberg and colleagues (1999), prevalence ranged from 2 to 13% (mean = 8.2%), and the male:female gender ratio ranged from 1.5 to 2.4 (mean = 1.8). As is the case for RD, gender ratios for PD are higher in referred samples. This study also found that about one-third of children with PD had SLI. Other studies of PD have found that it is also comorbid with ADHD (e.g., Beitchman, Hood, & Inglis, 1990). It is interesting that the gender ratio for PD is similar to that for RD, and that both are comorbid with ADHD and SLI.

Prevalence rates for SLI range from about 5% to 8%. In the Shriberg and colleagues (1999) study, the prevalence was 8.1%, with a male: female gender ratio of 1.25. Just as was true for RD and PD, the male: female gender ratio was higher in referred samples, about 3:1 (Smith et al., in press). Besides its comorbidities with RD and PD, SLI is also comorbid with ADHD (Beitchman et al., 1990).

In summary, RD, PD, and SLI are all comorbid with each other, and each is comorbid with ADHD. As we see next, there is evidence for shared genetic risk factors across these disorders.

Etiology

In the last two decades, our understanding of the etiology of dyslexia has increased considerably due to advances in both behavioral and molecular genetics. For 50 years after it was first described by Kerr (1897) and Pringle-Morgan (1896), evidence for recurrence of dyslexia in families was repeatedly documented in case reports, leading Hallgren (1950) to undertake a more formal genetic epidemiological study of a large sample of families. Besides conducting the first test of the mode of transmission, Hollgren's comprehensive monograph also documented several recently rediscovered characteristics of dyslexia: (1) The male: female ratio is nearly equal, about 1.5:1 (Shaywitz et al., 1990; Wadsworth, DeFries, Stevenson, Gilger, & Pennington, 1992), and (2) there is not a significant association between dyslexia and non-right-handedness (Pennington, Smith, Kimberling, Green, & Haith, 1987). Hallgren also documented co-occurrence of dyslexia with other language disorders.

Although Hallgren and his predecessors provided considerable evidence that dyslexia is familial, all of this data came from referred samples. Modern family studies using epidemiological samples have repeatedly confirmed the familiality of RD (Gilger et al., 1991). Roughly between 30% and 50% of the children of parents with RD will develop RD, a relative risk that is roughly four to eight times that found in controls (Gilger et al., 1991; Pennington & Lefly, 2001). It has taken modern twin studies to demonstrate that this familiality is substantially genetic, and modern linkage studies to begin actually to locate the genes involved. Unlike the situation in Hallgren's time, we now have very strong, converging evidence that dyslexia is both familial and heritable (see DeFries & Gillis, 1993, for a review). We can also reject the hypotheses of classic, X-linked or simple recessive autosomal transmission, at least in the vast majority of cases. There is also evidence that dyslexia is genetically heterogeneous. Perhaps most importantly, evidence supports Hallgren's observation that what looks like autosomal dominant transmission occurs in many families with dyslexia. So there do appear to be loci with sizable effects acting in a dominant or additive fashion on the transmission of reading problems.

However, we can place several important constraints on Hallgren's hypothesis of a monohybrid, autosomal dominant gene influencing dyslexia. First, it is very unlikely to be one gene, because of the evidence for genetic heterogeneity. Second, it may not be a gene influencing dyslexia per se, since the familiality, heritability, and transmission results for normal variations in reading skills are not clearly different from those for dyslexia (Gilger, Borecki, DeFries, & Pennington, 1994). The finding of a major locus effect on the transmission of normal reading skills, which acts to depress reading scores, suggests that the same loci may be involved in the transmission of both normal reading skills and dyslexia. If this is true, then people with dyslexia would just have more of the unfavorable alleles at these loci and/or more environmental risk factors, such that their reading scores were pushed beyond the cutoff for dyslexia. So reading skill is a quantitative trait that is likely influenced by multiple quantitative trait loci (QTLs); dyslexia, or RD, is just an extreme portion of the distribution of this quantitative trait. As we have seen, this view of the etiology of dyslexia is very consistent with that found for other psychopathologies.

In summary, several hypotheses about the transmission of dyslexia can be rejected on the basis of available data reviewed in Pennington (1994):

1. Dyslexia is not an X-linked disorder, and there is little evidence of parental gender effects on transmission. However, there is converging evidence for gender differences in penetrance, which would produce the slight preponderance of males that is often observed.

2. Simple polygenic/multifactorial transmission can be rejected, because there is a major locus effect in several samples that acts in an additive or dominant, but not in a recessive, fashion.

3. A monogenic hypothesis can be rejected, because dyslexia is genetically heterogeneous.

4. A necessary "disease" allele hypothesis can be rejected, because there is evidence for a major locus effect on the transmission of normal variation in reading skills.

A remaining hypothesis that fits these empirical data is that a small number of QTLs underlie the transmission of both dyslexia and normal variations in reading skills.

Given the strong possibility that the major loci contributing to dyslexia are QTLs, and given the evidence for genetic heterogeneity, traditional linkage analysis (of large, extended families with dyslexia) is not the most appropriate method to identify these loci. Instead, sibling-pair linkage analysis is more appropriate, as discussed earlier in the Genetic Methods section. By selecting sibling pairs in which at least one sibling has an extreme score, we can perform linkage analyses that screen for genetic loci influencing extreme scores on a continuous measure.

Using such a method, we found evidence for a QTL on the short arm of chromosome 6 across two independent samples of sib pairs and two sets of genetic markers (Cardon et al., 1994). Each sample provided significant evidence of a quantitative trail locus located in a 2-cM region of the interval between the D65105 and TNFB markers, which are situated in 6p21.3.

There have now been three replications of this finding (Fisher et al., 1999; Gayan et al., 1999; Grigorenko et al., 1997). So a QTL influencing dyslexia on chromosome 6p21.3 has now been found in five different samples by three independent laboratories. Grigorenko, Wood, Meyer, and Pauls (2000) expanded their sample and continued to find linkage to this region. However, two other studies failed to find linkage in this region, one in Canada (Field & Kaplan, 1998; Petryshen, Kaplan, Liu, & Field, 2000) and one in Germany (Nöthan et al., 1999). The reasons for these discrepant findings are unclear, but the distribution of risk alleles may vary across samples from different countries (i.e., genetic heterogeneity). A significant linkage has been found in the Canadian sample for markers on the *long* arm of chromosome 6, specifically on 6q13–16.2 (Petryshen, Kaplan, & Field, 1999).

In summary, the linkage between RD and the 6p21.3 region is one of the best replicated results in the genetics of complex behavioral disorders. Hence, it is quite likely that there is actually a gene in this region that influences reading skills. Work is proceeding to identify the gene. Two candidate genes in that region—a gene for GABA receptor (GABBR1), and a gene for myelin oligodendrocyte glycoprotein (MOG), both of which play a role in brain development—have now been excluded as the dyslexia locus (reviewed in Smith et al., in press).

Other replicated linkage regions for RD include 1p36, 2p15–16, and 15q21 (reviewed in Smith et al., 2001). In addition, a recently completed whole genome search of two separate samples identified the location of another likely QTL influencing RD on chromosome 18p (Fisher et al., 2002). Hence, at this point, it appears there are at least five QTLs that influence RD.

One of the most provocative conclusions of Grigorenko and colleagues (1997) is that cognitively dissociable components of the reading process are linked to separate genes, and that the mapping from genes to aspects of cognition may be quite close indeed. Besides replicating the 6p result, this study also found linkage for a different reading phenotype to 15q21. Specifically, Grigorenko and colleagues found that their single-word reading phenotype was significantly linked to 15q21, but that their phoneme segmentation phenotype was very significantly linked to 6p21.3. Their interpretation of these findings implied a genetic "double dissociation" between the genes influencing the two phenotypes, a somewhat bold conclusion, since the findings of differential linkage could be due to chance. But their general idea of differential genetic contributions to different cognitive components of a complex phenotype is well worth pursuing (Pennington, 1997).

As we see later, several cognitive components contribute to skill in printed word recognition. Although these components have substantial phenotypic and genetic covariance, there is also evidence for distinct genetic influences on some of these components, particularly orthographic and phonological coding. Orthographic coding involves lexical knowledge of the specific spelling of words (is it "rain" or "rane"?). Phonological coding involves using letter–sound correspondences to generate pronunciations of letter strings (does "rane" sound like a word?). So it is a reasonable hypothesis that different QTLs influencing reading skills might have differential effects on the development of orthographic and phonological coding.

Interestingly, the two recent replications of the chromosome 6 results (Fisher et al., 1999; Gayan et al., 1999) did not support this hypothesis. In these studies, deficits in both phonological and orthographic coding were linked to markers in the same region of chromosome 6. A later study by Grigorenko and colleagues (2000) found a similar result. So the jury is still out on the issue of differential genetic influences on different cognitive components of single-word reading skill. Work is under way to test more broadly for such differential effects using all five likely QTLs, and all the main cognitive components. This approach is highly relevant for the genetic dissection of the other complex behavioral phenotypes considered in this book.

Apart from the outcome of this issue, these exciting linkage findings for RD may eventually allow us to address how much variance in reading scores these genetic loci account for and, eventually, how frequently unaffected siblings have some unfavorable alleles at these loci, thus permitting the identification of protective factors. If a similar, sib-pair linkage study were conducted using probands selected for extremely *high* reading scores, we could determine whether different alleles at these same loci influence exceptionally good reading. If so, we could conclude that the same QTLs are affecting reading scores across the whole distribution. If not, then we would have direct evidence that dyslexia is etiologically distinct. Most importantly, once these genes are clearly identified, we can begin to trace the dynamic, developmental pathways that run from genes to brain to behavior.

There is also converging evidence that both SLI and PPD are familial and moderately heritable (see reviews in Bishop, 1997, and Smith et al., in press). Group heritability estimates (h^2_g) for SLI were .45 in the Tomblin and Buckwalter (1998) twin study and ranged from .47 to .93 for different SLI phenotypes in another twin sample (Bishop, North, & Donlan, 1995). PD is also moderately heritable (Bishop et al., 1995; Lewis & Thompson, 1992).

Researchers have begun to examine the etiological relations among RD, PD, and SLI. Lewis, Ekelman, and Aram (1989) found that PD is cofamilial with RD. Lewis (1992) found evidence for shared familial influences on PD and SLI; Bishop and colleagues (1995) provided evidence that the basis of this cofamiliality is in part genetic. But more research is needed to clarify the etiological relations among these three disorders. Obviously, progress in mapping QTLs for each disorder will greatly facilitate our understanding of both shared and distinct genetic influences on these three disorders, and on their relation to ADHD.

The main linkage result thus far for SLI and PD was first found in an interesting family (KE) with an autosomal dominant speech and language disorder. Their disorder was linked to markers on 7q31 (Fisher, Vargha-Khadem, Watkins, Monaco, & Pembrey, 1998). The phenotype in this family includes both a form of PD (severe oral–motor dyspraxia) and SLI (poor performance on a wide range of language measures), as well as somewhat lower IQ. Interestingly, this locus was *not* identified in a whole genome search for RD (Fisher et al., in press). The contribution of the known RD loci to both PD and SLI remains to be tested.

Since the heritabilities of all three disorders are roughly 50%, there must also be significant environmental risk factors for each. Candidates that have been explored include language input by caretakers and otitis media. However, only a threshold amount of language input from caretakers appears necessary for normal language development, so only an extreme reduction in language input is likely to be a risk factor for PD or SLI (see discussion in Bishop, 1997). Otitis media would also cause deprivation by producing a temporary conductive hearing loss; however, there is not a convincing association between otitis media and any of these three disorders (Bishop, 1997). It is well known that parents provide dramatic subcultural variations in the stimulation for early literacy skills (Pennington, 1991), including reading to children and playing rhyming games. It seems likely that these variations would affect literacy outcome, but this possibility has yet to be studied using a genetically sensitive design. In summary, more rigorous work is needed to identify environmental risk factors for these three disorders.

Brain Mechanisms

Structural Neuroimaging Studies

For RD, the main techniques utilized have been autopsy studies of a small number of cases and structural MRI studies. These studies of people with dyslexia have found size differences in the temporal lobe, especially the planum temporale (Galaburda, 1988; Hynd et al., 1990; Larsen, Høien, & Ödegaard, 1990; but see Schultz, Cho, Staib, Kier, &

Fletcher, 1994, and Rumsey et al., 1997a); insula (Hynd et al., 1990); corpus callosum (Duara, Kusch, & Gross-Glenn,1991; Hynd, Hall, Novey, & Eliopulos, 1995; Larsen, Høien, & Ödegaard, 1992); and thalamus (Galaburda & Livingstone, 1993; Jernigan, Hesselink, Stowell, & Tallal, 1991), although no finding for a given structure has been consistently replicated across studies. Moreover, samples in these studies were small and usually highly selected, and both anatomical definitions and methods of image acquisition varied across studies (Filipek, 1995). Two recent studies failed to replicate differences in the planum temporale found in the autopsy studies and some early MRI studies (Rumsey et al., 1997a; Schultz et al., 1994).

To test for brain size differences in RD, Pennington and colleagues (1999) examined cortical and subcortical brain structures in the largest dyslexic sample yet studied (75 individuals with RD and 22 controls). These subjects were single members of twin pairs from a large, population-based sample of twin pairs with and without RD. All analyses compared the dyslexic group and control groups, controlling for age, gender, and IQ. We found significant group-by-structure interactions for the major neocortical subdivisions. Although the overall volume of the neocortex did not differ by group, the insula and anterior superior neocortex were significantly smaller in the RD group, whereas the retrocallosal cortex was larger. In contrast, there was neither an overall group difference nor a group-by-structure interaction in the analysis of the subcortical structures. When subjects with ADHD were removed from the sample, the results were essentially the same. In summary, in this study, most brain structures did not differ in size in RD, but there were subtle differences in cortical development.

There do not appear to be structural studies of PD considered separately. The few structural studies of SLI also find altered symmetry relations in posterior temporal and anterior language regions, as well as more widespread volume reductions, including some subcortical structures, such as the thalamus (Jernigan, Hesselink, Sowell, & Tallal, 1991; Plante, Swisher, Vance, & Rapcsak, 1991). However, the samples are small in these studies of SLI. Hence, more work is needed to clarify the structural phenotype in SLI and PD, and to test for commonalities across RD, PD, and SLI. It is also noteworthy that early focal lesions to either hemisphere disrupt language development temporarily but do not produce SLI (Bates et al., 2001). Consequently, the structural basis of these three disorders is likely to be a more widespread change in brain development.

Functional Neuroimaging Studies

We were unable to find fMRI or PET studies of PD or SLI. Rumsey (1996) has reviewed studies of individuals with RD, which used a variety of reading and language tasks. All studies have found some differences in brain activity when individuals with dyslexia are compared to controls, but, again, the differences are found in multiple brain regions, arguing against a localized brain difference underlying dyslexia. Differences include (1) reduced activity in Wernicke's area accompanied by an increase in activity in a more posterior location, the temporoparietal junction; (2) increased metabolism in the lingual gyrus and greater symmetry of activation in lingual and prefrontal regions; (3) greater activation in the medial–temporal lobe bilaterally; and (4) reductions in left posterior–temporal cortex, near Wernicke's area, and left temporoparietal cortex, near the angular gyrus, during rhyme detection; but normal anterior–temporal and inferior–frontal activation during a syntactic task, as well as unexpected right-hemisphere reductions during a nonverbal tonal memory task.

Three later studies deserve mention. Paulesu and colleagues (1996) found reduced activity in the left insula in their dyslexic group, while activity in both posterior and anterior language areas was normal; they argue that this pattern of results suggests a disconnection syndrome. Rumsey, Nace, and colleagues (1997) used the same methodology as Rumsey and colleagues (1997b) to study adult males with dyslexia, who, like controls, showed similar locations of activity in response to both orthographic and phonological coding tasks. Hence, the predictions of dual-process theory do not fit with the patterns of brain activity for either normal readers or readers with dyslexia in these studies. Individuals with dyslexia did differ by having reduced blood flow in posterior perisylvian areas on all four tasks. These results are consistent with the first and fourth results in the previous list, but do not replicate the insula difference found by Paulesu and colleagues (1996). Finally, Eden and colleagues (1996) studied a subset of persons with dyslexia and controls from Rumsey, Nace, and colleagues (1997) on a visual motion sensitivity task; subjects with dyslexia performed more poorly on this task than controls and also showed activity reductions in part of the ventral visual pathway, specifically, area MT/V5. These results suggest possible visual processing deficits in both brain and behavior in persons with dyslexia who also have well-documented phonological processing differences in brain and behavior.

To summarize the functional neuroimaging studies of persons with dyslexia, some of the observed differences (i.e., greater activation) may reflect greater effort by the dyslexic group, while others may reflect a compensatory strategy (i.e., a posterior shift of activation), and still others, impaired processing capacity (i.e., decreased activation), but the studies do not experimentally establish which of these is the case. More generally, the causal relation between the observed brain imaging differences and the syndrome of dyslexia is ambiguous in these studies: The activity differences may cause dyslexia, or dyslexia may cause the activity differences (e.g., through a different history of print exposure), or both dyslexia and the activity differences may be caused by a third factor. So establishing causal links between brain and behavior is difficult because of possibly bidirectional causal influences.

Neuropsychology

This section first reviews the neuropsychology of RD and then considers PD and SLI. One key question concerns the degree of overlap among these three disorders at the neuropsychological level.

The recent advances in our understanding of the cognitive phenotype in dyslexia have built upon basic research focused on both human speech (Liberman, Cooper, Shankweiler, & Studdert-Kennedy, 1967) and skilled reading (Crowder, 1982; Just & Carpenter, 1987). Although the goal of reading is comprehension, which depends on many higher cognitive processes such as reasoning and memory, it turns out that a substantial proportion of the variation in reading comprehension, at least in children, can be accounted for by individual differences in the accuracy and speed of single printed word recognition (Perfetti, 1985).

To understand printed text, a reader must first be able to recognize individual words that compose the text and then understand them using many of the same comprehension processes that he or she would apply if the same message were spoken. A child brings to the task of learning to read considerable skill in listening comprehension, which has developed along with spoken language in the preschool years. Hence, it follows that the main thing the child needs to learn in order to comprehend text is to recognize single printed words. In fact, because using a spoken language is a species-typical human characteristic, virtually all children enter school with some degree of listening comprehension. There are obvious individual differences in children's listening comprehension that continue to develop, partly as a result of education (including reading itself), but children nonetheless enter school with a striking contrast between their skill in listening comprehension and lack of skill in printed-word recognition.

In contrast to spoken language, written language is a relatively recent cultural invention that is not universal across either spoken languages or individual humans; in fact, few spoken languages have scripts, and only a minority of the world's humans are literate. Moreover, because they are cultural inventions, scripts vary more in their conventions (e.g., the printed characters in orthography can stand for words, syllables, or phonemes) than do spoken languages, all of which combine phonemes to make words (Liberman & Liberman, 1990). A child must be explicitly taught to learn a written language, which is not the case for spoken language. Learning to speak is easy, but learning to read is hard. In fact, as I discuss later, part of what makes speaking easy—coarticulation—makes learning to read difficult.

Gough has formulated "the simple view of reading" (Gough & Walsh, 1991), in which reading comprehension (RC) equals the product of single printed-word recognition (WR) and listening comprehension (LC), or RC = WR × LC. There is considerable empirical support for this simple model of reading development. For example, Gough and Walsh (1991) found that in children the product of WR and LC correlates highly with RC (.84). Moreover, given that virtually all children begin school with some LC skills, we should expect that for early readers, the main contributor to individual RC differences is skill in WR. Consistent with this expectation, Curtis (1980) found that among second graders, the correlation between WR and RC is .78, whereas, LC had a negligible relation. She also found that by fifth grade, the balance between these two factors had shifted considerably; the correlation for WR was now .45, whereas LC had increased to .74. In other words, by fifth grade, most students had developed enough WR skill that individual LC differences emerged as the major factor limiting RC, but individual WR differences still played a substantial role. However, despite instruction, some children do not develop WR skill, so their LC continues to exceed considerably their WR ability. These are the children who have dyslexia, or RD.

Gough's view of reading is so simple that we might wonder who could disagree with it. A legitimate disagreement is that the comprehension processes used in reading text are more demanding than those used in LC. Written texts are longer and more complicated than most oral discourse, so they exert greater demands on working memory. In addition, the context to which they refer is not in the immediate environment, so the reader must construct a mental model of the written text's context.

A very different disagreement with Gough's simple view of reading is embodied in a highly influential but controversial view of reading development. Goodman (1986) has argued that learning to read could be as easy as learning to talk (a maturational view of reading), if only reading were taught in a way that makes it similarly meaningful. Instead, Goodman argues, traditional reading instruction has made learning to read difficult "by breaking whole (natural) language into bite-size, abstract little pieces" (Goodman, 1986, qtd. in Liberman & Liberman, 1990, p. 54). He argues that comprehending a text is a "psycholinguistic guessing game" in which a skilled reader only decodes some words and uses context and previous word knowledge to infer the meaning of the rest. Goodman's view of skilled reading has led to an instructional emphasis on guessing from context in the whole language approach.

The validity of this competing view can be evaluated by empirical research on what skilled readers actually do. Contrary to Goodman's (1986) theory, studies of eye movements during reading demonstrate that skilled readers fixate on virtually all content words in a text (Rayner & Pollatesek, 1989), decoding each word's phonology and meaning as they go (Share & Stanovich, 1995; Van Orden, Pennington, & Stone, 1990) . The few skipped words are highly predictable function words, such as "the," "and," "of," and "to" (O'Regan, 1979). Regardless of whether printed words are presented in isolation or in connected text, skilled readers identify them with similar speed and accuracy. This finding also argues against the use of context by skilled readers to guess the meaning of printed words (Adams, 1990). In fact, literate adults are actually much less likely than less literate adults to use guessing as a strategy (Perfetti & Lesgold, 1979). Only poor readers with faulty word recognition skills have to rely on guessing. There is an excellent reason why good readers do not use the guessing strategy: It does not work very well and often leads to major errors (Gough, Alford, & Holly-Wilcox, 1981). Guessing on content words is only correct about 10% of the time, whereas the predictability of function words (the only words that skilled readers are likely to skip) is much higher, about 40% (Gough, 1983). These function words are the most frequently occurring words in text (e.g., "the," the most frequently encountered word in English, accounts for 7.3% of the words in text). If we had beginning readers memorize by rote the 100 or so most frequently occurring words in the language, those words would account for about one-half of the words they encounter in typical school texts. Unfortunately, the remaining one-half of words they encounter varies enormously in frequency, with less frequently encountered words occurring fewer than 10 times in a whole year of reading. However, the less frequently a word occurs, and the harder it is to guess, the *more* the meaning of a passage depends on its correct interpretation (Torgesen, 1997). Consequently, a skilled reader needs some strategy besides either rote memorization or guesswork to ensure that these crucial, less frequently encountered words are recognized correctly.

The foregoing discussion clarifies why word recognition skill is crucial to reading comprehension, and why deficits in word recognition undermine reading development. But why do some children (i.e., those with dyslexia) have these deficits? To answer this question, we have to consider the cognitive mechanisms involved in WR, both in skilled reading and in reading development. It turns out that research on these mechanisms provides an important example of how intuitions about skilled performance in adults match neither the actual cognitive mechanism used by adults or those mechanisms important in development. In fact, a better understanding of reading development has contributed to a clearer understanding of adult performance.

So what happens cognitively when a skilled reader recognizes a printed word? A standard view has been that there is a rapid look-up procedure in a mental lexicon that contains the word's meaning and pronunciation. This procedure has been termed "direct access," and corresponds to our intuition of immediate and effortless recognition of printed words. According to this view, words are visual objects that we recognize in much the same manner as other visual objects in the world, such as chairs, tables, and cars. Of course, some printed words, like some objects, are unfamiliar. How do we recognize those? We can often derive the name for an unfamiliar printed word, unlike the case for objects, by "sounding it out," that is, by using our understanding of letter–sound correspondences to work out its pronunciation. This procedure for naming a printed word has been called "indirect," because it involves converting letters to sounds (i.e., graphemes to phonemes.) If we add the assumptions that direct access is the faster, preferred route for WR, that it does not involve phonological mediation, and that the slower, indirect route is more important in reading development when fewer words are recognized automatically, then we have the standard dual-route model of WR. Another important feature is that this model deals naturally with how we successfully read and understand homophones (we distinguish "four" from "for," and "knot" from "not,") and how we can pronounce unfamiliar words or even pseudowords.

This intuitively plausible and beguilingly simple model of WR has been the subject of considerable investigation and debate. How one conceptualizes the mechanisms used in the direct and indirect routes generally depends on fundamental issues in psycholinguistics and cognitive science. A good place to begin this story is with the adult patient GR (Marshall & Newcombe, 1966), who, after a gunshot wound to the head, had severe aphasia and dyslexia. The pattern of reading deficits exhibited by GR has come to be called "deep dyslexia." GR, who could not read nonwords, had a deficit in grapheme–phoneme conversion, also called "phonological coding." When he attempted to read real words, he sometimes made semantic errors, such as saying "vase" for "antique," apparently indicating some access to printed-word meaning despite impaired phonological coding (although the errors exhibited by GR and others with deep dyslexia indicate some minimal, residual phonological coding). This dissociation between phonological coding and semantics falsified an earlier, widely prevalent but very simple, serial, single-route model of WR. According to this model, a printed word is first converted to an abstract graphemic representation, then into a sequence of phonemes that in turn access meaning in the same fashion as a spoken word. Since GR could access meaning from printed words but could not perform grapheme–phoneme conversion (phonological coding), it was necessary to add a second direct route to this simple model, making it the standard, dual-route model I have just described. The new route provided "direct access" to word meaning from the abstract graphemic representation, bypassing the grapheme–phoneme conversion route. As I already mentioned, even without the data from GR, the revision of the simple, single-route model would have been necessary to deal with homophones and strange or exception words such as "yacht," whose pronunciation cannot be derived from the usual relations between letters and sounds.

Other patients like GR were found (Coltheart, Patterson, & Marshall, 1980), as well as patients with a cleaner selective deficit in phonological coding, called "phonological dyslexia." Most interesting were patients with an opposite performance profile: intact nonword reading but impaired reading of exception words. These patients were said to have a "surface dyslexia" (Patterson, Marshall, & Coltheart, 1985). The double dissociation between phonological and surface dyslexia was taken as very strong evidence in favor of the dual-route model of WR, which became the standard model of both normal and abnormal adult reading. Consistent with much linguistic theory at the time, this model assumed that grapheme–phoneme conversion depends on an abstract set of rules, similar to propositions in a logical system. Once the knowledge involved in grapheme–phoneme conversion was conceptualized in this fashion, then the necessity for a second, separate route or mechanism to deal with exceptions was inevitable. Similar dual-route models were postulated for other linguistic domains, such as forming the past tense of verbs. Many (regular) verbs conform to a rule—for example, "talk"–"talked" and "jump"–"jumped," but other (irregular) verbs do not—for example, "go"–"went" and "hit"–"hit."

This dual-route model of mature reading led to a similar model of normal and abnormal reading development (e.g., Frith, 1985) in which phonological coding was viewed as an earlier and slower strategy for recognizing words. Although normal children passed through this stage in their reading development, it was thought they eventually reached a mature strategy that relied almost exclusively on the faster, direct route that bypassed phonology. Children with reading problems were conceptualized as being "stuck" at different points in this sequence of stages. Hence, children with developmental phonological dyslexia were described as unable to master the phonological coding stage, whereas those with developmental surface dyslexia were thought of as stuck at the later, second stage: They had mastered phonological coding but could not master the direct-route strategy. In summary, the dual-route theory appeared to be comprehensive; it explained normal and abnormal adult reading, as well as normal and abnormal reading development.

However, closer examination of both skilled reading and reading development produced findings that did not fit the theory. In the case of skilled reading, evidence accumulated that virtually every instance of WR involved phonological activation, which happened very quickly, perhaps before the activation of spelling knowledge or meaning (Frost, 1998; Van Orden et al., 1990). So contrary to the theory, phonology was not bypassed in mature reading, and the time course of phonological coding was not slow.

In the case of reading development, examination of the developmental relations between reading nonwords and exception words revealed a closer connection than would be predicted if the two types of words were handled by independent mechanisms. Moreover, these findings were true for both normal children and those with developmental dyslexia. For example, Gough and Walsh (1991) found that in young, normal readers, the correlation between nonword and exception word reading was between .66 and .90, much higher than one would predict if the two kinds of stimuli were handled by separate mechanisms. They also found that some degree of skill in reading nonwords was necessary for any skill in reading exception words; all the children who read more than a few exception words correctly also displayed an ability to read nonwords, whereas the opposite was not the case. In other words, some proficiency in nonword reading appeared to be a prerequisite for reading exception words, again implying that some kind of common mechanism was involved in dealing with both kinds of stimuli.

Similar relations are also seen in developmental dyslexia. Extensive research has documented that persons with dyslexia read pseudowords (phonological coding) less accurately than even younger, normal readers matched on single, real-word reading accuracy (Rack, Snowling, & Olson, 1992). And consistent with Gough and Walsh's (1991) findings, people with dyslexia lag behind normal readers in speed and accuracy of reading both regular and exception words. So many persons with dyslexia have a deficit in phonological coding that at least partially explains a key defining symptom of their disorder: slower and less accurate recognition of both regular and exception words. Phonological coding skill underlies both normal and abnormal reading development, and reading both regular and exception words, which leads to the next question: What is the developmental precursor of phonological coding?

To answer this question, I need to say more about the speech sounds that the phonological code represents. A skilled reader knows that the spoken word "bag" is spelled with three letters, and that these letters correspond to the three "speech sounds" in the spoken word (Liberman, Shankweiler, Fischer, & Carter, 1974). However, because of the phenomenon of coarticulation, a sound spectrograph of this or other spoken words will not reveal discrete speech sounds; the articulatory gestures for each speech sound overlap in their production, allowing us to talk much faster than would be the case if we produced each speech sound separately. Linguists call these speech sounds "phonemes," explicit awareness of which is called "phoneme awareness," which can be measured by tasks that require a subject to count or manipulate the phonemes in a word. Interestingly, we can learn to talk without phoneme awareness, because spoken language can be processed in larger "chunks," such as words or syllables. But we cannot learn to read unless the language is a syllabary, such as Japanese Kana. Linguistic theory predicts (Mattingly, 1972), and extensive empirical research has confirmed (Wagner & Torgesen, 1987), that the ability to segment these phonemes in spoken speech is a prerequisite for learning to read an alphabetic language such as English. If the alphabet is a code, and if the letters correspond to phonemes, then how could we understand that code without phoneme awareness?

Thus, we might expect that deficiencies in phoneme awareness underlie the problems in phonological coding that characterize many persons with dyslexia, which is what numerous studies have found. Across the lifespan, groups of people with dyslexia have been shown to have deficits in phoneme awareness (Liberman, Shankweiler, Fischer, & Carter, 1974; Pennington, Van Orden, Smith, Green, & Haith, 1990). Recent evidence from our laboratory indicates that deficits in phoneme awareness are present before kindergarten and predict later dyslexia among children of parents with dyslexia (Pennington & Lefly, 2001), although these children also exhibit deficits in some other phonological skills. So the spoken language deficit in dyslexia is not restricted to phoneme awareness. Moreover, nondyslexic children of parents with dyslexia also have some milder phonological differences relative to otherwise similar children of nondyslexic parents, a result consistent with the view that familial risk for dyslexia is continuous, not discrete. In passing, I should also acknowledge that the relation between reading and phoneme awareness is reciprocal; while phoneme awareness is a prerequisite for normal reading, reading experience also facilitates phoneme awareness (Morais, Cary, Algeria, & Bertelson, 1979).

These facts about normal and dyslexic reading development question the dual-route model, because phonology is more central to reading than the model assumes, and because the putative, direct route is not independent of phonological coding. Therefore, we should question the validity of developmental dyslexia syndromes based on dual-route theory.

As already mentioned, following the standard dual-process account of both normal adult reading and acquired dyslexias, at least two developmental analogues have been postulated—developmental phonological dyslexia and developmental surface dyslexia (Frith, 1985; Temple, 1985)—due, respectively, to selective impairment in the phonological (or sublexical) versus lexical routes for word pronunciation. Case studies have reported relatively "pure" cases of developmental phonological dyslexia (Temple & Marshall, 1983) or developmental surface dyslexia

(Coltheart, Masterson, Byng, Prior, & Riddoch, 1983). However, the existence of pure cases does not prove the underlying theory, since the definition of a pure case involves a double circularity: (1) Different processing theories will identify different cases as "pure," so there is not a theory-neutral way of defining pure cases; and (2) the notion of a pure case itself presupposes some form of modularity (Van Orden, Pennington, & Stone, 2001).

Moreover, among normally developing readers, Bryant and Impey (1986) found many of the errors supposedly diagnostic of developmental surface dyslexia among younger, normal readers, questioning its validity as a distinct, developmental dyslexia syndrome. Hence, an epidemiological rather than a selective case study approach provides a better test of the separability of the hypothesized dual processes in normal and abnormal reading development.

Castles and Coltheart (1993) conducted such a study and found that among 53 children with dyslexia, 60% were significantly below age level on both nonword and exception word reading, whereas only about 20%, respectively, were selectively impaired on either; hence, the combined, pure subtypes (40%) occurred somewhat less frequently than the mixed subtype. This study indicates that, among persons with developmental dyslexia, pure cases are somewhat rarer than mixed ones. The predominance of mixed cases is problematic for the dual-process theory discussed earlier. Since the theory postulates that the lexical and sublexical processes are separate, it must postulate two deficits, one in the development of each process, in the mixed cases. (A modified dual-process theory in which both routes interact in development would be better able to explain mixed cases.)

In order to address this and other issues, Manis, Seidenberg, Doi, McBride-Chang, and Petersen (1996) conducted a replication study and considered how the connectionist framework developed by Seidenberg and McClelland (1989) could account for the results from both studies.

In their replication study, Manis and colleagues (1996) also found a similar predominance of the mixed subtype. In addition, like Bryant and Impey (1986), they found that subjects with a surface profile were similar to younger, normal readers, whereas those with a phonological profile were not, suggesting that the surface subtype represents a general developmental delay in word recognition, whereas the phonological subtype represents a specific deficit in phonological processing. These authors argue that to explain these two characteristics of the data, the dual-route theory must introduce additional assumptions.

So we have a paradox: The earlier, simple, single-route model of WR has been rejected, but its dual-route replacement does not completely fit the data either. To resolve this paradox, researchers have either modified the dual-route model (to allow interaction between routes) or turned to a different kind of cognitive model of reading, a connectionist one (Seidenberg & McClelland, 1989). Here, I present the connectionist alternative. Although not composed of separate routes or processes, a connectionist model can capture both rule-like and item-specific processing within the same mechanism. In this model, the development of visual word pronunciation is modeled by a three-layer neural network in which the input layer corresponds to graphemes, the output layer corresponds to phonemes, and the "hidden" or middle layer makes it possible to learn the complex, quasi-regular covariation between letters and sounds in English words. Through repeated training trials with feedback, the network gradually adjusts the weights on the connections between layers, until it reaches near-optimal performance in generating the pronunciation of single printed words. Although the network does not contain any explicit pronunciation rules, it can generalize from its training corpus to new exemplars, including pronounceable pseudowords. Because the correspondence between print and pronunciation in English is only quasi-regular, and the spelling of some words (e.g., "yacht") is unlike that of any others, the network must strike a balance between encoding rule-like and word-specific information. If it becomes too rule-like, then the network will mispronounce exception words on which it was trained (no network or human can pronounce a given exception word without training on that particular item). On the other hand, if it becomes too word-specific, the network will be unable to generalize and thus read either new words or pseudowords poorly.

Manis and colleagues (1996) discussed how such a connectionist model can explain the development of the three dyslexia subtypes observed in both their study and that of Castles and Coltheart (1993). Essentially, they explain the mixed and phonological types as arising from degraded phonological representations that impair nonword reading the most, exception word reading the next most, and regular word reading the least. Depending on the degree of phonological degradation, either a mixed or phonological subtype is observed. This is obviously a more parsimonious explanation than is provided by the dual-process account, which must explain in the mixed subtype the combination of impaired nonword and exception word reading, with dysfunction in two separate processes instead of by degrees of dysfunction in the same underlying mechanism. To explain the rarer surface subtype and its similarity to younger, normal readers, Manis and colleagues postulate a different alteration in the model: a reduced number of hidden units. With fewer hidden units, the model can learn (albeit less efficiently) the rule-like regularities in the input (rendering it able to pronounce regular words and nonwords), but such a model lacks the representational resources to learn word-specific patterns (such as are found in exception words). This account explains not only why people with surface dyslexia perform poorly on particular exception words, but also why they are rarely completely normal with regular and nonwords; once again, the single-process account is more parsimonious than the dual-route model. In addition, because learning word-specific patterns takes more trials for even a normal network to learn, this network's pattern of errors should resemble that of a "younger" normal network, just as children with the surface profile resemble younger, normal readers. (See also the reanalysis of these two studies by Stanovich, Siegel, & Gottardo, in press, who found that the surface subtype disappeared when reading level instead of chronological-age-level controls were used.)

This connectionist reinterpretation of subtypes of developmental dyslexia extends an earlier use of connectionist principles to critique the standard dual-process account of both mature reading and the acquired dyslexias (Plaut, 1995; Plaut, McClelland, Seidenberg, & Patterson, 1996; Seidenberg & McClelland, 1989; Van Orden et al., 1990, 2001). One basic criticism is the same as that discussed earlier, namely, that there are single-process accounts that explain the relevant reading phenomena as well as dual-route accounts; hence, they are preferable on the basis of parsimony. Both frequency and regularity or consistency effects can be produced by the same mechanism, whereas each effect is due to separate processes in a dual-route account. A second criticism is based on the empirical result that phonological mediation of mature reading is virtually ubiquitous and occurs very early in the time course of word recognition, neither of which is predicted by dual-route accounts discussed earlier, which hold that phonological mediation is optional and slow in mature word recognition. (There are other dual-route models in which both routes are always activated and may interact; which route predominates in performance is the result of a "horse race." But even these dual-route models do not deal with all the criticisms discussed here.) Perhaps most telling is the finding that virtually identical damage to a single, interdependent network can, on different runs, produce an apparent double dissociation of the sort that has been taken as strong confirmation of the hypothesized dual processes (Plaut, 1995).

At a more general level, these connectionist results question the transparency of the mapping from the symptoms of dyslexia, whether acquired or developmental, to underlying processing mechanisms. Hence, the connectionist results question the modularity and localizability of the cognitive components of reading, an issue that I also discussed in the section on Neuroimaging.

In summary, I have shown how a model based on intuitions about skilled performance in adults, and on data from lesion patients with acquired dyslexias, matched neither the actual cognitive mechanisms used by adult readers nor those used by normal children or children with dyslexia learning to read. So data from normal and abnormal development helped change the cognitive theory of mature performance.

Finally, although there have been attempts to simulate developmental dyslexia in a connectionist network, these attempts until recently (see Harm & Seidenberg, 1999) have started with the task of learning to read. A realistic simulation needs to start earlier in the developmental process, focusing initially on the development of phonological representations themselves, and showing how a network can be altered in such a way that speech imitation is fairly normal but phoneme awareness is impaired. It then needs to show that a network with immature phonological representations has trouble learning to read in the same ways as do individuals with dyslexia (which seems likely, given the arguments presented by Manis et al., 1996). In other words, we need a computational account of phonological development that will allow us to test the kinds of perturbations that will lead both to the later developmental differences that characterize dyslexia and to other disturbances of speech and language development. This account would then be a comprehensive model of normal and abnormal development in this domain, which is the long-term goal of cognitive theory and research. The next step toward a comprehensive understanding of dyslexia would be to understand the biological influences on these cognitive mechanisms.

I now turn to the neuropsychology of PD and SLI. Harm and Seidenberg (1999), whose modeling results provide a good transition to this topic, went beyond earlier connectionist models of reading and dyslexia by considering how the quality of phonological representations in the model affects speech perception. Deficits on standard speech perception tasks are found in some individuals with RD (Harm & Seidenberg, 1999), as well as in those with SLI and PD. Problems in speech perception very likely interfere with the development of both speech production and language comprehension, so a neuropsychological deficit that affects speech perception could be a common phenotype across all three disorders. Harm and Seidenberg found that a milder degradation of the quality of the phonological representations in their model affected only reading, not speech perception. With greater degradation, both speech perception and reading development were affected.

Their results support both a *phonological* and a *severity* hypothesis regarding the neuropsychological relation among these three disorders. The phonological hypothesis holds that the primary deficit in most RDs and at least some PDs and SLIs is immature or deficient phonological representations. The severity hypothesis holds that there is a continuum of severity of this deficit across these three disorders: RD only is least severe, RD + PD is more severe, and RD + PD + SLI is the most severe. These hypotheses cannot account for (1) the few individuals with developmental surface dyslexia, (2) individuals with PD but not RD or SLI, or (3) individuals with SLI but not PD or RD. So a necessary corollary of these hypotheses is that there must be neuropsychologically distinct subtypes of RD, PD, and SLI that have no deficit in phonological representations.

The next logical question follows: How much evidence is there for a phonological deficit in PD and SLI? Research has focused on two kinds of tasks, both of which arguably depend on the quality of underlying phonological representations: phoneme awareness and nonword repetition tasks. As we have seen, groups with RD are clearly impaired on not only phoneme awareness tasks but also nonword repetition tasks (Brady, 1997; Snowling, 1981).

Children with both PD and PD + SLI perform more poorly on phoneme awareness tasks than age-and nonverbal-IQ-matched controls but do not differ with respect to each other (Bird, Bishop, & Freeman, 1995). Research with adults has also provided evidence that individuals with a history of PD continue to have difficulties on phoneme awareness tasks compared to control subjects, despite the fact their speech disorder has resolved (Lewis & Freebairn, 1992). These results document phoneme awareness deficits in PD, with or without SLI. The hypotheses discussed earlier predict that such deficits should not be found in children with PD but not RD, or in children with SLI but not PD, but to my knowledge, there are no studies that test these predictions.

Research has also revealed that children with SLI tend to have deficits in nonword repetition ability, which has been posited to measure phonological short-term memory (Gathercole & Baddeley, 1990). Since this task requires children to repeat nonsense words that must be encoded and recalled using their phonological representations, it is also an indirect measure of the quality of those representations. Research by Gathercole and Baddeley (1990) revealed that children with SLI perform significantly worse on a nonword repetition task than language-matched control subjects. They reported a disproportionate deficit in nonword repetition abilities in the SLI group, such that children were 20 months below age expectations on the language measures used to assess SLI, and 48 months below age expectations on the nonword repetition task. Bishop and colleagues (1995) confirmed this nonword repetition deficit in SLI; they also demonstrated that children with resolved SLI continue to have a deficit in nonword repetition abilities, arguing that this deficit is not just a result of SLI. Finally, Dollaghan and Campbell (1998) replicated these findings with a different measure of nonword repetition that provided better controls for lexical effects on nonword repetition.

In summary, nonword repetition deficits beyond what reading or language levels would predict are robust correlates of RD, PD, and SLI. Because nonword repetition tasks tap both the quality of phonological representations and the capacity of phonological memory, among other things, we do not know for certain if each group is impaired for the same reason. The same applies for the deficit in phoneme awareness shared by all three groups. So more research is needed to answer this question. Nonetheless, deficits in either phonological representations or phonological memory (which are clearly related) are appealing candidates for a neuropsychological deficit common to all three language disorders. For example, as discussed in the MR section of this chapter, we have evidence across syndromes for a relation between phonological memory and the development of syntax.

Other hypotheses regarding the underlying neuropsychological deficit in SLI are reviewed in Bishop (1997) and Leonard (2000), and include (1) the *auditory* hypothesis, (2) a deficit in *grammatical* knowledge, and (3) a limitation in *general processing* capacity. I discuss these hypotheses in turn.

The auditory hypothesis (see, e.g., Tallal, Stark, & Mellits, 1985) holds that children with SLI are unable to process brief auditory events, and that this deficit undermines the development of speech perception, which then interferes with other aspects of language development. The phonological and auditory hypotheses are not mutually exclusive, since an auditory deficit could undermine phonological development. If this were shown to be the case, the phonological hypothesis would be reduced to the auditory hypothesis. However, recent tests of the auditory hypothesis raise significant questions about its validity (e.g., Bishop et al., 1999a; Bishop, Carlyon, Deaks, & Bishop, 1999b). Bishop and colleagues (1999a) used a twin design to test the heritability of auditory deficits in an SLI sample and their coheritability with nonword repetition deficits. Whereas deficits in nonword repetition were heritable and coheritable with SLI itself, deficits in rapid auditory processing were not heritable.

Grammatical knowledge hypotheses of SLI (e.g., Rice & Oetting, 1993; van der Lely, 1994) posit that particular grammatical rules are absent from the underlying linguistic competence of children with this disorder. A strength of this approach is that grammatical theory is rich enough to derive very specific predictions about normal and abnormal aspects of surface language performance, depending on which grammatical rules are absent. But this general approach has several significant weaknesses: (1) It assumes that grammatical knowledge is innate and therefore does not offer a developmental account of how particular grammatical deficits arise (see Bishop, 1997); (2) the predictions of these theories do not hold up well across languages; different aspects of grammar are difficult for SLI children depending on which language they speak (Leonard, 2000); and (3) there are alternative, processing accounts of why particular aspects of grammar are more or less difficult to acquire. For example, a deficit in phonological representations or memory could account for these grammatical deficits.

General processing hypotheses of SLI (e.g., Kail, 1994) posit a reduction in some general cognitive resource, such that children with SLI are slower at processing all kinds of information. For example, Kail found evidence for a generalized slowing of reaction times (RTs) in children with SLI. To explain why some aspects of grammar are more difficult than others in children with SLI, a second postulate is needed, namely, that some aspects of linguistic form are more vulnerable than others and will be "the first to go" if processing capacity is reduced. Data from normal adult speakers in dual-task conditions and computer simulations with degraded connections support this postulate for English (Leonard, 2000). In other words, those same aspects of linguistic form that are deficient in English-speaking children with SLI are also deficient in normal adults or computer simulations with reduced processing resources. This kind of hypothesis would also explain the diversity of problems found in children with SLI across languages; different aspects of linguistic form are vulnerable in different languages. One of the more serious challenges to this theory comes from MR syndromes, notably, Williams syndrome. Individuals with MR have reduced processing resources and slowing of RTs across tasks, probably more so than that observed in SLI, yet they vary considerably in grammatical competence. Imagine a thought experiment in which we match RTs of individuals with Down syndrome, Williams syndrome, and SLI. Would we then predict equivalent grammatical competence? General processing hypotheses of SLI need to be refined so that they can account for variations in grammatical development across syndromes that have a similar speed of processing. A phonological representation or memory hypothesis could be a more refined version of the general processing hypothesis; as we have seen, ability of phonological memory varies across MR syndromes and covaries with grammatical ability.

In summary, although there is evidence to support each of these other hypotheses, none accounts for all the phenomena encompassed by SLI (Leonard, 2000). It is possible that each different hypothesis may in fact be correct for a different subtype of SLI. It is also clear that more research is needed to clarify neuropsychological relations among subtypes of RD, PD, and SLI.

Treatment

Treatment of dyslexia comprises two parts: remediation and compensation. Remediation involves intensive training of the weak phonological skills, since it is impossible to bypass phonics completely in learning to read, particularly in English. At this time, multisensory approaches, such as Orton–Gillingham and systematic training on letter-to-sound correspondences, are favored by the International Dyslexia Association (IDA) and many other experts.

Several therapies lack scientific support or require further research (Silver, 1995), including tinted lenses training, visual training, patterning, auditory processing training, and use of various nutritional additives or adjustments.

Compensation for a specific reading disability involves strategies that both the child and educators can use to work around some of the problems posed by this disorder. For example, reduced time pressure, marking but not penalizing for spelling errors, not asking a child to read aloud in class, and possible waiver of foreign language requirements, may all be provided in the school environment to help children with dyslexia perform to their greatest potential. Children can use spell checkers (including handheld models), calculators to check computation, and tape recorders or other aids for note taking. Dyslexia can easily lead to secondary emotional problems, and children need to be monitored carefully by both teachers and parents.

Significant support for families and individuals with dyslexia comes from organizations such as the IDA (formerly the Orton Dyslexia Society), which has branches in many states (*www.interdys.org*).

Treatment of SLI and PD is reviewed in Leonard (2000). A variety of approaches, including imitation, modeling, focused stimulation, and milieu teaching, provide children with SLI- or PD-targeted exposure to, and practice with, the linguistic forms in which they are deficient. In other words, these therapies provide a more intensive and focused "dose" of some of the things parents and other adults naturally do to stimulate language development. Evaluation of these various approaches indicates gains relative to either untreated controls or untreated linguistic forms in the child's repertoire. Such interventions have also been shown to increase the rate of language development and transfer to spontaneous speech.

Despite these optimistic outcomes from research on the treatment of PD and SLI, there are some caveats. First, just as in psychotherapy outcome studies, many forms of speech and language therapy appear to work to about an equal extent (see meta-analysis by Nye, Foster, & Seaman, 1987). The treatment provided by clinicians using different approaches may nonetheless share some common elements, but these elements have not been clearly delineated. A second caveat is that long-term follow-up studies of treated children find that initial severity of SLI (or PD) predicts language outcome, but duration of treatment does not (Aram & Nation, 1980; Bishop & Edmundson, 1987). Although these were not treatment studies per se, since the treatment would ordinarily have occurred in community settings, no evidence of a dose–response relation for duration of treatment is a point of concern. Moreover, since there is wide range of normal variation in speech and language development in the young children, some children identified as having PD or SLI and given treatment would likely have developed normally anyway. Other children have more persistent problems; the critical question is how much treatment helps those children.

Finally, treatment does not cure SLI or PD. As we have seen, adults treated for PD as children still have phoneme awareness deficits and reading problems (Lewis & Freebairn, 1992). Follow-up of SLI children into adolescence (Snowling, Bishop, & Stothard, 2000) or young adulthood (Rutter & Mahwood, 1991) finds that a sizable proportion of subjects have declined in reading IQ, language, and even social skills. Language skills are so important to development that it is not surprising that a persistent language impairment would exact greater and greater costs. Just as the social deficit in autism deprives a child of important inputs for development, so does persistent language impairment.

Chapter 6

Conclusions

In this final chapter, I discuss the main conclusions that can be drawn from the foregoing chapters, including directions for future research. This discussion is organized into five sections: (1) fundamental issues revisited, (2) etiology, (3) brain mechanisms, (4) neuropsychology, and (5) prevention and treatment.

FUNDAMENTAL ISSUES REVISITED

The main goals of this book have been to propose a unified framework for studying the development of psychopathologies and to examine the current state of empirical knowledge about the development of various psychopathologies in light of this framework. This multilevel, interactionist framework stresses the importance of neuroscience for understanding psychopathology and at the same time resists reductionistic or dogmatic claims about the priority of a given level over others. Again and again, I have stressed the *bidirectional* nature of the relations between levels. Both bottom-up and top-down influences are important.

At this point, the reader might ask several questions. Is this just a loose framework or the beginnings of a unified theory? Just how much is research at various levels constrained by other levels? How will such a framework change our classification system for psychopathologies? How will it change public understanding of normal and abnormal behavior? These are the questions I consider.

Loose Framework or Unified Theory?

The roughly 100-year history of the field of psychology is partly a story of the failures of grand theories. Psychoanalysis, behaviorism and what might be called "symbolic cognitivism" each aspired to universal explanations and was then replaced by the next paradigm. Hence, contemporary psychologists are rightly skeptical of universal theories. Many feel it is better to focus narrowly on a particular empirical problem at a particular level of analysis than to engage in theory building or cross-level integration. So one might ask whether a neuroscience approach is any different from these previous paradigms. If so, how is it different?

One of the reasons for failure is that these earlier paradigms in psychology did not consider other levels of analysis or other scientific fields. As knowledge accumulated at these other levels or fields, the shortcomings of these paradigms became apparent. A neuroscience approach is different in that it is explicitly a multilevel approach that aspires to integrate psychology with the rest of science.

How successful that integration will be remains to be seen. A fair amount of autonomy is characteristic of scientific work at different levels of analysis and is in many ways a good thing. In terms of psychopathology, there is not a clear a priori reason for saying which level of analysis—cultural, social/interpersonal, neuropsychological, neurocomputational, neurobiological, or genetic—should receive priority. Important insights might come from any of these levels. The important point of a neuroscience approach is that work at each of these levels should be *mutually constraining*. It is axiomatic in the so-called "hard sciences" that everything known at one level of analysis is utilized as a constraint on other levels of analysis. Physics constrains chemistry, and chemistry constrains biology. Although there are many branches of biology, all are constrained by evolutionary theory. Mathematical advances in the analysis of the behavior of complex systems are now serving as both a tool and a constraint across many scientific fields. The principle of mutual constraint, also called "conceptual integration" or "vertical integration" (Barkow, Cosmides, & Tooby, 1992), is actually quite a powerful constraint that can save a lot of time. A chemist or biologist would never dream of developing a theory that violates the laws of physics or some other aspect of natural science. Consequently, the search space for new hypotheses is narrowed considerably. Unfortunately, conceptual integration has not been characteristic of the social sciences. As Barkow and colleagues (1992, p. 4) point out, "Evolutionary biology, psychology, psychiatry, anthropology, sociology, history, and economics largely live in glorious isolation from one another." Workers in each field routinely posit mechanisms known to be impossible (or at least very improbable) by workers in other social science disciplines.

The social sciences have for a long time been able to proceed in seeming safety on the assumption that the genome and the brain were "black boxes." So little was known about them that they provided few constraints on theories of behavior and culture. But new technologies, such as molecular genetics and neuroimaging, have changed all that. As the reviews in this book make clear, there is a virtual avalanche of new findings from the applications of such technologies to psychopathologies. In fact, the pace of new knowledge is so rapid that perhaps many of the findings reported here will be somewhat out of date by the time this book is published. But my overall point is that the neuroscience framework will not become outdated with such new findings. Instead, it will be increasingly needed to integrate findings from different levels of analysis.

So a neuroscience approach is not a call for scientific imperialism or just the most recent grand paradigm in psychology. Actually much less ambitious than that, it simply says that the principle of mutual constraint or conceptual integration needs to be taken seriously by the social sciences and that, especially with continuing advances in genetics and neuroscience, the social sciences cannot develop in isolation from the natural sciences. Just how much integration will occur is an empirical matter. Based on what has happened in the natural sciences, it seems likely that there will remain important, emergent phenomena specific to different disciplines and levels of analysis.

Whither DSM?

As discussed earlier, current taxonomies of psychopathologies, such as DSM-IV-TR, are descriptive and based on the symptom level of analysis. Progress in modern psychiatry has depended crucially on having reliable diagnoses. At the same time, it is widely understood that such behaviorally defined diagnoses are provisional and somewhat crude. Most researchers expect that there are valid subtypes of schizophrenia, autism, CD, ADHD, and most other psychopathologies. There is also accumulating evidence that some diagnostic distinctions are misleading, such as the one between mood and anxiety disorders.

One of the points of a neuroscience approach, and of the neuropsychological systems approach to psychopathologies taken here, is that a goal for psychopathology research is to develop a classification system based on underlying causal processes to replace the current, purely descriptive taxonomies. We need to understand psychopathology at the level of what is called "pathogenesis" or "pathophysiology." In internal medicine, multifactorial conditions, such as ischemic heart disease, are diagnosed and classified based on pathophysiology, not on the basis of either symptoms or etiology (Rutter, 2001). Each such multifactorial condition has multiple symptoms and etiologies but a single pathophysiological mechanism. So explanation and treatment are simplified by focusing on this level of analysis (whereas prevention focuses on the etiological level by reducing smoking, cholesterol levels, and other risk factors). Medical diagnoses have not always been based on pathophysiology. For much of the history of medicine, too little was known about pathophysiology for there to be valid diagnostic categories at this level of analysis. For example, in the 19th century, there was a detailed taxonomy of fevers based on their time course (e.g., diurnal fevers, nocturnal fevers, quotidian fevers, etc.). As the pathophysiology of fever became understood, these reified categories simply disappeared. Such, too, will be the fate of some of the diagnostic distinctions we currently defend with great tenacity!

So what corresponds to pathophysiology in psychiatry? The approach I take here proposes the neuropsychological or neurocomputational level. In other words, once we have a systems neuroscientific understanding of the development of psychopathological symptoms, our classification system will shift to that level of analysis, and the boundaries among psychopathologies will shift as well. This book provides a very preliminary idea of how such a classification system will look.

What Becomes of Folk Psychology?

The genetic and neuroscientific discoveries catalogued in this book are already raising profound questions about our understanding of human nature. One has only to look at the recent debate about embryonic stem cells to see an example of how fundamental assumptions about the nature of human life can clash with scientific advances. If a frozen embryo is already a person or an embodied soul, then experimenting on it seems unethical, even if the potential benefits are enormous. If a frozen embryo is just a collection of cells, and if personhood and what we call a "soul" emerge as part of a protracted developmental process, then the ethical implications are different.

As we learn more about the genome and the brain, and their roles in psychopathology, we will increasingly run into similar clashes with folk psychology. The public's fear is that such advances will be used in a dehumanizing way. Certainly that is always a risk; scientists, policymakers, and the public need continually to be watchful for misuse of discoveries.

At the same time, improved understanding of mental illnesses is potentially liberating and, in that sense, humanizing. Such an improved understanding will lessen stigma and free many sufferers from the constraints that mental illness imposes on their development. The more accurate our understanding of human nature, the better we can operate within the scope and limits it imposes.

We now turn to conclusions regarding etiology, brain mechanisms, neuropsychology, and treatment and prevention. To help focus these parts of the discussion, Table 3 lists main findings regarding the disorders reviewed in this book.

ETIOLOGY

One broad conclusion is that the etiology of all the behaviorally defined disorders in this book includes both genetic and environmental influences. On the genetic side, the one gene, one disorder (OGOD) hypothesis has been thoroughly rejected, as have deterministic notions of genetic influence. Instead, the genetic influences on these disorders involve multiple genes, which may be best conceptualized as quantitative trait loci (QTLs). QTLs act probabilistically with environmental factors to increase or decrease risk for a given developmental outcome, and no single QTL is either necessary or sufficient to produce a given developmental outcome. Another possibility is that *some* of these multiple genes are necessary and have a more categorical or interactive effect. Still another possibility is that the risk alleles for psychopathology will turn out to be quite common in the population; some may even have allele frequencies greater than 50%. In such a case, the risk allele would

TABLE 3. Summary of the Neuroscience of Psychopathologies

	Etiology		Brain findings			Neuropsychology
	Genes	Environment	Neurochemical	Structural	Functional	
Motivation						
Depression	5-HT transporter?	Loss, stress	Cortisol, NE, 5-HT	FL, BG	HPA, Amyg, PFC, ACG	Dysregulated stress response
Anxiety	5-HT transporter	Threat, stress	NE, 5-HT, GABA, CCK	—	Amyg, PFC	Conditioned fear response
PTSD	?	Trauma	Cortisol, opiates	HC	Amyg, OFC, ACG	Conditioned fear response?
Bipolar disorder	18p, q; 21q	Stress	DA, NE, GABA	WM, cortex	PFC	Overactive approach system
Action selection						
Attention-deficit/ hyperactivity disorder	DRD4; DAT1	FAS, CHI	DA	PFC, BG, CC	PFC, BG	Executive inhibition
Conduct disorder	MAOA, TPH	Harsh parenting; abuse	5-HT	PFC	PFC, Amyg	Inhibition, low autonomic arousal
Tourette syndrome	4q, 8p	Strep infection	DA	BG	BG, OFC, ACG	Inhibition?
Obsessive–compulsive disorder	5-HT transporter?	Strep infection	DA	BG	OFC, CN, ACG	Inhibition?
Schizophrenia	6p, 8p, 22q, 15q	OCs, viral infection	DA, GABA, glutamate, Ach	Ventricles, TL, Thal	PFC	Low IQ, WM, LTM
Language and cognition						
Autism	7q	Extreme neglect?	5-HT	Large brain	P300, OFC, FG	EF, ToM, praxis, emotional processing?
Down syndrome	Trisomy 21	—	Ach?	Small brain, HC, cerebellum, PFC	—	Verbal STM, syntax, LTM
Fragile X syndrome	FMR1	—	—	Large brain	—	Pragmatic language, EF
Williams syndrome	7p microdeletion	—	—	Small brain	—	Spatial deficit, language strengths
Dyslexia	1p, 2p, 6p, 15q, 18p	?	—	Language cortex	—	Phonological

Note. Neurotransmitters: NE, norepinephrine; 5-HT, serotonin; DA, dopamine; Ach, acetylcholine; GABA, gamma-aminobutyric acid; CCK, cholecystokinin. *Brain regions:* FL, frontal lobes; BG, basal ganglia; HPA, hypothalamic–pituitary–adrenal axis; Amyg, amygadala; ACG, anterior cingulate gyrus; PFC, prefrontal cortex; OFC, orbitofrontal cortex; WM, white matter; HC, hippocampus; CN, caudate nucleus; TL, temporal lobes; Thal, thalamus; FG, fusiform gyrus; CC, corpus callosum. *Other:* DRD4, dopamine receptor 4; DAT1, dopamine transporter 1; TPH, tryptophan hydroxylase; MAOA, monoamine oxidase A; FAS, fetal alcohol syndrome; CHI, closed head injury; Strep, streptococcus; OCs, obstetrical complications; ToM, theory of mind; WM, working memory; LTM, long-term memory; STM, short-term memory; EF, executive function; FMR1, fragile X mental retardation gene 1; P300, a component of the evoked response.

be "normal," and abnormality would arise because of its interaction with other risk alleles and environmental risk factors. These empirical issues will be settled by more research.

In any case, these genetic effects are probabilistic rather than deterministic, because the developmental process is a complex, dynamic system characterized by many epigenetic interactions. Therefore, the relation between an etiological input and an eventual phenotypic output is nonlinear. In some cases, small differences in initial conditions may lead to large deviations in the developmental trajectory. In other cases, larger differences in initial conditions may lead to no detectable phenotypic effect, because those initial differences were offset by later interactions. Another important consequence of this view of development is that some of the variance in behavioral outcomes will *not* be explicable in terms of individual differences in genes or environment, and will instead be due to variations in the developmental process itself (Finch & Kirkwood, 2000; Molenaar et al., 1993). Another important corollary of this view is that without understanding the developmental process, we cannot understand why a risk factor increases the probability of a given behavioral outcome. So the explanation of any psychopathology has to include development.

Molecular methods have begun to identify the locations and, in some cases, the identity of these QTLs, but much work remains to be done. In Table 3, we already see fairly convincing evidence for discriminant validity of these diagnostic constructs at the genetic level. For the most part, different disorders have different genetic risk factors. The main exceptions at this point are depression and anxiety, which may have a common risk factor, an allele of the serotonin transporter gene. But we would expect shared QTLs for these two disorders given their comorbidity, cofamiliality, and very high genetic correlation. As the molecular work progresses, it is very likely that other, shared QTLs will emerge to help account for the comorbidity and genetic correlation between other disorders. For example, we recently found that the QTL on 6p that influences reading disability also influences comorbid ADHD (Willcutt et al., in press). Once we have a more complete list of the specific and shared QTLs influencing psychopathologies, diagnostic definitions will very likely change.

We might ask at this point whether we can expect to obtain an exhaustive list of the QTLs influencing psychopathologies or, for that matter, any complex behavior. Since the statistical power to find QTLs depends on their effect sizes, and since it is very likely that QTLs for a given trait will exhibit a wide range of effect sizes, we will probably never obtain an exhaustive list. For example, many QTLs affecting complex traits will have effect sizes much less than 1%. Although it may be realistic to find QTLs with effect sizes of 1%, the ratio of return to investment gets exponentially less favorable as we move to increasingly smaller effect sizes. So it remains an open empirical question of how much genetic variance for each psychopathology will be due to identifiable QTLs, and how much to QTLs with very small effects.

Nonetheless, we have begun to identify the approximate locations of QTLs influencing many disorders and, in a few cases, we know the actual genes involved (e.g., the serotonin transporter gene, DRD4, and DAT1). Within the next decade, more actual genes influencing psychopathologies will be identified. These discoveries will permit much more discerning studies of how these genes influence brain development (one example of what is called "functional genomics").

On the environmental side, we have already learned a great deal about environmental correlates of psychopathologies, but it has been more difficult to nail down the environmental correlates that actually play a causal role, and the variance for which they account. One of the key points of this book is that a neuroscience approach does *not* mean that we embrace reductionism or biological determinism. We have learned that the development of the human brain depends crucially on environmental input, much of which is conveyed through social relations. The plasticity and protracted development of the human brain allow culture to play a greater role in human development than is true for any other species. Because of this, the flexibility and adaptability of human behavior is greater than that of any other species. At the same time, this plasticity is an Achilles' heel: If the environmental input is missing or aberrant, then brain and behavioral development can be changed irreversibly. Early stress, social deprivation, or abuse can all produce such irreversible effects, as can certain toxins (e.g., lead and alcohol).

These and other points are documented in a recent report from the National Academy of Sciences, *From Neurons to Neighborhoods* (Shonkoff & Phillips, 2000), that summarizes what is known and not known about the influence of early experiences on brain and behavioral development, and makes public policy recommendations based on that knowledge, some of which I return to in a later discussion of prevention. One exciting aspect is that this report demonstrates how a science of early environmental influences on development is emerging from work with both humans and animals at different levels of analysis. As I discussed earlier, researchers interested in early and later social influences on development are using much more sophisticated designs to determine which of these influences actually play a *causal* role in changing developmental trajectories (Collins et al., 2000).

As discussed by Rutter (2001), needed now is more research aimed at understanding the underlying mechanisms through which such risk factors work and the reasons for both vulnerability and resilience across individuals exposed to the same risk factor. Both genetics and brain development will be key to this understanding. Certain environmental risk factors now treated as unitary may actually be a bundle of more specific risk factors, each with specific effects. As Rutter discusses, we know that the risks posed by cigarette smoking work in this way. Smoking exposes one to tars, nicotine, and carbon monoxide, which in turn have links to various specific diseases, including lung cancer, heart disease, osteroporosis, and premature aging of the skin. Certain social–environmental risk factors, such as an abusive parent, a poor neighborhood, or a deviant peer group, may similarly bundle together a range of disparate, specific risk factors, but the details of what they are and how they influence brain and behavioral development remain to be fully worked out.

Once we identify actual genes influencing disorders, we can study more precisely the environmental risk and protective factors that are important for each disorder at specific points in development. Of very great interest will be studies of how the environment influences gene expression, and how gene–environment interactions actually work. Such research will allow us to fill in details of how the diathesis–stress model works. Although this model appears to apply in broad terms to many psychopathologies, we know very little about the specific diatheses or which stresses interact with them.

BRAIN MECHANISMS

In Table 3, we find less evidence for discriminant validity across disorders at the level of brain mechanisms. Some of the same neurotransmitters (e.g., norepinephrine, serotonin, and dopamine) and brain structures (e.g., amygdala, anterior cingulate, orbitofrontal, and other parts of prefrontal cortex) play a major role in many disorders. Other neurotransmitters (e.g., histamine and glycine) and brain structures (e.g., occipital and parietal cortices) seem much less important for psychopathology. These results are consistent with the earlier claim that the action selection and motivation systems of the brain are important for psychopathology, whereas the perception system is not. It is also clear in Table 3 that all disorders appear to have multiple neurotransmitter and structural correlates. So once again, the hypothesis of single causes for disorders, this time at the level of brain, is untenable.

One limitation in our current understanding of brain mechanisms is the sensitivity of the methods available for examining these mechanisms in humans. Although current methods, such as PET and fMRI, are much more sophisticated than methods available only a decade ago, their spatial and temporal resolution does not allow us to discriminate between separate circuits within the same structure. So while different disorders may share fMRI or PET activity differences in the amygdala, basal ganglia, or orbitofrontal cortex, the actual circuits involved may be distinct. As the sensitivity of methods increases, we should find more evidence for discriminant validity across disorders in terms of brain mechanisms. Nonetheless, it remains likely that some of the neural circuits will be shared across disorders.

Much more work is needed to sort out the relations between these various brain findings and particular disorders. As discussed earlier, some brain findings may be primary and pathogenetic, others may be secondary, and still others may be correlated. Once we have a better handle on the actual genes that constitute genetic risk for a disorder, animal models that manipulate these genes can help us understand which aspects of brain development are most directly affected. So advances in understanding genetic and environmental risk factors will provide invaluable information about how aspects of brain development are involved in different disorders.

Another overall lesson from the work on brain mechanisms in psychopathology is recognition of the need for a closer integration between molecular neuroscience and systems neuroscience. We can easily feel overwhelmed by the list of neurobiological correlates of a given disorder, partly because much of the existing research is descriptive. We lack strong theories for evaluating the significance of a particular finding, or for predicting new findings. One promising direction in systems neuroscience is neurocomputational modeling, but such models have only been applied to a few psychopathologies (e.g., dyslexia and schizophrenia). As these models become increasingly realistic, it will be possible to predict which brain correlates to expect and not expect in a given disorder. Another goal for this work will be to explain how partly shared neurotransmitters and neural circuits give rise to different symptom complexes.

One partly unfulfilled goal of this book is to understand how psychosocial factors alter brain development and thereby contribute to psychopathology. I have discussed results from animal models that demonstrate how early psychosocial stress can permanently alter the hypothalamic–pituitary–adrenal axis, partly by changing gene expression. But we need a much more comprehensive account of how various psychosocial factors alter brain functions and development. For example, one pathway is by explicit, cortical learning of new expectations and social skills; we assume this kind of learning occurs in psychotherapy. How do these new expectations and skills get implemented in the brain, and by what brain mechanisms do they affect mood?

NEUROPSYCHOLOGY

One of the main goals of this book has been to take a neuropsychological perspective on psychopathology. Ironically, many aspects of behavior that are best understood by neuropsychology are the least relevant for psychopathology. The cognitive neuroscience of perception, memory, and language is much more mature than the cognitive neuroscience of action selection, emotion regulation, or social cognition. So we are much closer to a neuropsychological explanation for some disorders, such as dyslexia, than we are for others, such as autism. We really do not have neuropsychological theories of disorders such as bipolar disorder or PTSD.

So there is a pressing need for better neuropsychological models of motivation, emotion regulation, and social cognition. We have also seen the close interaction between the motivation system and the action selection system in many disorders, and that interaction will also need to be incorporated into models of these two systems. Derryberry and Rothbart (1997) provide a nice account of how interactions between these two systems shape the development of temperament. Individual differences in the motivation system provide biases for behavioral tendencies (such as approach or avoidance), but these biases in turn influence cortical development and shape representations (expectations) about self and the world. At the same time, development of the executive and attentional systems permits top-down, effortful control of such behavioral tendencies. But most neuropsychological theories do not incorporate motivational influences—or psychosocial influences, for that matter. A canonical neuropsychological explanation for an individual's deficit on a given task is a problem with the cognitive computations intrinsic to the task; that is, the relevant neural networks that map input conditions onto outputs are either damaged or have failed to develop properly. But, obviously, deficits in performance can arise even when the networks necessary for these intrinsic cognitive computations are intact, if motivational state is altered. Beliefs, expectations, and social relationships all impact an individual's motivational state. So at the levels of both actual brain mechanisms and neurocomputation, we need to understand how motivational and psychosocial influences change what the brain is doing.

Another general point concerns what we can learn from these disorders about normal neuropsychological development. The neuropsychological associations and dissociations found across the disorders reviewed in this book provide clues about some of the main dimensions of neuropsychological development. For example, language skill is dissociable from spatial cognition, and structural language is dissociable from pragmatic language. We would like to know how many dimensions of neuropsychological development there are, how many of these are needed to account for the psychopathologies considered here, and the developmental relations among these dimensions. We could argue that focusing research on the development of psychopathology per se is a mistake. Instead, we should focus research on the normal development of these dimensions of individual differences, and that research will inform us about how extreme points (i.e., psychopathologies) arise on those dimensions. Some disorders may be simple (e.g., dyslexia), in that they represent an extreme position on a single, underlying neuropsychological dimension (phonological skill). Other disorders may be complex (e.g., CD), in that they require extremes on more than one dimension (e.g., inattention and emotion regulation). Obviously, it would be much more intellectually satisfying to have a comprehensive model of normal neuropsychological development that also accounts for extreme outcomes. Too much of our current theorizing begins with the disorder itself and focuses on only one disorder at a time.

Developmental relations among some dimensions appear to be competitive. Language and spatial development appear to have a competitive relation, especially if there is a limitation in cortical capacity. We saw evidence for this competitive relation across MR syndromes. If something interferes with language development, then overdevelopment of spatial cognition (as is true in autism or even Down syndrome) may occur. An overall limitation in cortical capacity, but nothing that blocks language development, may lead to underdevelopment of spatial cognition (as is true in Williams syndrome). This way of thinking about the neuropsychological profile in developmental disorders is very different from a static, neuropsychological approach that assumes the profile of a given disorder is fairly constant across development (see Oliver et al., 2000).

So we need better developmental models of altered developmental pathways. The initial conditions for a psychopathology may be only a slight deviation in some dimension of development but have many later and larger consequences for other dimensions.

PREVENTION AND TREATMENT

For many of the disorders considered here, both medication and psychotherapy have been demonstrably efficacious, which helps to illustrate a more general point: The etiology of a disorder does not necessarily dictate its treatment. Psychosocial interventions can be very helpful for highly heritable disorders, such as autism, and medications can be beneficial for disorders whose etiology is mainly environmental, such as PTSD. We also saw evidence from studies of obsessive–compulsive disorder that either medication or psychotherapy may impact the function of the same brain regions (Schwartz et al., 1996). As we try to develop an integrated model of how both genetic and psychosocial factors influence brain development, such treatment studies could be particularly informative.

In terms of prevention, what we *already* know about certain environmental risk and protective factors could be used to reduce the prevalence of psychopathologies. The policy recommendations that flow from this knowledge are discussed in the recent report from the National Academy of Sciences (Shonkoff & Phillips, 2000). Reducing exposure to environmental toxins such as lead and alcohol, reducing social environmental risk factors such as harsh parenting and abuse, improving prenatal and postnatal health care, and improving day care and early childhood education would reduce the rates of psychopathologies. I also reviewed earlier the promising approaches for preventing depression and anxiety in Chapter 3. Refining and implementing these approaches broadly would be a way to reduce the rates of two of the most common psychopathologies. A few prevention programs, such as the Elmyra project (Olds et al., 1998), with demonstrated *long-term* efficacy, are also cost-effective. If a program can reduce the rates of psychopathologies *and* produce a net savings, it should appeal to policymakers regardless of their political orientation.

In recent decades, for some disorders, such as major depression, there is clear evidence of increasing prevalence and younger age of onset. This disturbing secular trend is telling us that something about modern life is bad for mental health. As Rutter (2001) points out, the last 50 years have witnessed a paradoxical combination of not only unprecedented gains in the physical health of children (and adults) but also a dramatic increase in psychosocial disorders among young people. "If we had a proper understanding of why society had been so spectacularly successful in making things psychologically worse for children and young people, we might have a better idea of how we could make things better in the future" (p. 32). One possibility is reduced social support. There is evidence that community involvement has declined over the last few decades. Perhaps many people get less social support from their communities or families than once was the case. However, much more work is needed to test this hypothesis, and how to reverse this trend is not straightforward.

Obviously, future research on genetic and environmental risk and protective factors will eventually permit more precise early identification and treatment of individuals at risk. Since most of the disorders we have considered represent the output of a developmental process that exacerbates an initial vulnerability, early preventive treatment could be much more effective and less expensive than later interventions. So the neuroscience approach advocated in this book will not only increase scientific understanding of how psychopathology develops, but it will also lead to important advances in prevention and treatment.

References

Abell, F., Krams, M., Ashurner, J., Passingham, R., Friston, K., Frackowiak, R., Happe, F., Frith, C., & Frith, U. (1999). The neuroanatomy of autism: A voxel-based whole brain analysis of structural scans. *Cognitive Neuroscience, 10,* 1647–1651.

Abramson, L. Y., Seligman, M. E. P., & Teasdale, J. D. (1978). Learned helplessness in humans: Critique and reformulation. *Journal of Abnormal Psychology, 87,* 49–74.

Achenbach, T. M. (1982). *Developmental psychopathology.* New York: Wiley.

Achenbach, T. M. (1991). The derivation of taxonomic constructs: A necessary stage in the development of developmental psychopathology. In D. Cicchetti & S. L. Toth (Eds.), *Models and integrations* (pp. 43–74). Rochester, NY: University of Rochester Press.

Adams, M. (1990). *Beginning to read: Learning and thinking about print.* Cambridge, MA: MIT Press.

Aldridge, M. A., Stone, K. R., Sweeney, M. H., & Bower, T. G. R. (2000). Preverbal children with autism understand the intentions of others. *Developmental Science, 3*(3), 294–301.

Alexander, G. E. (1995). Basal ganglia. In M. A. Arbib (Ed.), *The handbook of brain theory and neural networks* (pp. 139–149). Cambridge, MA: MIT Press.

Alsobrook, J. P., II, & Pauls, D. L. (1999). Molecular genetics of childhood psychiatric disorders. In D. S. Charney, E. J., Nestler, & B. S. Bunney (Eds.), *Neurobiology of mental illness* (pp. 749–760). New York: Oxford University Press.

Altemus, M., Murphy, D., Greenberg, B., & Lesch, K. (1996). Intact coding region of the serotonin transporter gene in obsessive–compulsive disorder. *American Journal of Medical Genetics, 67*(4), 409–411.

Aman, C. J., Roberts, R. J., & Pennington, B. F. (1998). A neuropsychological examination of the underlying deficit in attention deficit hyperactivity disorder: Frontal lobe versus right parietal lobe theories. *Developmental Psychology, 34,* 956–969.

325

Amen, D. G., Paldi, J. H., & Thisted, R. A. (1993). Brain SPECT imaging. *Journal of the American Academy of Child and Adolescent Psychiatry, 32,* 1080–1081.

American Psychiatric Association. (1980). *Diagnostic and statistical manual of mental disorders.* Washington, DC: Author.

American Psychiatric Association. (1994). *Diagnostic and statistical manual of mental disorders* (4th ed). Washington, DC: Author.

American Psychiatric Association. (2000). *Diagnostic and statistical manual of mental disorders* (4th ed., rev.). Washington, DC: Author.

Anderson, M. (2001). Annotation: Conceptions of intelligence. *Journal of Child Psychology and Psychiatry, 42,* 287–298.

Anderson, M., O'Connor, N., & Hermelin, B. (1998). A specific calculating ability. *Intelligence, 26,* 383–403.

Angold, A., & Rutter, M. (1992). Effects of age and pubertal status on depression in a large clinical sample. *Development and Psychopathology, 4,* 5–28.

Aram, D., & Nation, J. (1980). Preschool language disorders and subsequent language and academic difficulties. *Journal of Communication Disorders, 13,* 159–170.

Arbib, M. A. (1989). *The metaphorical brain 2.* New York: Wiley.

Asherson, P., Virdee, V., Curran, S., Ebersole, S., Freeman, B., Craig, I., Simonoff, E., Eley, T., Plomin, R., & Taylor, E. (1998). Association of DSM-IV-TR attention deficit hyperactivity disorder and monoamine pathway genes [Abstract]. *American Journal of Medical Genetics, 81,* 549.

Asperger, H. (1991). "Autistic psychopathy" in childhood. In U. Frith (Ed. & Trans.), *Autism and Asperger syndrome* (pp. 37–92). Cambridge, UK: Cambridge University Press. (Original work published 1944)

Aylward, E. H., Minshew, N. J., Goldstein, G., Honeycutt, N. A., Augustine, A. M., Yates, K. O., Barta, P. E., & Pearlson, G. D. (1999). MRI volumes of amygdala and hippocampus in non-mentally retarded autistic adolescents and adults. *Neurology, 53,* 2145–2150.

Aylward, E. H., Reiss, A. L., Reader, M. J., Singer, H. S., Brown, J. E., & Denckla, M. B. (1996). Basal ganglia volumes in children with attention-deficit hyperactivity disorder. *Journal of Child Neurology, 11,* 112–115.

Bailey, A., LeCouteur, A., Gottesman, I., Bolton, P., Simonoff, E., Yuzda, F. Y., & Rutter, M. (1995). Autism as a strongly genetic disorder: Evidence from a British twin study. *Psychological Medicine, 25,* 63–77.

Bailey, A., Phillips, W., & Rutter, M. (1996). Autism: Towards an integration of clinical, genetic, neuropsychological, and neurobiological perspectives. *Journal of Psychology and Psychiatry, 37,* 89–126.

Ball, D., Hill, L., Freeman, B., Eley, T. C., Strelau, J., Riemann, R., Sinath, F. M., Angleitner, A., & Plomin, R. (1997). The serotonin transporter gene and peer-rated neuroticism. *Neuro-Report, 8,* 1301–1305.

Barker, P. (1994). *The eye in the door.* New York: Penguin Books.

Barkley, R. A. (1996). Attention-deficit/hyperactivity disorder. In E. J. Mash & R. A. Barkley (Eds.), *Child psychopathology* (pp. 63–112). New York: Guilford Press.

Barkley, R. A. (1997). Behavioral inhibition, sustained attention, and executive functions: Constructing a unifying theory of ADHD. *Psychological Bulletin, 121,* 65–94.

Barkley, R. A. (1998). *Attention-deficit/hyperactivity disorder: A handbook for diagnosis and treatment* (2nd ed.). New York: Guilford Press.

Barkley, R. A., Grodzinsky, G., & DuPaul, G. (1992). Frontal lobe functions in attention deficit disorder with and without hyperactivity: A review and research report. *Journal of Abnormal Child Psychology, 20,* 163–188.

Barkow, J. H., Cosmides, L., & Tooby, J. (1992). *The adapted mind.* New York: Oxford University Press.

Barlow, D. H. (2002). *Anxiety and its disorders* (2nd ed.). New York: Guilford Press.

Baron-Cohen, S., Leslie, A. M., & Frith, U. (1985). Does the autistic child have a "theory of mind"? *Cognition, 21*, 37–46.

Baron-Cohen, S., Leslie, A. M., & Frith, U. (1986). Mechanical, behavioral and intentional understanding of picture stories in autistic children. *British Journal of Developmental Psychology, 4*, 113–125.

Baron-Cohen, S., Ring, H. A., Bullmore, E. T., Wheelwright, S., Ashwin, C., & Williams, S. C. R. (2000). The amygdala theory of autism. *Neuroscience and Biobehavioral Reviews, 24*, 355–364.

Baron-Cohen, S., Ring, H., Wheelwright, S., Bullmore, E., Brammer, M., Simmons, A., & Williams, S. (1999). Social intelligence in the normal and autistic brain: An fMRI study. *European Journal of Neuroscience, 11*, 1891–1898.

Barondes, S. H. (1993). *Molecules and mental illness*. New York: Freeman.

Bates, E., Reilly, J., Wulfeck, B., Dronkers, N., Opie, M., Fenson, J., Kriz, S., Jeffries, R., Miller, L., & Herbst, K. (2001). Differential effects of unilateral lesions on language production in children and adults. *Brain and Language, 79*(2), 223–265.

Baum, A., Gatchel, R. J., & Schaeffer, M. A. (1983). Emotional, behavioral, and physiological effects of chronic stress at Three Mile Island. *Journal of Consulting and Clinical Psychology, 51*, 565–572.

Bauman, M. L., & Kemper, T. L. (1994). *Neurobiology of autism*. Baltimore: Johns Hopkins University Press.

Baumgardner, T. L., Singer, H. S., Denckla, M. B., Rubin, M. A., Abrams, M. T., Colli, M. J., & Reiss, A. L. (1996). Corpus callosum morphology in children with Tourette syndrome and attention deficit hyperactivity disorder. *Neurology, 4*, 477–482.

Baxter, L. R., Jr. (1999). Functional imaging of brain systems mediating obsessive–compulsive disorder. In D. S. Charney, E. J. Nestler, & B. S. Bunney (Eds.), *Neurobiology of mental illness* (pp. 534–547). New York: Oxford University Press.

Beck, A. T. (1987). Cognitive models of depression. *Journal of Cognitive Psychotherapy, 1*(1), 5–37.

Beidel, D. C., & Turner, S. M. (1997). At risk for anxiety: I. Psychopathology in the offspring of anxious parents. *Journal of the American Academy for Child Adolescent Psychiatry, 36*, 918–924.

Beitchman, J. H., Hood, J., & Inglis, A. (1990). Psychiatric risk in children with speech and language disorders. *Journal of Abnormal Child Psychology, 18*(3), 283–296.

Bellugi, U., Mills, D., Jernigan, T., Hickok, G., & Galaburda, A. (1999). Linking cognition, brain structure, and brain function in Williams syndrome. In H. Tager-Flusberg (Ed.), *Neurodevelopmental disorders* (pp. 111–136). Cambridge, MA: MIT Press.

Belmont, J. M., & Butterfield, E. C. (1971). Learning strategies as determinants of memory deficiencies. *Cognitive Psychology, 2*, 411–420.

Bench, C. J., Frackowiak, R. S. J., & Dolan, R. J. (1995). Changes in regional cerebral blood flow on recovery from depression. *Psychological Medicine, 25*, 247–251.

Benjamin, J., Li, L., Patterson, C., Greenberg, B. D., Murphy, D., & Hamer, D. (1996). Population and family association between the D4 dopamine receptor gene and measures of novelty seeking. *Nature Genetics, 12*, 81–84.

Bennetto, L., & Pennington, B. F. (1996). The neuropsychology of fragile X syndrome. In R. J. Hagerman & A. Cronister (Eds.), *Fragile X syndrome* (pp. 210–248). Baltimore: John Hopkins University Press.

Bennetto, L., & Pennington, B. F. (in press). The neuropsychology of fragile x syndrome. In R. J. Hagerman & P. J. Hagerman (Eds.), *The fragile X syndrome: Diagnosis, treatment and research* (3rd ed.). Baltimore: Johns Hopkins University Press.

Bennetto, L., Pennington, B. F., Porter, D., Taylor, A. K., & Hagerman, R. J. (2001). Profile of cognitive functioning in women with fragile X mutation. *Neuropsychology,* *15,* 290–299.

Benton, A. L., & Pearl, D. (1978). *Dyslexia.* New York: Oxford University Press.

Berkson, J. (1946). Limitations of the application of fourfold table analysis to hospital data. *Biometrics, 2,* 47–51.

Berman, K. F., & Weinberger, D. R. (1999). Neuroimaging studies of schizophrenia. In D. S. Charney, E. J. Nestler, & B. S. Bunney (Eds.), *Neurobiology of mental illness* (pp. 246–257). New York: Oxford University Press.

Bernstein, G. A., & Borchardt, C. M. (1991). Anxiety disorders of childhood and adolescence: A critical review. *Journal of Child and Adolescent Psychiatry, 30*(4), 519–532.

Bernstein, G. A., Garfinkel, B. D., & Hoberman, H. M. (1989). Self-reported anxiety in adolescents. *American Journal of Psychiatry, 146,* 384–386.

Berrettini, W. (1998). Progress and pitfalls: Bipolar molecular linkage studies. *Journal of Affective Disorders, 50*(2–3), 287–297.

Berrettini, W. H., Ferraro, T. N., Goldin, L. R., Detrea-Wadleigh, S. D., Choi, H., Muniec, D., Guroff, J. J., Kazuba, D. M., Nurnberger, J. I., Jr., Hsieh, W. T., Hoehe, M. R., & Gershon, E. S. (1997). A linkage study of bipolar illness. *Archives of General Psychiatry, 54,* 27–35.

Berridge, K. C., & Winkielman, P. (in press). What is an unconscious emotion? *Cognition and Emotion.*

Bertrand, J., & Mervis, C. B. (1996). Longitudinal analysis of drawings by children with Williams syndrome: Preliminary results. *Visual Arts Research, 22,* 19–34.

Bertrand, J., Mervis, C. B., & Eisenberg, J. D. (1997). Drawing by children with Williams syndrome: A developmental perspective. *Developmental Neuropsychology, 13,* 41–67.

Bettelheim, B. (1967). *The empty fortress.* New York: Free Press.

Biederman, J., Faraone, S. V., Keenan, K., Benjamin, J., Krifcher, B., Moore, C., Sprich-Buckminster, S., Ugalglia, K., Jelinek, M. S., Steingard, R., Spencer, T., Norman, D., Kolodny, R., Draus, I., Perrin, J., Keller, M. B., & Tsuang, M. T. (1992). Further evidence for family–genetic risk factors in attention deficit hyperactivity disorder: Patterns of comorbidity in probands and relatives in psychiatrically and pediatrically referred samples. *Archives of General Psychiatry, 49,* 728–738.

Biederman, J., Faraone, S. V., Keenan, K., Knee, D., & Tsuang, M. T. (1990). Family–genetic and psychosocial risk factors in DSM III attention deficit disorder. *Journal of the American Academy of Child and Adolescent Psychiatry, 29,* 526–533.

Biederman, J., Rosenbaum, J. F., Boldue-Murphy, E. A., Faraone, S. V., Chaloff, J., Hirshfeld, D. R., & Kagan, J. (1993). A three year follow-up of children with and without behavioral inhibition. *Journal of the American Academy of Child and Adolescent Psychiatry, 32,* 814–821.

Bierut, L. J., Heath, A. C., Bucholz, K. K., Dinwiddie, S. H., Madden, P. A., Statham, D. J., Dunne, M. P., & Martin, N. G. (1999). Major depressive disorder in a community-based twin sample: Are there different genetic and environmental contributions for men and women? *Archives of General Psychiatry, 56,* 557–563.

Billet, E. A., Richter, M. A., King, N., Heils, A., Lesch, K. P., & Kennedy, J. L. (1997). Obsessive compulsive disorder: Response to serotonin reuptake inhibitors and the serotonin transporter gene. *Molecular Psychiatry, 2,* 403–406.

Bird, J., Bishop, D. V., & Freeman, N. H. (1995). Phonological awareness and literacy development in children with expressive phonological impairments. *Journal of Speech and Hearing Research, 38*(2), 446–462.

Bishop, D. V. M. (1997). *Uncommon understanding: Development and disorders of language comprehension in children.* Cambridge, UK: Psychology Press.

Bishop, D. V. M., Bishop, S. J., Bright, P., James, C., Delaney, T., & Tallal, P. (1999a). Different origin of auditory and phonological processing problems in children with language impairment: Evidence from a twin study. *Journal of Speech, Language, and Hearing Research, 42,* 155–168.

Bishop, D. V. M., Carlyon, R. P., Deeks, J. M., & Bishop, S. J. (1999b). Auditory temporal processing impairment: Neither necessary nor sufficient for causing language impairment in children. *Journal of Speech, Language, and Hearing Research, 42,* 1295–1310.

Bishop, D. V. M., & Edmundson, A. (1987). Language-impaired 4-year-olds: Distinguishing transient from persistent impairment. *Journal of Speech and Hearing Disorders, 52,* 156–173.

Bishop, D. V. M., North, T., & Donlan, C. (1995). Genetic basis of specific language impairment: Evidence from a twin study. *Developmental Medicine and Child Neurology, 37,* 56–71.

Blair, R. J. R. (1995). A cognitive developmental approach to morality: Investigating the psychopath. *Cognition, 57,* 1–29.

Blair, R. J. R., Jones, L., Clark, F., & Smith, M. (1997). The psychopath: A lack of responsiveness to distress cues? *Psychophysiology, 34,* 192–198.

Blashfield, R. K., & Livelsey, J. W. (1999). Classification. In T. Millon & P. H. Blaney (Eds.), *Oxford textbook of psychopathology* (pp. 3–28). New York: Oxford University Press.

Bleuler, E. (1950). *Dementia praecox or a group within the schizophrenias* (J. Zinkin, Trans.). New York: International Universities Press. (Original work published 1911)

Boetsch, E. A. (1996). *A longitudinal study of the relationship between dyslexia and socioemotional functioning in young children.* Unpublished doctoral dissertation, University of Denver.

Bolton, P., & Griffiths, P. (1997). Association of tuberous sclerosis of temporal lobes with autism and atypical autism. *Lancet, 349,* 392–395.

Bolton, P., Macdonald, H., Pickles, A., Rios, P., Goode, S., Crowson, M., Bailey, A., & Rutter, M. (1994). A case–control family history study of autism. *Journal of Child Psychology and Psychiatry, 35,* 877–900.

Bookheimer, S. Y. (2000, September). *fMRI of emotional processing in autism.* Paper presented at the Collaborative Programs of Excellence in Autism meeting, Denver, CO.

Booth, R. J., & Pennebaker, J. W. (2000). Emotions and immunity. In M. Lewis & J. M. Haviland-Jones (Eds.), *Handbook of emotions* (2nd ed., pp. 558–570). New York: Guilford Press.

Borger, N., van der Meere, J. J., Ronner, A., Alberts, A., Geuze, R., & Bogte, H. (1999). Heart rate variability and sustained attention in ADHD. *Journal of Abnormal Child Psychology, 27,* 25–33.

Bownds, M. D. (1999). *Biology of mind.* Bethesda, MD: Fitzgerald Science Press.

Brady, S. A. (1997). Ability to encode phonological representations: An underlying difficulty of poor readers. In B. A. Blachman (Ed.), *Foundations of reading acquisition and dyslexia: Implications for early intervention* (pp. 21–47). Mahwah, NJ: Erlbaum.

Brainard, S. S., Schreiner, R. A., & Hagerman, R. J. (1991). Cognitive profiles of the adult carrier fra(X) female. *American Journal of Medical Genetics, 38,* 505–508.

Brennan, P. A., Raine, A., Schulsinger, F., Kirkegaard-Sorensen, L., Knop, J., Hutchings, B., Rosenberg, R., & Mednick, S. A. (1997). Psychophysiological protective factors for male subjects at high risk for criminal behavior. *American Journal of Psychiatry, 154,* 853–855.

Breslau, N., Davis, G. C., Andreski, P., & Peterson, E. (1991). Traumatic events and posttraumatic stress disorder in an urban population of young adults. *Archives of General Psychiatry, 48,* 216–222.

Brestan, E. V., & Eyberg, S. M. (1998). Effective psychosocial treatments of conduct-disordered children and adolescents: 29 years, 82 studies, and 5,272 kids. *Journal of Clinical Child Psychology, 27*(2), 180–189.

Brown, G. L., Goodwin, F. K., & Ballenger, J. C. (1979). Aggression in humans correlates with cerebrospinal fluid amine metabolites, *Psychiatry Research, 1*, 131–139.

Brown, G. W., & Harris, T. O. (1978). *Social origins of depression: A study of psychiatric disorders in women.* New York: Free Press.

Brown, R., Hobson, R. P., & Lee, A. (1997). Are there autistic-like features in congenitally blind children? *Journal of Child Psychology and Psychiatry, 38*, 693–703.

Brown, T. A. (1999). Generalized anxiety disorder and obsessive-compulsive disorder. In T. Millon, P. H. Blaney, & R. D. Davis (Eds.), *Oxford textbook of psychopathology* (pp. 114–143). New York: Oxford University Press.

Brunner, H. G., Nelen, M., Breakfield, X. O., Ropers, H. H., & Van Oost, B. A. (1993). Abnormal behavior associated with a point mutation in the structural gene for monoamine oxidase A. *Science, 262*, 578–580.

Bryant, P., & Impey, L. (1986). The similarity between normal readers and developmental and acquired dyslexics. *Cognition, 24*, 121–137.

Bryson, S. E., & Smith, I. M. (1998). Epidemiology of autism: Prevalence, associated characteristics, and implications for research and service delivery. *Mental Retardation and Developmental Disabilities Research Reviews, 4*, 97–103.

Burton, R. (1948). *The anatomy of melancholy.* New York: Tudor. (Original work published 1621)

Byne, W., Kemether, E., Jones, L., Haroutunian, V., & Davis, K. L. (1999). The neurochemistry of schizophrenia. In D. S. Charney, E. J. Nestler, & B. S. Bunney (Eds.), *Neurobiology of mental illness* (pp. 236–245). New York: Oxford University Press.

Byrum, C. E., Ahearn, E. P., & Krishnan, K. (1999). A neuroanatomic model for depression. *Progress in Neuropsychopharmacology and Biological Psychiatry, 23*(2), 175–193.

Cadoret, R. J., Yates, W. R., Troughton, E., Woodworth, G., & Stewart, M. A. (1995). Genetic–environmental interaction in the genesis of aggressivity and conduct disorders. *Archives of General Psychiatry, 52*, 916–924.

Caine, E., McBride, M., Chiverton, P., Bamford, K., Rediess, S., & Shiao, J. (1988). Tourette's syndrome in Monroe County school children. *Neurology, 38*, 472–475.

Caldji, C., Tannenbaum, B., Sharma, S., Francis, D., Plotsky, P. M., & Meaney, M. J. (1998). Maternal care during infancy regulates the development of neural systems mediating the expression of fearfulness in the rat. *Proceedings of the National Academy of Sciences of the United States of America, 95*(9), 5335–5340.

Caltagirone, C, Nocentini, U., & Vicari, S. (1990). Cognitive functions in adult Down's syndrome. *International Journal of Neuroscience 54*, 221–230.

Campbell, D. T., & Stanley, J. C. (1966). *Experimental and quasi-experimental designs for research.* Chicago: Rand McNally.

Canli, T., Zhao, Z., Desmond, J. E., Kang, E., Gross, J., & Babrieli, J. D. E. (2001). An fMRI study of personality influences on brain reactivity to emotional stimuli. *Behavioral Neuroscience, 115*, 33–42.

Cardon, L. R., DeFries, J. C., Fulker, D. W., Kimberling, W. J., Pennington, B. F., & Smith, S. D. (1994). Quantitative trait locus for reading disability on chromosome 6. *Science, 265*, 276–279.

Carey, G., & Gottesman, I. I. (1981). Twin and family studies of anxiety, phobic and obsessive disorders. In D. F. Klein & J. Rabkin (Eds.), *Anxiety: New research and changing concepts* (pp. 117–136). New York: Raven Press.

Carlesimo, G. A., Marotta, L., & Vicari, S. (1997). Long-term memory in mental retardation: Evidence for a specific impairment in subjects with Down's syndrome. *Neuropsychologia, 35*(1), 71–79.

Carlson, G. A. (1990). Annotation: Child and adolescent mania—diagnostic considerations. *Journal of Child Psychology and Psychiatry, 31*, 331–341.

Caron, C., & Rutter, M. (1991). Comorbidity in child psychopathology: Concepts, issues and research strategies. *Journal of Child Psychology and Psychiatry and Allied Disciplines, 32*(7), 1063–1080.

Carpenter, M., Pennington, B. F., & Rogers, S. J. (2001). Understanding of others' intentions in children with autism. *Journal of Autism and Developmental Disorders, 31*, 589–599.

Carter, A. S., Pauls, D. L., & Leckman, J. F. (1995). The development of obsessionality: Continuities and discontinuities. In D. Cicchetti & D. J. Cohen (Eds.), *Developmental psychopathology* (pp. 609–632). New York: Wiley.

Casey, B. J., Castellanos, F. X., Giedd, J. N., Marsh, W. L., Hamburger, S. D., Schubert, A. B., Vauss, Y. C., Vaituzis, A. C., Dickstein, D. P., Sarfatti, S. E., & Rapoport, J. L. (1997). Implication of right frontostriatal circuitry in response inhibition and attention deficit hyperactivity disorder. *Journal of the American Academy of Child and Adolescent Psychiatry, 36*, 374–383.

Casey, B. J., Durston, S., & Fossella, J. (2001). A mechanistic model of cognitive control: Clinical, neuroimaging, and lesion studies. *Clinical Neuroscience Research, 1*, 267–282.

Castles, A., & Coltheart, M. C. (1993). Varieties of developmental dyslexia. *Cognition, 47*, 149–180.

Caspi, A., & Moffitt, T. E. (1995). The continuity of maladaptive behavior: From description to understanding in the study of antisocial behavior. In D. Cicchetti & D. J. Cohen (Eds.), *Developmental psychopathology* (Vol. 2, pp. 472–511). New York: Wiley.

Caspi, A., Taylor, A., Moffitt, T. E., & Plomin, R. (2000). Neighborhood deprivation affects children's mental health: Environmental risks identified in a genetic design. *Psychological Science, 11*, 338–342.

Castellanos, F. X., Giedd, J. N., Marsh, W. L., Hamburger, S. D., Vaituzis, A. C., Dickstein, D. P., Sarfatti, S. E., Vauss, Y. C., Snell, J. W., Lange, N., Kaysen, D., Krain, A. L., Ritchie, G. F., Rajapakse, J. C., & Rapoport, J. L. (1996). Quantitative brain magnetic resonance imaging in attention-deficit/hyperactivity disorder. *Archives of General Psychiatry, 53*, 607–616.

Castellanos, F. X., Lau, E., Tayebi, N., Lee, P., Long, R. E., Giedd, J. N., Sharp, W., Marsh, W. L., Walter, J. M., Hamburger, S. D., Ginns, E. I., Rapoport, J. L., & Sidransky, E. (1998). Lack of an association between a dopamine-4 receptor polymorphism and attention-deficit/hyperactivity disorder: Genetic and brain morphometric analyses. *Molecular Psychiatry, 3*, 431–434.

Catalano, M., Sciuto, G., DiBella, D., Novella, E., Nobile, M., & Bellodi, L. (1994). Lack of association between obsessive–compulsive disorder and the dopamine D3 receptor gene: some preliminary considerations. *American Journal of Medical Genetics, 54*(3), 232–253.

Changeaux, J. P. (1985). *Neuronal man.* New York: Oxford University Press.

Chapman, L. J., & Chapman, J. P. (1973). Problems in the measurement of cognitive deficit. *Psychological Bulletin, 79*, 380–385.

Chapman, R. S. (1999). Language and cognitive development in children and adolescents with Down syndrome. In J. F. Miller, L. A. Leavitt, & M. Leddy (Eds.), *Improving the communication of people with Down syndrome* (pp. 41–60). Baltimore: Brookes.

Chemtob, C., Roitblatt, H. L., Hamada, R. S., Carlson, J. G., & Twentyman, C. T. (1988). A cognitive action theory of post-traumatic stress disorder. *Journal of Anxiety Disorders, 2*, 253–275.

Chess, S. (1977). Follow-up report on autism in congenital rubella. *Journal of Autism and Childhood Schizophrenia, 7*, 69–81.

Chhabildas, N., Pennington, B. F., & Willcutt, E. G. (in press). A comparison of the cognitive deficits in the DSM-IV subtypes of ADHD. *Journal of Abnormal Child Psychology.*

Chrousos, G. P., & Gold, P. W. (1992). The concepts of stress and stress system disorders. *Journal of the American Medical Association, 267,* 1244–1252.

Churchland, P. M. (1988). *Matter and consciousness.* Cambridge, MA: MIT Press.

Churchland, P. M. (1995). *The engine of reason, the seat of the soul.* Cambridge, MA: MIT Press.

Cicchetti, D., & Toth, S. (1995). Developmental psychopathology and disorders of affect. In D. Cicchetti & D. J. Cohen (Eds.), *Developmental psychopathology* (pp. 369–420). New York: Wiley.

Clark, L. A., & Watson, D. (1991). Tripartite model of anxiety and depression: Psychometric evidence and taxonomic implications. *Journal of Abnormal Psychology, 100,* 316–336.

Clifford, C. A., Murrary, R. M., & Fulker, D. W. (1984). Genetic and environmental influences on obsessional traits and symptoms. *Psychological Medicine, 14,* 791–800.

Cloninger, C. R., Sigvardsson, S., Bohman, M., & von Knorring, A. L. (1982). Predisposition to petty criminality in Swedish adoptees: II. Cross-fostering analysis of gene–environment interaction. *Archives of General Psychiatry, 39,* 1242–1247.

Cohen, I. L., Vietze, P. M., Sudhalter, V., Jenkins, E. C., & Brown, W. T. (1989). Parent–child dyadic gaze patterns in fragile X males and in non-fragile X males with autistic disorder. *Journal of Child Psychology and Psychiatry, 30*(6), 845–856.

Cohen, J. D., Noll, D. C., & Schneider, W. (1993). Functional magnetic resonance imaging: Overview and methods for psychological research. *Behavior Research Methods, Instruments and Computers, 25,* 101–113.

Cohen, J. D., & Servan-Schreiber, D. (1992). Context, cortex, and dopamine: A connectionist approach to behavior and biology in schizophrenia. *Psychological Review, 99,* 45–77.

Cohn, J. F., Campbell, S. B., Matias, R., & Hopkins, J. (1990). Face-to-face interactions of postpartum depressed and nondepressed mother–infant pairs at two months. *Developmental Psychology, 26,* 15–23.

Collier, D. A., Arranz, M. J., Sham., P., & Battersby, S. (1996). The serotonin transporter is a potential susceptibility factor for bipolar affective disorder. *Neuroreport: An International Journal for the Rapid Communication of Research in Neuroscience, 7*(10), 1675–1679.

Collins, W. A., Maccoby, E. E., Steinberg, L., Hetherington, E. M., & Bornstein, M. H. (2000). Contemporary research on parenting: The case for nature and nurture. *American Psychologist, 55,* 218–232.

Coltheart, M. C., Masterson, J., Byng, S. Prior, M., & Riddoch, J. (1983). Surface dyslexia. *Quarterly Journal of Experimental Psychology, 37A,* 469–495.

Coltheart, M., Patterson, K. E., & Marshall, J. C. (1980). *Deep dyslexia.* London: Routledge & Kegan Paul.

Conners, C. K., & Wells, K. C. (1986). *Hyperkinetic children: A neuropsychological approach.* Beverly Hills, CA: Sage.

Cook, E. H., Stein, M. A., Krasowski, M. D., Cox, N. J., Olkon, D. M., Kieffer, J. E., & Leventhal, B. L. (1995). Association of attention deficit disorder and the dopamine transporter gene. *American Journal of Human Genetics, 56,* 993–998.

Cornblatt, B. A., Green, M. F., & Walker, E. F. (1999). Schizophrenia: Etiology and neurocognition. In T. Millon, P. H. Blaney, & R. D. Davis (Eds.), *Oxford textbook of psychopathology* (pp. 277–310). New York: Oxford University Press.

Costello, E. J., & Angold, A. (1995). Developmental epidemiology. In D. Cicchetti & D. J. Cohen (Eds.), *Developmental psychopathology: Vol 1. Theory and methods* (pp. 23–56). New York: Wiley.

Courchesne, E., Yeung-Courchesne, R., Press, G. A., Hesselink, J. R., & Jernigan, T. L. (1988). Hypoplasia of cerebellar vermal lobules VI and VII in autism. *New England Journal of Medicine, 318,* 1349–1354.

Cox, A., Klein, K., Charman, T., Baird, G., Baron-Cohen, S., Swettenham, J., Drew, A., & Wheelwright, S. (1999). Autism spectrum disorders at 20 and 42 months of age: Stability of clinical and ADI-R diagnosis. *Journal of Child Psychology and Psychiatry, 40,* 719–732.

Cox, B. J., & Taylor, S. (1999). Anxiety disorders: Panic and phobias. In T. Millon, P. H. Blaney, & R. D. Davis (Eds.), *Oxford textbook of psychopathology* (pp. 81–113). New York: Oxford University Press.

Crick, N. R., & Dodge, K. A. (1994). A review and reformulation of social information processing mechanisms in children's social adjustment. *Psychological Bulletin, 115,* 74–101.

Cronbach, L. J., & Meehl, P. E. (1955). Construct validity in psychological tests. *Psychological Bulletin, 52,* 281–302.

Crnic, L. S., & Pennington, B. F. (2000). Down syndrome: Neuropsychology and animal models. In C. Rovee-Collier, L. P. Lipsitt, & H. Hayne (Eds.), *Progress in infancy research, Vol. I* (pp. 69–111). Mahwah, NJ: Erlbaum.

Crow, T. J. (1980). Molecular pathology of schizophrenia: More than one disease process? *British Medical Journal, 280,* 66–68.

Crowder, R. G. (1982). *The psychology of reading: An introduction.* New York: Oxford University Press.

Crowe, R. R. (1999). Molecular genetics of anxiety disorders. In D. S. Charney, E. J. Nestler, & B. S. Bunney (Eds.), *Neurobiology of mental illness* (pp. 451–462). New York: Oxford University Press.

Csibra, G., Gergely, G., Biro, S, Koos, O., & Brockbank, M. (1999). Goal attribution without agency cues: The perception of "pure reason" in infancy. *Cognition, 72,* 237–267.

Curtis, M. E. (1980). Development of components of reading skill. *Journal of Educational Psychology, 72,* 656–669.

Dadds, M. R., Holland, D. E., Laurens, K. R., Mullins, M., Barrett, P. M., & Spence, S. H. (1999). Early intervention and prevention of anxiety disorders in children: Results at 2-year follow-up. *Journal of Consulting and Clinical Psychology, 67,* 145–150.

Damasio, A. R. (1994). *Descartes' error.* New York: Putnam's Sons.

Davidson, R. J., Abercrombie, H., Nitschke, J. B., & Putnam, K. (1999). Regional brain function, emotion and disorders of emotion. *Current Opinion in Neurobiology, 9*(2), 228–234.

Davidson, R. J., Putnam, K. M., & Larson, C. L. (2000). Dysfunction in the neural circuitry of emotion regulation: A possible prelude to violence. *Science, 289,* 591–594.

Dawson, G., & Osterling, J. (1997). Early intervention in autism: Effectiveness and common elements of current approaches. In M. J. Guralnick (Ed.), *The effectiveness of early intervention* (pp. 307–325). Baltimore: Brookes.

DeFries, J. C., & Fulker, D. W. (1988). Multiple regression analysis of twin data: Etiology of deviant scores versus individual differences. *Acta Geneticae Medicae et Gemellologiae, 37,* 205–216.

DeFries, J. C., & Gillis, J. J. (1993). Genetics of reading disability. In R. Plomin & G. E. McClearn (Eds.), *Nature, nurture and psychology* (pp. 121–145). Washington, DC: American Psychological Association.

Dennett, D. C. (1987). *The intentional stance.* Cambridge, MA: MIT Press.

Depue, R. A., & Iacono, W. G. (1989). Neurobehavioral aspects of affective disorders. *Annual Review of Psychology, 40,* 457–492.

Derryberry, D., & Rothbart, M. K. (1997). Reactive and effortful processes in the organization of temperament. *Development and Psychopathology, 9,* 633–652.

Detterman, D. K., & Daniel, M. H. (1989). Correlations of mental tests with each other and with cognitive variables are highest for low IQ groups. *Intelligence, 13,* 349–359.

Devenny, D. A., Hill, A. L., Patxot, O., Silverman, W. P., & Wisniewski, K. E. (1992). Aging in higher functioning adults with Down's syndrome: An interim report in a longitudinal study. *Journal of Intellectual Disability Research, 36,* 241–250.

Diamond, A., Prevor, M. B., Callender, G., & Druin, D. P. (1997). Prefrontal cortex cognitive deficits in children treated early and continuously for PKU. *Monographs of the Society for Research in Child Development, 62*(4), 1–205.

DiLalla, L. F., & Gottesman, I. I. (1989). Heterogeneity of causes for delinquency and criminality: Lifespan perspectives. *Development and Psychopathology, 1,* 339–349.

Dingman, H. F., & Tarjan, G. (1960). Mental retardation and the normal distribution curve. *American Journal of Mental Deficiency, 64,* 991–994.

Dishion, T. J., French, D. C., & Patterson, G. R. (1995). The development and ecology of antisocial behavior. In D. Cicchetti & D. J. Cohen (Eds.), *Developmental psychopathology* (Vol. 2, pp. 421–471). New York: Wiley.

Dishion, T. J., Patterson, G. R., & Kavanagh, K. A. (1992). An experimental test of the coercion model: Linking theory, measurement, and intervention. In J. McCord & R. E. Tremblay (Eds.), *Preventing antisocial behavior: Interventions from birth through adolescence* (pp. 253–282). New York: Guilford Press.

Dodge, K. A., Bates, J., & Pettit, G. S. (1990). Mechanisms in the cycle of violence. *Science, 250,* 1678–1683.

Dollaghan, C., & Campbell, T. F. (1998). Nonword repetition and child language impairment. *Journal of Speech, Language and Hearing Research, 41*(5), 1136–1146.

Douglas, V. I. (1983). Attention and cognitive problems. In M. Rutter (Ed.), *Developmental neuropsychiatry* (pp. 280–329). New York: Guilford Press.

Douglas, V. I. (1988). Cognitive deficits in children with attention deficit disorder with hyperactivity. In L. M. Bloomingdale & J. Sergeant (Eds.), *Attention deficit disorder: Criteria, cognition, intervention* (pp. 65–81). Elmsford, NY: Pergamon Press.

Douglas, V. I. (1989). Can Skinnerian theory explain attention deficit disorder?: A reply to Barkley. In L. M. Bloomingdale & J. A. Sergeant (Eds.), *Attention deficit disorder: Current concepts and emerging trends in attentional and behavioral disorders of childhood* (pp. 235–254). Elmsford, NY: Pergamon Press.

Down, J. L. N. (1866). Observations on ethnic classification of idiots. *Mental Science, 13,* 121–128.

Downey, G., & Coyne, J. C. (1990). Children of depressed parents: An integrative review. *Psychological Bulletin, 108,* 50–76.

Duara, R., Kushch, A., & Gross-Glenn, K. (1991). Neuroanatomic differences between dyslexic and normal readers on magnetic resonance imaging scans. *Archives of Neurology, 48,* 410–416.

Dubovsky, S. L., & Buzan, R. (1999). Mood disorders. In R. E. Hales, J. C. Yudofsky, & J. A. Talbott (Eds.), *Textbook of psychiatry* (3rd ed., pp. 479–565). Washington, DC: American Psychiatric Press.

Dugdale, R. L. (1877). *The jukes.* New York: Putnam.

Dunmore, E., Clark, D. M., & Ehlers, A. (1999). Cognitive factors involved in the onset and maintenance of posttraumatic stress disorder (PTSD) after physical or sexual assault. *Behaviour Research and Therapy, 37*(9), 809–829.

Dunst, C. J. (1990). Sensorimotor development of infants with Down syndrome. In D. Cicchetti & M. Beeghly (Eds.), *Children with Down syndrome* (pp. 180–230). New York: Cambridge University Press.

Dykens, E. M., Hodapp, R. M., & Leckman, J. F. (1987). Strengths and weaknesses in the intellectual functioning of males with fragile X syndrome. *American Journal of Medical Genetics, 28,* 13–15.

Eaves, L., Silberg, J., Meyer, J., Maes, H., Simonoff, E., Pickles, A., Rutter, M., Neale, M., Reynolds, C., Erickson, M., Heath, A., Loeber, R., Truett, K., & Hewitt, J. (1997). Genetics and developmental psychopathology. 2: The main effects of genes and environment on behavioral problems in the Virginia Twin Study of Adolescent Behavioral Development. *Journal of Child Psychology and Psychiatry, 38,* 965–980.

Eaves, L. J., Eysenck, H. J., & Martin, N. G. (1989). *Genes, culture, and personality.* San Diego, CA: Academic Press.

Ebstein, R. P., Gritsenko, I., Nemanov, L., Frisch, A., Osher, Y., & Belmaker, R. H. (1997). No association between the serotonin transporter gene regulatory region polymorphism and the Tridimensional Personality Questionnaire (TPQ) temperament of harm avoidance. *Molecular Psychiatry, 2,* 224–226.

Ebstein, R. P., Novick, O., Umansky, R., Priel, B., Osher, Y., Blaine, D., Bennett, E., Nemanov, L., Katz, M., & Belmaker, R. (1996). Dopamine D4 receptor (D4DR) exon III polymorphism associated with the human personality trait of novelty seeking. *Nature Genetics, 12,* 78–80.

Edelman, G. M. (1987). *Neural Darwinism.* New York: Basic Books.

Eden, G. F., VanMeter, J. W., Rumsey, J. M., Maisog, J. M., Woods, R. P., & Zeffiro, T. A. (1996). Abnormal processing of visual motion in dyslexia revealed by functional brain imaging. *Brain, 382,* 66–69.

Egeland, J. A., Hostetter, A. M., & Eshleman, S. K. (1983). Amish study III: The impact of cultural factors on the diagnosis of bipolar illness. *American Journal of Psychiatry, 140,* 67–71.

Ehrenkranz, J., Bliss, E., & Sheard, M. H. (1974). Plasma testosterone: Correlation with aggressive behavior and social dominance in man. *Psychosomatic Medicine, 36*(6), 469–475.

Einfeld, S., Maloney, H., & Hall, W. (1989). Autism is not associated with the fragile X syndrome. *American Journal of Medical Genetics, 34,* 187–193.

Eley, T. C., Bishop, D. V. M., Dale, P. S., Oliver, B., Petrill, S. A., Price, T. S., Purcell, S., Saudino, K., Simonoff, E., Stevenson, J., & Plomin, R. (1999a). Genetic and environmental origins of verbal and performance components of cognitive delay in two-year-olds. *Developmental Psychology, 35,* 1122–1131.

Eley, T. C., Lichtenstein, P., & Stevenson, J. (1999b). Sex differences in the etiology of aggressive and nonaggressive antisocial behavior: Results from two twin studies. *Child Development, 70*(1), 155–168.

Eley, T. C., & Stevenson, J. (1999). Using genetic analysis to clarify the distinction between depressive and anxious symptoms in children. *Journal of Abnormal Child Psychology, 27,* 105–114.

Eley, T. C., & Stevenson, J. (2000). Specific life events and chronic experiences differentially associated with depression and anxiety in young twins. *Journal of Abnormal Child Psychology, 28,* 383–394.

Ellis, N. R. (1963). The stimulus trace and behavioral inadequacy. In N. R. Ellis (Ed.), *Handbook of mental deficiency, psychological theory and research* (pp. 134–158). New York: McGraw-Hill.

Ellis, N. R., Woodley-Zanthos, P., & Dulaney, C. L. (1989). Memory for spatial location in children, adults, and mentally-retarded persons. *American Journal on Mental Retardation, 93,* 521–527.

Elman, J. L., Bates, E. A., Johnson, M. H., Karmiloff-Smith, A., Parisi, D., & Plunkett, K. (1996). *Rethinking innateness: A connectionist perspective on development.* Cambridge, MA: MIT Press.

Epstein, C. J. (1989). Down syndrome. In C. R. Scriver, A. L. Beaudet, W. S. Sly, & P. Valle (Eds.), *The metabolic basis of inherited disease* (pp. 291–396). New York: McGraw-Hill.

Evans, D. W., King, R. A., & Leckman, J. F. (1996). Tic disorders. In E. J. Mash & R. A. Barkley (Eds.), *Child psychopathology* (pp. 436–454). New York: Guilford Press.

Ewart, A. K., Jin, W., Atkinson, D., Morris, C. A., & Keating, M. T. (1994). Supravalvular aortic stenosis associated with a deletion disrupting the elastin gene. *Journal of Clinical Investigation, 93,* 1071–1077.

Ewart, A. K., Morris, C. A., Atkinson, D., Jin, W., Sternes, K., Spallone, P., Stock, A. D., Leppert, M., & Keating, M. T. (1993a). Hemizygosity at the elastin locus in a developmental disorder, Williams syndrome. *Nature Genetics, 5,* 11–16.

Ewart, A. K., Morris, C. A., Ensing, G. J., Loker, J., Moore, C., Leppert, M., & Keating, M. T. (1993b). A human vascular disorder, supravalvular aortic stenosis, maps to chromosome 7. *Proceedings of the National Academy of Sciences of the United States of America, 90,* 3226–3230.

Falk, C. T., & Rubinstein, P. (1987). Haplotype relative risks: An easy reliable way to construct a proper control sample for risk calculations. *Annals of Human Genetics, 51,* 227–233.

Fannon, D., Chitnis, X, Doku, V., Tennakoon, L., O'Ceallaigh, S., Soni, W., Sumich, A., Lowe, J., Santamarie, M., & Sharma, T. (2000). Features of structural brain abnormality detected in first episode psychosis. *American Journal of Psychiatry, 157*(11), 1829–1834.

Faraone, S., Biederman, J., Chen, W. J., Krifcher, B., Moore, C., Sprich, S., & Tsuang, M. (1992). Segregation analysis of attention deficit hyperactivity disorder: Evidence for single major gene transmission. *Psychiatric Genetics, 2,* 257–275.

Faraone, S., Biederman, J., Keenan, K., & Tsuang, M. T. (1991). A family genetic study of girls with DSM-III attention deficit disorder. *American Journal of Psychiatry, 148,* 112–117.

Faraone, S., Kremen, W., & Tsuang, M. (1990). Genetic transmission of major affective disorders: Quantitative models and linkage analyses. *Psychological Bulletin, 108,* 109–127.

Faraone, S. V., Biederman, J., Weiffenbach, B., Chu, M. P., Weaver, A., Spencer, T. J., Wilens, T. E., Frazier, J., Cleves, M., & Sakai, J. (1999a). Dopamine D4 gene 7–repeat allele and attention-deficit hyperactivity disorder. *American Journal of Psychiatry, 156,* 768–770.

Faraone, S. V., Tsuang, M. T., & Tsuang, D. W. (1999b). *Genetics of mental disorders: A guide for students, clinicians, and researchers.* New York: Guilford Press.

Fein, D., Pennington, B. F., Markowitz, P., Braverman, M., & Waterhouse, L. (1986). Towards a neuropsychological model of infantile autism: Are the social deficits primary? *Journal of the American Academy of Child Psychiatry, 25,* 198–212.

Fenichel, O. (1945). *The psychoanalytic theory of neuroses.* New York: Norton.

Ferguson, H. B., & Rappaport, J. L. (1983). Nosological issues and biological validation. In M. Rutter (Ed.), *Developmental neuropsychiatry* (pp. 369–384). New York: Guilford Press.

Feshbach, N. D. (1989). The construct of empathy and the phenomenon of physical maltreatment of children. In D. Cicchetti & V. Carlson (Eds.), *Child maltreatment: Theory and research on the causes and consequences of child abuse and neglect* (pp. 349–373). New York: Cambridge University Press.

Field, L. L., & Kaplan, B. J. (1998). Absence of linkage of phonological coding dyslexia to chromosome 6p23–p21.3 in a large family data set. *American Journal of Human Genetics, 63,* 1448–1456.

Filipek, P. A. (1995). Neurobiologic correlates of developmental dyslexia: How do dyslexics' brains differ from those of normal readers? *Journal of Child Neurology, 10,* S62–S69.

Filipek, P. A., Richelme, C., Kennedy, D. M., Rademacher, J., Pitcher, D. A., Zidel, S., & Caviness, V. S. (1992). Morphometric analysis of the brain in developmental language disorders and autism. *Annals of Neurology, 32,* 475.

Filipek, P. A., Semrud-Clikeman, M., Steingard, R. J., Renshaw, P. F., Kennedy, D. N., & Biederman, J. J. (1997). Volumetric MRI analysis comparing attention deficit hyperactivity disorder with normal controls. *Neurology, 48,* 589–601.

Finch, C. E., & Kirkwood, T. B. L. (2000). *Chance, development, and aging.* New York: Oxford University Press.

Fisher, S. E., Francks, C., Marlow, A. J., MacPhie, I. L., Newbury, D. F., Cardon, L. R., Ishikawa-Brush, Y., Richardson, A. J., Talcott, J. B., Gayan, J., Olson, R. K., Pennington, B. F., Smith, S. D., DeFries, J. C., Stein, J. F., & Monaco, A. P. (2002). Independent genome-wide scans identify a chromosome 18 quantitative-trait locus influencing dyslexia. *Nature Genetics, 30,* 86–91.

Fisher, S. E., Marlow, A. J., Lamb, J., Maestrini, E., Williams, D. F., Richardson, A. J., Weeks, D. E., Stein, J. F., & Monaco, A. P. (1999). A quantitative-trait locus on chromosome 6p influences different aspects of developmental dyslexia. *American Journal of Human Genetics, 64,* 146–156.

Fisher, S. E., Vargha-Khadem, F., Watkins, K. E., Monaco, A. P., & Pembrey, M. E. (1998). Localization of a gene implicated in a severe speech and language disorder. *Nature Genetics, 18,* 168–170.

Fleming, K., Goldberg, T., Gold, J., & Weinberger, D. (1995). Verbal working memory dysfunction in schizophrenia: Use of a Brown–Peterson paradigm. *Psychiatry Research, 56,* 155–161.

Fletcher, J. M. (1985). External validation of learning disability typologies. In B. P. Rourke (Ed.), *Neuropsychology of learning disabilities: Essentials of subtype analysis* (pp. 187–211). New York: Guilford Press.

Fletcher, J. M., Foorman, B. R., Shaywitz, S. E., & Shaywitz, B. A. (1999). Conceptual and methodological issues in dyslexia research: A lesson for developmental disorders. In H. Tager-Flusberg (Ed.), *Neurodevelopmental disorders* (pp. 271–305). Cambridge, MA: MIT Press.

Flint, J. (1999). The genetic basis of cognition. *Brain, 122,* 2015–2031.

Foa, E. B., Dancu, C. V., Hembree, E. A., Jaycox, L. H., Meadows, E. A., & Street, G. P. (1999). A comparison of exposure therapy, stress inoculation training, and their combination for reducing posttraumatic stress disorder in female assault victims. *Journal of Consulting and Clinical Psychology, 67*(2), 194–200.

Foa, E. B., Hearst-Ikeda, D., & Perry, K. J. (1995). Evaluation of a brief cognitive-behavioral program for the prevention of chronic PTSD in recent assault victims. *Journal of Consulting and Clinical Psychology, 63*(6), 948–955.

Foa, E. B., & Riggs, D. S. (1995). Posttraumatic stress disorder following assault: Theoretical considerations and empirical findings. *Current Directions in Psychological Sciences, 4,* 61–65.

Foa, E. B., Steketee, G., & Olasov-Rothbaum, B. (1989). Behavioral/cognitive conceptualizations of post-traumatic stress disorder. *Behavior Therapy, 20,* 155–176.

Foa, E. B., Zinbarg, R., & Olasov-Rothbaum, B. (1992). Uncontrollability and unpredictability in post-traumatic stress disorder: An animal model. *Psychological Bulletin, 112,* 218–238.

Fodor, J. A. (1983). *The modularity of mind.* Cambridge, MA: MIT Press.

Foley, D. L., Neale, M. C., & Kendler, K. S. (1998). Reliability of a lifetime history of major depression: Implications for heritability and co-morbidity. *Psychological Medicine, 28,* 857–870.

Folstein, S., & Rutter, M. (1977). Genetic influences and infantile autism, *Nature, 265,* 726–728.

Fowler, A. E. (1998). Language in mental retardation: Associations with and dissociations from general cognition. In J. A. Burack, R. M. Hodapp, & E. Zigler (Eds.), *Handbook of mental retardation and development* (pp. 290–333). Cambridge, UK: Cambridge University Press.

Fowler, A. E., Gelman, R., & Gleitman, L. R. (1994). The course of language learning in children with Down syndrome: Longitudinal and language level comparisons with young normally developing children. In H. Tager-Flusberg (Ed.), *Constraints on language acquisition* (pp. 91–140). Hillsdale, NJ: Erlbaum.

Frangiskakis, J. M., Ewart, A. K., Morris, C. A., Mervis, C. B., Bertrand, J., Robinson, B. F., Klein, B. P., Ensing, G. J., Everett, L. A., Green, E. D., Proschel, C., Gutowski, N., Noble, M., Atkinson, D. L., Odelberg, S. J., & Keating, M. T. (1996). LIM-kinase1 hemizygosity implicated in impaired visuospatial constructive cognition. *Cell, 86,* 59–69.   ,

Frank, E., Hlastala, S., Ritenour, A., Houck, P., Tu, X. M., Monk, T. H., Mallinger, A. G., & Kupfer, D. J. (1997). Inducing lifestyle regularity in recovering bipolar disorder patients: Results from the maintenance therapies in bipolar disorder protocol. *Biological Psychiatry, 41,* 1165–1173.

Freedman, R. C. H., Myles-Worsley, M., Orr-Urteger, A., Oliney, A., Davis, A., Polymeropoulos, M., Holik, J., Hopkins, J., Hoff, M., Rosenthal, J., Waldo, M., Reimherr, F., Wender, P., Yaw, J., Young, D. A., Breese, C. R., Adams, C., Patterson, D., Adler, L. E., Kruglyak, L., Leonard, S., & Byerly, W. (1997). Linkage of a neurophysiological deficit in schizophrenia to a chromosome 15 locus. *Proceedings of the National Academy of Sciences of the United States of America, 94,* 587–592.

Freud, S. (1963). Mourning and melancholia. In J. Strachey (Ed. & Trans.), *The standard edition of the complete psychological works of Sigmund Freud* (Vol. 14, pp. 237–260). London: Hogarth Press. (Original work published 1915)

Freund, I. S., & Reiss, A. I. (1991). Cognitive profiles associated with the fra(X) syndrome in males and females. *American Journal of Medical Genetics, 38,* 542–547.

Friston, K. J., & Frith, C. D. (1995). Schizophrenia: A disconnection syndrome? *Clinical Neuroscience, 3,* 89–97.

Frith, U. (1985). Beneath the surface of developmental dyslexia. In K. E. Patterson, J. C. Marshall, & M. Coltheart (Eds.), *Surface dyslexia: Neuropsychological and cognitive studies of phonological reading* (pp. 301–330). Hillsdale, NJ: Erlbaum.

Frombonne, E. (2001). Is there an epidemic of autism? *Pediatrics, 107,* 411–412.

Frost, R. (1998). Toward a strong phonological theory of visual word recognition: True issues and false trails. *Psychological Bulletin, 123,* 71–99.

Fulker, D. W., Cherny, S. S., & Cardon, L. R. (1995). Multipoint interval mapping of quantitative trait loci using sib pairs. *American Journal of Human Genetics, 56,* 1224–1233.

Fuster, J. M. (1989). *The prefrontal cortex: Anatomy, physiology and neuropsychology of the frontal lobe* (2nd ed.). New York: Raven Press.

Galaburda, A. M. (1988). The pathogenesis of childhood dyslexia. *Research in Nervous Mental Disorders, 66,* 127–138.

Galaburda, A. M., & Livingstone, M. (1993). Evidence for a magnocellular defect in developmental dyslexia. *Annals of New York Academy of Science, 682,* 70–82.

Galton, F. (1892). *Hereditary genius: An inquiry into its laws and consequences.* New York: Macmillan.

Ganzini, L., McFarland, B. H., & Cutler, D. (1990). Prevalence of mental disorders after catastrophic financial loss. *Journal of Nervous and Mental Disease, 178,* 680–685.

Gathercole, S. E., & Baddeley, A. D. (1990). Phonological memory deficits in language disordered children: Is there a causal connection? *Journal of Memory and Language, 29*, 336–360.

Gayan, J., Smith, S. D., Cherny, S. S., Cardon, L. R., Fulker, D. W., Brower, A. M., Olson, R. K., Pennington, B. F., & DeFries, J. C. (1999). Quantitative-trait locus for specific language and reading deficits on chromosome 6p. *American Journal of Human Genetics, 64*, 157–164.

Ge, X., Conger, R. D., Cadoret, R. J., Neiderhiser, J. M., Yates, W. R., Troughton, E., & Steward, M. A. (1996). The developmental interface between nature and nurture: A mutual influence model of child antisocial behavior and parent behaviors. *Developmental Psychology, 32*(4), 574–589.

Gelernter, J., Kranzler, H., Coccaro, E. F., Siever, L. J., & New, A. S. (1998). Serotonin transporter protein gene polymorphism and personality measures in African American and European American subjects. *Psychiatric Genetics, 8*, 1332–1338.

Gernsbacher, M. A., & Goldsmith, H. H. (in press). Toward a dyspraxic subtype of autism spectrum disorder: A research hypothesis. *Journal of Autism and Developmental Disorders.*

Gibson, D. (1978). *Down syndrome: The psychology of mongolism.* London: Cambridge University Press.

Giedd, J. N., Castellanos, F. X., Casey, B. J., Kozuch, P., & King, A. C. (1994). Quantitative morphology of the corpus callosum in attention deficit hyperactivity disorder. *American Journal of Psychiatry, 151*, 665–669.

Gilger, J., Pennington, B. F., & DeFries, J. C. (1991). Risk for reading disability as a function of parental history in three family studies. *Reading and Writing, 3*, 205–217.

Gilger, J. W., Borecki, I. B., DeFries, J. C., & Pennington, B. F. (1994). Commingling and segregation analysis of reading performance in families of normal reading. *Behavior Genetics, 24*, 345–355.

Gill, M., Daly, G., Heron, S., Hawi, Z., & Fitzgerald, M. (1997). Confirmation of association between attention deficit hyperactivity disorder and a dopamine transporter polymorphism. *Molecular Psychiatry, 2*, 311–313.

Gilles de la Tourette, G. (1885). Etude sur une affection nerveuse caractisée par de l'incoordination motrice accompagnée d'écholalie et de coprolalie. *Archives of Neurology, 9*, 158.

Gillis, J. J., Gilger, J. W., Pennington, B. F., & DeFries, J. C. (1992). Attention deficit disorder in reading-disabled twins: Evidence for a genetic etiology. *Journal of Abnormal Child Psychology, 20*(3), 303–315.

Gittelman, R., Mannuzza, S., Shenker, R., & Gonagura, N. (1985). Hyperactive boys almost grown up. *Archives of General Psychiatry, 42*, 937–947.

Gjane, H., Stevenson, J., & Sundet, J. (1996). Genetic influence on parent-reported attention-related problems in a Norweigian general population twin sample. *Journal of the American Academy of Child and Adolescent Psychiatry, 35*, 588–596.

Goddard, H. H. (1912). *The Kallikak family: A study in the heredity of feeble-mindedness.* New York: Macmillan.

Goetz, R., Klein, D., Gully, R., Kahn, J., Leibowitz, M., Fyer, A., & Gorman, J. (1993). Panic attacks during placebo procedures in the laboratory. *Archives of General Psychiatry, 50*, 280–295.

Gold, P., Goodwin, F., & Chrousos, G. (1988a). Clinical and biochemical manifestations of depression: Relation to the neurobiology of stress (Part I). *New England Journal of Medicine, 319*, 348–353.

Gold, P., Goodwin, F., & Chrousos, G. (1988b). Clinical and biochemical manifestations of depression: Relation to the neurobiology of stress (Part II). *New England Journal of Medicine, 319*, 413–420.

Goldberg, J., True, W. R., Eisen, S. A., & Henderson, W. G. (1990). A twin study of the effects of the Vietnam War on posttraumatic stress disorder. *Journal of the American Medical Association, 263,* 1227–1232.

Goldman-Rakic, P. S. (1987a). Development of cortical circuitry and cognitive function. *Child Development, 58,* 601–622.

Goldman-Rakic, P. S. (1987b). Circuitry of primate prefrontal cortex and regulation of behavior by representational memory. In V. B. Mountcastle, F. Plum, & S. R. Geiger (Eds.), *Handbook of physiology: The nervous system* (pp. 373–417). Bethesda, MD: American Physiological Society.

Goldstein, R. B., Wickramaratne, P. J., Horwath, E., & Weissman, M. M. (1997). Familial aggregation and phenomenology of "early" onset (at or before age 20 years) panic disorder. *Archives of General Psychiatry, 54,* 271–278.

Goodman, K. S. (1986). *What's whole in whole language: A parent–teacher guide.* Portsmouth, NH: Heinemann.

Gottesman, I. I. (1991). *Schizophrenia genetics: The origins of madness.* New York: Freeman.

Gottlieb, G. (1991). Experimental canalization of behavioral development: Theory. *Developmental Psychology, 27*(1), 4–13.

Gottlieb, G. (1998). Normally occurring environmental and behavioral influences on gene activity: From central dogma to probabilistic epigenesis. *Psychological Review, 105,* 792–802.

Gough, P. B. (1983). Context, form, and interaction. In K. Rayner (Ed.), *Reading: Perceptual and language processes.* New York: Academic Press.

Gough, P. B., Alford, J. A., Jr., & Holly-Wilcox, P. (1981). Words and contexts. In O. J. L. Tzeng & H. Singer (Eds.), *Perception of print: Reading research in experimental psychology.* Hillsdale, NJ: Erlbaum.

Gough, P. B., & Walsh, M. A. (1991). Chinese, phoenicians, and the orthographic cipher of English. In S. A. Brady & D. P. Shankweiler (Eds.), *Phonological processes in literacy* (pp. 199–209). Hillsdale, NJ: Erlbaum.

Grandin, T. (1995). *Thinking in pictures: And other reports from my life with autism.* New York: Doubleday,

Greenough, W. T., Black, J. E., & Wallace, C. S. (1987). Experience and brain development. *Child Development, 58,* 539–559.

Grice, D., Leckman, J., Pauls, D., Kurlan, R., Kidd, K., Pakstis, A., Chang, F., Buxbaum, J., Cohen, D., & Gelernter, J. (1996). Linkage disequilibrium between an allele at the dopamine D4 receptor locus and Tourette syndrome, by the transmission–disequilibrium test. *American Journal of Human Genetics, 59,* 644–652.

Griffith, E. M., Pennington, B. F., Wehner, E. A., & Rogers, S. J. (1999). Executive functions in young children with autism. *Child Development, 70,* 817–832.

Grigorenko, E. L., Wood, F. B., Meyer, M. S., Hart, L. A., Speed, W. C., Shuster, A., & Pauls, D. L. (1997). Susceptibility loci for distinct components of developmental dyslexia on chromosome 6 and 15. *American Journal of Human Genetics, 60,* 27–39.

Grigorenko, E. L., Wood, F. B., Meyer, M. S., & Pauls, D. L. (2000). Chromosome 6p influences on different dyslexia-related cognitive processes: Further confirmation. *American Journal of Human Genetics, 66*(2), 715–723.

Grillon, C., Dierker, L., & Merikangas, K. R. (1997). Startle modulation in children at risk for anxiety disorders and/or alcoholism. *Journal of the American Academy of Child and Adolescent Psychiatry, 36*(7), 925–932.

Gualtieri, C. T., & Hicks, R. E. (1985). Neuropharmacology of methylphenidate and an neural substrate for childhood hyperactivity. *Psychiatric Clinics of North America, 6,* 875–892.

Haaga, D. A., Dyck, M. J., & Ernst, D. (1991). Empirical status of cognitive theory of depression. *Psychological Bulletin, 110,* 215–236.

Hagerman, R. J. (1987). Fragile X syndrome. *Current Problems in Pediatrics, 7,* 627–674.

Hagerman, R. J. (1996). Physical and behavioral phenotype. In R. J. Hagerman & A. Cronister (Eds.), *Fragile X syndrome: Diagnosis, treatment, and research* (2nd ed., pp. 3–87). Baltimore: Johns Hopkins University Press.

Hagerman, R. J. (1999). Clinical and molecular aspects of fragile X syndrome. In H. Tager-Flusberg (Ed.), *Neurodevelopmental disorders* (pp. 27–42). Cambridge, MA: MIT Press.

Hagerman, R. J., Jackson, C., Amin, K., Silverman, A. C., O'Connor, R., & Sobesky, W. (1992). Girls with fragile X syndrome: Physical and neurocognitive status and outcome. *Pediatrics, 89,* 395–400.

Hagerman, R. J., Kemper, M., & Hudson, M. (1985). Learning disabilities and attentional problems in boys with the fragile X syndrome. *American Journal of Disabled Children, 139*(7), 674–678.

Hagnell, O., Lanke, J., Rorsman, B., & Ojesjo, L. (1982). Are we entering an age of melancholy? Depressive illnesses in a prospective epidemiological study over 25 years: The Lundby Study, Sweden. *Psychological Medicine, 12,* 279–289.

Hahn, W. E., Van Ness, J., & Maxwell, I. H. (1978). Complex population of mRNA sequences in large polydenylated nuclear RNA molecules. *Proceedings of the National Academy of Science, 75*(11), 5544–5547.

Hallgren, B. (1950). Specific dyslexia (congenital word-blindness): A clinical and genetic study. *Acta Psychiatrica et Neurologica Supplement, 65,* 1–287.

Halperin, J., Wolfe, L., Pascualvaca, D., Newcorn, J., Healy, J., O'Brien, J., Morgenstein, A., & Young, J. (1988). Differential assessment of attention and impulsivity in children. *Journal of the American Academy of Child and Adolescent Psychiatry, 27,* 326–329.

Hamilton, S. P., Heiman, G. A., Haghighi, F., Mick, S., Klein, D. F., Hodge, S. E., Weissman, M. M., Fyer, A. J., & Knowles, J. A. (1999). Lack of genetic linkage or association between a functional serotonin transporter polymorphism and panic disorder. *Psychiatric Genetics, 9,* 1–6.

Hammen, C., & Rudolph, D. D. (1996). Childhood depression. In E. J. Mash & R. A. Barkley (Eds.), *Child psychopathology* (pp. 153–195). New York: Guilford Press.

Hanson, D. M., Jackson, A. W., & Hagerman, R. J. (1986). Speech disturbances (cluttering) in mildly impaired males with the Martin–Bell fragile X syndrome. *American Journal of Medical Genetics, 7,* 471–489.

Harcherick, D. F., Cohen, D. J., Ort, S., Paul, R., Shaywitz, B. A., Volkman, F. R., Rothman, S. L. G., & Leckman, T. F. (1985). Computed tomographic brain scanning in four neuropsychiatric disorders of childhood. *American Journal of Psychiatry, 142,* 731–737.

Hare, R. D. (1965). Temporal gradient of fear arousal in psychopaths. *Journal of Abnormal Psychology, 70,* 442–445.

Hare, R. D. (1982). Psychopathy and physiological activity during anticipation of an aversive stimulus in a distraction paradigm. *Psychophysiology, 19,* 266–271.

Hare, R. D., Frazell, J., & Cox, D. N. (1978). Psychopathy and physiological responses to threat of an aversive stimulus. *Psychophysiology, 15,* 165–172.

Harm, M. W., & Seidenberg, M. S. (1999). Phonology, reading acquisition, and dyslexia: Insights from connectionist models. *Psychological Review, 106*(3), 491–528.

Harrington, R. (1992). Annotation: The natural history and treatment of child and adolescent affective disorders. *Journal of Child Psychology and Psychiatry, 33*(8), 1287–1302.

Harrington, R., Fudge, H., Rutter, M., Pickles, A., & Hill, J. (1990). Adult outcomes of childhood depression: Psychiatric status. *Archives of General Psychiatry, 47,* 465–473.

Harrington, R., Fudge, H., Rutter, M., Pickles, A., & Hill, J. (1991). Adult outcomes of childhood and adolescent depression: II. Risk for antisocial disorders. *Journal of American Academy of Child and Adolescent Psychiatry, 30,* 434–439.

Hattori, M., Fujiyama, A., Taylor, T. D., Watanabe, H., Yada, T., Park, H. S., Toyoda, A., Ishii, K., Totoki, Y., Choi, D. K., Soeda, E., Ohki, M., Takagi, T., Sakaki, Y., Taudien, S., Blechschmidt, K., Polley, A., Menzel, U., Delabar, J., Kumpf, K., Lehmann, R., Patterson, D., Reichwald, K., Rump, A., Schillhabel, M., Schudy, A., Zimmermann, W., Rosenthal, A., Kudoh, J., Schibuya, K., Kawasaki, K., Asakawa, S., Shintani, A., Sasaki, T., Nagamine, K., Mitsuyama, S., Antonarakis, S. E., Minoshima, S., Shimizu, N., Nordsiek, G., Hornischer, K., Brant, P., Scharfe, M., Schon, O., Desario, A., Reichelt, J., Kauer, G., Blocker, H., Ramser, J., Beck, A., Klages, S., Hennig, S., Riesselmann, L., Dagand, E., Haaf, T., Wehrmeyer, S., Borzym, K., Gardiner, K., Nizetic, D., Francis, F., Lehrach, H., Reinhardt, R., & Yaspo, M. L. (2000). The DNA sequence of human chromosome 21. *Nature, 405,* 311–319.

Heaton, R. K., Baade, L. E., & Johnson, K. L. (1978). Neuropsychological test results associated with psychiatric disorders in adults. *Psychology Bulletin, 85,* 141–162.

Heninger, G. R. (1999). Special challenges in the investigation of the neurobiology of mental illness. In D. S. Charney, E. J. Nester, & B. S. Bunney (Eds.), *Neurobiology of mental illness* (pp. 89–99). New York: Oxford University Press.

Hinshaw, S. P., & Anderson, C. A. (1996). Conduct and oppositional defiant disorders. In E. J. Mash & R. A. Barkley (Eds.), *Child psychopathology* (pp. 113–149). New York: Guilford Press.

Hobson, R. P. (1989). Beyond cognition: A theory of autism. In G. Dawson (Ed.), *Autism: Nature, diagnosis, and treatment* (pp. 22–48). New York: Guilford Press.

Hobson, R. P. (1993). Understanding persons: The role of affect. In S. Baron-Cohen, H. Tager-Flusberg, & D. J. Cohen (Eds.), *Understanding other minds* (pp. 204–227). Oxford, UK: Oxford University Press.

Hobson, R. P., & Lee, A. (1999). Imitation and identification in autism. *Journal of Child Psychology and Psychiatry, 40,* 649–659.

Hodapp, R. M., Burack, J. A., & Zigler, E. (1998). Developmental approaches to mental retardation: A short introduction. In J. A. Burack, R. M. Hodapp, & E. Zigler (Eds.), *Handbook of mental retardation and development* (pp. 3–19). Cambridge, UK: Cambridge University Press.

Hodapp, R. M., & Dykens, E. M. (1996). Mental retardation. In R. J. Mash & R. A. Barkley (Eds.), *Child psychopathology* (pp. 362–389). New York: Guilford Press.

Hodapp, R. M., Leckman, J. F., Dykens, E. M., Sparrow, S., Zelinsky, D., & Ort, S. (1992). K-ABC profiles in children with fragile X syndrome, Down syndrome, and nonspecific mental retardation. *American Journal on Mental Retardation, 97,* 39–46.

Hodapp, R. M., & Zigler, E. (1990). Applying the developmental perspective to individuals with Down syndrome. In D. Cicchetti & M. Beeghly (Eds.), *Children with Down syndrome* (pp. 1–28). New York: Cambridge University Press.

Hodge, S. E. (1993). Linkage analysis versus association analysis: distinguishing between two models that explain disease–marker associations. *American Journal of Human Genetics, 53*(2), 367–384.

Hoffman, H. (1845). *Der Struwwelpeier: Oder lustige Geschichien unddrollige Bilder.* Leipzig: Insel-Verlag.

Hollander, E., Simeon, D., & Gorman, J. M. (1999). Anxiety disorders. In R. E. Hales, S. C. Yudofsky, & J. A. Talbott (Eds.), *Textbook of psychiatry* (pp. 567–633). Washington, DC: American Psychiatric Press.

Holmes, D. S. (1997). *Abnormal psychology.* New York: Longman.

Hooley, J. M., & Candela, S. F. (1999). Interpersonal functioning in schizophrenia. In T. Millon, P. H. Blaney, & R. D. Davis (Eds.), *Oxford textbook of psychopathology* (pp. 311–338). New York: Oxford University Press.

Hounsfield, G. N. (1979). Computed medical imaging. Nobel lecture, December 8, 1979. *Journal of Computer Assisted Tomography, 4*(5), 665–674.

Howland, R. H., & Thase, M. E. (1999). Affective disorders: Biological aspects. In T. Millon, P. H. Blaney, & R. D. Davis (Eds.), *Oxford textbook of psychopathology* (pp. 166–202). New York: Oxford University Press.

Hughlings-Jackson, J. (1931). *Selected writings* (J. Taylor, Ed.). London: Hodder & Stoughton.

Hulme, C., & Mackenzie, S. (1992). *Working memory and severe learning difficulties.* Hove, UK: Erlbaum.

Hynd, G. W., Hall, J., Novey, E. S., & Eliopulos, D. (1995). Dyslexia and corpus callosum morphology. *Archives of Neurology, 52,* 32–38.

Hynd, G. W., Hern, K. L., Novey, E. S., & Eliopulos, D., Marshall, R., Gonzalez, J. J., & Voeller, K. K. S. (1993). Attention deficit hyperactivity disorder and asymmetry of the caudate nucleus. *Journal of Child Neurology, 8,* 339–347.

Hynd, G. W., Semrud-Clikeman, M., Lorys, A. R., Novey, E. S., Eliopulas, D. (1990). Brain morphology in developmental dyslexia and attention deficit disorder/hyperactivity. *Archives of Neurology, 47,* 919–926.

Hynd, G. W., Semrud-Clikeman, M., Lorys, A. R., Novey, E. S., Eliopulos, D., & Lyytinen, H. (1991). Corpus callosum morphology in attention-deficit hyperactivity disorder: Morphometric analysis of MRI. *Journal of Learning Disabilities, 24,* 141–146.

Ingram, J. L., Stodgell, C. J., Hyman, S. L., Figlewicz, D. A., Weitkamp, L. R., & Rodier, P. M. (2000). Discovery of allelic variants of HOXA1 and HOXB1: Genetic susceptibility to autism spectrum disorders. *Teratology, 62,* 393–405.

International Molecular Genetic Study of Autism Consortium. (1998). A full genome screen for autism with evidence for linkage to a region on chromosome 7q. *Human Molecular Genetics, 7,* 571–578.

International Molecular Genetic Study of Autism Consortium. (2001). A genomewide screen for autism: Strong evidence for linkage to chromosomes 2q, 7q, and 16p. *American Journal of Human Genetics, 69,* 570–581.

Jamison, K. R. (1993). *Touched with fire: Manic depressive illness and the artistic temperment.* New York: Free Press.

Jamison, K. R. (1995). *An unquiet mind.* New York: Knopf.

Jernigan, T. L., Bellugi, U., Sowell, E., Doherty, S., & Hesselink, J. R. (1993). Cerebral morphologic distinctions between Williams and Down syndromes. *Archives of Neurology, 50*(2), 186–191.

Jernigan, T., Hesselink, J. R., Sowell, E., & Tallal, P. (1991). Cerebral structure on magnetic resonance imaging in language- and learning-impaired children. *Archives of Neurology, 48,* 539–545.

Johnson, S. L., & Roberts, J. E. (1995). Life events and bipolar disorder: Implications for biological theories. *Psychological Bulletin, 117*(3), 434–449.

Just, M. A., & Carpenter, P. A. (1987). *The psychology of reading and language comprehension.* Boston: Allyn & Bacon.

Kagan, J., Reznick, J. S., & Gibbons, J. (1989). Inhibited and uninhibited types of children. *Child Development, 60,* 838–845.

Kail, R. (1994). A method of studying the generalized slowing hypothesis in children with specific language impairment. *Journal of Speech and Hearing Research, 37,* 418–421.

Kanner, L. (1943). Autistic disturbances of affective contact. *Nervous Child, 2,* 217–250.

Kanner, L. (1945). *Child psychiatry.* Springfield, IL: Thomas.

Kaplan, H. I., & Sadock, B. J. (1988). *Synopsis of psychiatry* (5th ed.). Baltimore: Williams & Wilkins.

Karayiorgou, M., Altemus, M., Galke, B. L., Goldman, D., Murphy, D. L., Ott, J., &

Gogos, J. A. (1997). Genotype determining low catechol-O-methyltransferase activity as a risk factor for obsessive-compulsive disorder. *Proceedings of the National Academy of Science USA, 94,* 4572–4575.

Kashani, J. H., & Orvaschel., H. (1990). A community study of anxiety in children and adolescents. *American Journal of Psychiatry, 147,* 313–318.

Kashani, J. H., Vaidya, A. F., Soltys, S. M., Dandoy, A. C., Katz, L. M., & Reid, J. C. (1990). Correlates of anxiety in psychiatrically hospitalized children and their parents. *American Journal of Psychiatry, 147,* 319–323.

Katsuragi, S., Kunugi, H., Sano, A., Tsutsumi, T., Isogawa, K., Nanko, S., & Akiyoshi, J. (1999). Association between serotonin transporter gene polymorphism and anxiety-related traits. *Biological Psychiatry, 45,* 368–370.

Kelley, A. E. (1987). Dopamine and mental illness: Phenomenological and anatomical considerations. Open peer commentary to: N. R. Swerdlow & G. F. Koob (1987). [Dopamine, schizophrenia, mania, and depression: Toward a unified hypothesis of cortico–strito–pallido–thalamic function.] *Behavioral and Brain Science, 10,* 197–245.

Kelsoe, J. R. (1997). The genetics of bipolar disorder. *Psychiatric Annals, 27,* 557–566.

Kemper, M. B., Hagerman, R. J., Ahmad, R. S., & Mariner, R. (1986). Cognitive profiles and the spectrum of clinical manifestations in heterozygous fra(X) females. *American Journal of Medical Genetics, 23,* 139–156.

Kemper, M. B., Hagerman, R. J., & Altshul-Stark, D. (1988). Cognitive profiles of boys with the fragile X syndrome. *American Journal of Medical Genetics, 30,* 191–200.

Kendler, K. S. (1999). Molecular genetics of schizophrenia. In D. S. Charney, E. J. Nestler, & B. S. Bunney (Eds.), *Neurobiology of mental illness* (pp. 203–213). New York: Oxford University Press.

Kendler, K. S., & Gardner, C. O., Jr. (1998). Boundaries of major depression: An evaluation of DSM-IV criteria. *American Journal of Psychiatry, 155,* 172–177.

Kendler, K. S., Heath, A. C., Martin, N. G., & Eaves, L. J. (1987). Symptoms of anxiety and depression and generalized anxiety disorder: Same genes, (partly) different environments? *Archives of General Psychiatry, 44,* 451–457.

Kendler, K. S., Karkowski, L. M., & Prescott, C. A. (1999). Causal relationship between stressful life events and the onset of major depression. *American Journal of Psychiatry, 156,* 837–848.

Kendler, K. S., Neale, M. C., Kessler, R. C., Heath, A. C., & Eaves, L. J. (1992a). Generalized anxiety disorder in women: A population-based twin study. *Archives of General Psychiatry, 49,* 267–272.

Kendler, K. S., Neale, M. C., Kessler, R. C., Heath, A. C., & Eaves, L. J. (1992b). Major depression and generalized anxiety disorder: Same genes, (partly) different environments? *Archives of General Psychiatry, 49,* 716–722.

Kendler, K. S., Neale, M. C., Kessler, R. C., Heath, A. C., & Eaves, L. J. (1992c). A population-based twin study of major depression in women. *Archives of General Psychiatry, 49,* 257–266.

Kendler, K. S., Neale, M. C., Kessler, R. C., Heath, A. C., & Eaves, L. J. (1993a). Panic disorder in women: A population-based twin study. *Psychological Medicine, 23,* 397–406.

Kendler, K. S., Neale, M. C., Kessler, R. C., Heath, A. C., & Eaves, L. J. (1993b). A twin study of recent life events and difficulties. *Archives of General Psychiatry, 50,* 789–796.

Kendler, K. S., Walters, E. E., Neale, M. C., Kessler, R. C., Heath, A. C., & Eaves, L. J. (1995). The structure of the genetic and environmental risk factors for six major psychiatric disorders in women: Phobia, generalized anxiety disorder, panic disorder, bulimia, major depression, and alcoholism. *Archives of General Psychiatry, 52,* 374–383.

Kerr, J. (1897). School hygiene, in its mental, moral, and physical aspects. *Journal of the Royal Statistical Society, 60,* 613–680.

Kerr, M., Tremblay, R. E., Pagani, L., & Vitaro, F. (1997). Boys' behavioral inhibition and the risk of later delinquency. *Archives of General Psychiatry, 54,* 809–816.

Kesslak, J. P., Nagata, S. F., Lott, I., & Nalcioglu, O. (1994). Magnetic resonance imaging analysis of age-related changes in the brains of individuals with Down's syndrome. *Neurology, 44,* 1039–1045.

Kessler, R. C., McGonagle, K. A., Zhao, S., Nelson, C. B., Hughes, M., Eshleman, S., Wittchen, H., & Kendler, K. S. (1994). Lifetime and 12–month prevalence of DSM-III-R psychiatric disorders in the United States. *Archives of General Psychiatry, 51,* 8–19.

Kessler, R. C., Sonnega, A., Bromet, R., Hughes, M., & Nelson, C. B. (1995). Posttraumatic stress disorder in the National Comorbidity Survey. *Archives of General Psychiatry, 52,* 1048–1060.

Kidd, K. K. (1993). Associations of disease with genetic markers: Déjà vu all over again. *American Journal of Medical Genetics (Neuropsychiatric Genetics), 48,* 71–73.

Klein, D. F. (1993). False suffocation alarms, spontaneous panics, and related conditions: An integrative hypothesis. *Archives of General Psychiatry, 50,* 306–317.

Klerman, G. L., & Weissman, M. M. (1989). Increasing rates of depression. *Journal of the American Medical Association, 261,* 2229–2235.

Klinger, L. G., & Dawson, G. (1996). Autistic disorder. In E. J. Mash & R. A. Barkley (Eds.), *Child psychopathology* (pp. 311–339). New York: Guilford Press.

Knowles, J. A., Kaufmann, C. A., & Rieder, R. O. (1999). Genetics. In R. E. Hales, S. C. Yudofsky, & J. A. Talbott (Eds.), *Textbook of psychiatry* (pp. 35–82). Washington, DC: American Psychiatric Press.

Kobayashi, R., Murata, T., & Yoshinaga, K. (1992). A follow-up study of 201 children with autism in Kyushu and Yamaguchi areas, Japan. *Journal of Autism and Developmental Disorders, 22,* 395–411.

Kolb, B., & Whishaw, I. Q. (1990). *Fundamentals of human neuropsychology* (3rd ed.). New York: Freeman.

Kovacs, M., Akiskal, H. S., Gatsonis, C., & Parrone, P. L. (1994). Childhood-onset dysthymic disorder: Clinical features and prospective naturalistic outcome. *Archives of General Psychiatry, 51,* 365–374.

Kovacs, M., Gatsonis, C., Paulaskas, S. L., & Richards, C. (1989). Depressive disorders in childhood: IV. A longitudinal study of comorbidity with and risk for anxiety disorders. *Archives of General Psychiatry, 46*(9), 776–782.

Kraepelin, E. (1971). *Dementia praecox and paraphrenia.* Huntington, NY: Krieger. (Original work published 1919)

Kramer, P. D. (1993). *Listening to Prozac.* New York: Viking Press.

Kruesi, M. J., Hibbs, E. D., Zahn, T. P., Keysor, C. S., Hamburger, S. D., Bartko, J. J., & Rapoport, J. L. (1992). A 2–year prospective follow-up study of children and adolescents with disruptive behavior disorders: Prediction by cerebrospinal fluid 5–hydroxyindoleacetic acid, homovanillic acid, and autonomic measures? *Archives of General Psychiatry, 49,* 429–435.

Kuntsi, J., Osterlaan, J., & Stevenson, J. (2001). Psychological mechanisms in hyperactivity: I. Response inhibition deficit, working memory impairment, delay aversion, or something else? *Journal of Child Psychology and Psychiatry, 42,* 199–210.

Kuntsi, J., & Stevenson, J. (2001). Psychological mechanisms in hyperactivity: II. The role of genetic factors. *Journal of Child Psychology and Psychiatry, 42,* 211–219.

Kutcher, S. P. (1998). Affective disorders in children and adolescents: A critical clinically relevant review. In B. T Walsh (Ed.), *Child psychopharmacology* (pp. 91–114). Washington, DC: American Psychiatric Press.

LaBar, K. S., & LeDoux, J. E. (1997). Emotion and the brain: An overview. In T. E. Feinberg & M. J. Farah (Eds.), *Behavioral neurology and neuropsychology* (pp. 675–689). New York: McGraw-Hill.

Lachiewicz, A. M., Spiridigliozzi, G. A., Gullion, C. M., & Ransford, S. N. (1994). Aberrant behaviors of young boys with fragile X syndrome. *American Journal on Mental Retardation, 98*(5), 567–579.

LaHoste, G., Wigal, S., Glabe, C., Cook, E., Kennedy, J., & Swanson, J. (1995, November). *Dopamine related genes and attention deficit hyperactivity disorder.* Paper presented at the annual meeting of the Society for the Neurosciences, San Diego, CA.

Lainhart, J. E., Piven, J., Wzorek, M., Landa, R., Santangelo, S. L., Coon, H., & Folstein, S. E. (1997). Macrocephaly in children and adults with autism. *Journal of the American Academy of Child and Adolescent Psychiatry, 36*(2), 282–292.

Lamb, J. A., Moore, J., Bailey, A., & Monaco, A. P. (2000). Autism: Recent molecular genetic advances. *Human Molecular Genetics, 9,* 861–868.

Lapouse, R. L., & Monk, M. A. (1958). An epidemiologic study of behavior characteristics in children. *American Journal of Public Health, 48,* 1134–1144.

Larsen, J. P., Høien, T., & Ödegaard, H. (1990). MRI evaluation of the size and symmetry of the planum temporale in adolescents with developmental dyslexia. *Brain and Language, 39,* 289–301.

Last, C. G., Hersen, M., Kazdin, A. E., Orvaschel, H., & Perrin, S. (1991). Anxiety disorders in children and their families. *Archives of General Psychiatry, 48,* 928–934.

LeJeune, J., Gautier, M., & Turpin, R. (1959). Etudes des chromosomes somatiques de neuf enfants mongoliens. *Comptes Rendus de l'Académie des Sciences, 48,* 1721.

Leonard, L. B. (2000). *Children with specific language impairment.* Cambridge, MA: MIT Press.

Leonard, S., Gault, J., Moore, T., Hopkins, J., Robinson, D., Olincy, A., Adler, L. E., Cloninger, C. R., Kaufmann, D., Tsuang, M. T., Faraone, S. V., Malaspina, D., Svrakic, F., & Freedman, R. (1998). Further investigation of a chromosome 15 locus in schizophrenia: analysis of affected sibpairs from the NIMH genetics initiative. *American Journal of Medical Genetics (Neuropsychiatric Genetics), 81,* 308–312.

Lesch, K. P., Bengel, D., Heils, A., Sabol, S. Z., Greenberg, B. D., Petri, S., Benjamin, J., Muller-Reible, C. R., Hamer, D. H., & Murphy, D. L. (1996). A gene regulatory region polymorphism alters serotonin transporter expression and is associated with anxiety-related personality traits. *Science, 274,* 1527–1531.

Levin, H. S., Eisenberg, H. M., & Benton, A. L. (1991). *Frontal lobe function and dysfunction.* New York: Oxford University Press.

Levy, F., Hay, D., McStephen, M., Wood, C., & Waldman, I. (1997). Attention-deficit hyperactivity disorder: A category or a continuum? A genetic analysis of a large-scale twin study. *Journal of the American Academy of Child and Adolescent Psychiatry, 36,* 737–744.

Lewinsohn, P. M. (1974). A behavioral approach to depression. In R. J. Friedman & M. M. Katz (Eds.), *The psychology of depression: Contemporary theory and research* (pp. 157–185). Washington, DC: Winston/Wiley.

Lewinsohn, P. M., Rohde, P. D., Seeley, J. R., & Fischer, S. A. (1993). Age-cohort changes in the lifetime occurrence of depression and other mental disorders. *Journal of Abnormal Psychology, 102,* 110–120.

Lewinsohn, P. M., Steinmetz, J. L., Larson, D. W., & Franklin, J. (1981). Depression-related cognitions: Antecedent or consequence? *Journal of Abnormal Psychology, 90,* 213–219.

Lewis, B. (1992). Pedigree analysis of children with phonology disorders. *Journal of Learning Disabilities, 25,* 586–597.

Lewis, B., Ekelman, B., & Aram, D. (1989). A family study of severe phonological disorders. *Journal of Speech and Hearing Research, 32,* 713–724.

Lewis, B., & Thompson, L. A. (1992). A study of developmental speech and language disorders in twins. *Journal of Speech and Hearing Research, 35,* 1086–1094.

Lewis, B. A., & Freebairn, L. (1992). Residual effects of preschool phonology disorders in grade school, adolescence, and adulthood. *Journal of Speech and Hearing Research, 35*(4), 819–831.

Liberman, A. M., Cooper, F. S., Shankweiler, D. P., & Studdert-Kennedy, M. (1967). Perception of the speech code. *Psychological Review, 74*(6), 431–461.

Liberman, I. Y., & Liberman, A. M. (1990). Whole language vs. code emphasis: Underlying assumptions and their implications for reading instruction. *Annals of Dyslexia, 40,* 51–76.

Liberman, I. Y., Shankweiler, D., Fischer, F. W., & Carter, B. (1974). Reading and the awareness of linguistic segments. *Journal of Experimental Child Psychology, 18,* 201–212.

Liu, D., Korio, J., Tannenbaum, B., Caldji, C., Francis, D., Freedman, A., Sharma, S., Pearson, S., Plotsky, P. M., & Meaney, M. J. (1997). Maternal care, hippocampal glucocorticoid receptors, and hypothalmic–pituitary–adrenal responses to stress. *Science, 277,* 1659–1662.

Loeber, R. (1990). Development and risk factors of juvenile antisocial behavior and delinquency. *Clinical Psychology Review, 10,* 1–41.

Loeber, R., Wung, P., Keenan, K., Giroux, B., Stouthamer-Loeber, M., Van Kammen, W. B., & Maughan, B. (1993). Developmental pathways in disruptive child behavior. *Development and Psychopathology, 5,* 103–133.

Logan, G., Schachar, R., & Tannock, R. (1997). Impulsivity and inhibitory control. *Psychological Science, 8,* 60–64.

Logan, G. D., Cowan, W. B., & Davis, K. A. (1984). On the ability to inhibit simple and choice reaction time responses: A model and a method. *Journal of Experimental Psychology: Human Perception and Performance, 10,* 276–291.

Lögdberg, B., & Brun, A. (1993). Prefrontal neocortical disturbances in mental retardation. *Journal of Intellectual Disability Research, 37,* 459–468.

Lombroso, P. J., & Leckman, J. F. (1999). The neurobiology of Tourette's syndrome and tic-related disorders in children. In D. S. Charney, E. J. Nestler, & B. S. Bunney (Eds.), *Neurobiology of mental illness* (pp. 779–787). New York: Oxford University Press.

Lord, C., Rutter, M., & LeCouteur, A. (1994). Autism Diagnostic Interview—Revised: A revised version of a diagnostic interview for caregivers of individuals with possible pervasive developmental disorders. *Journal of Autism and Developmental Disorders, 24,* 659–685.

Losier, B., McGrath, P., & Klein, R. (1996). Error patterns on the continuous performance test in non-medicated and medicated samples of children with and without ADHD: A meta-analytic review. *Journal of Child Psychology and Psychiatry, 37,* 971–987.

Lou, H. C., Henriksen, L., & Bruhn, P. (1984). Focal cerebral hypoperfusion in children with dysphasia and/or attention deficit disorder. *Archives of Neurology, 41,* 825–829.

Lou, H. C., Henriksen, L., & Bruhn, P. (1989). Strial dysfunction in attention deficit and hyperkinetic disorder. *Archives of Neurology, 46,* 48–52.

Lovaas, O. I. (1987). Behavioral treatment and normal educational and intellectual functioning in young autistic children. *Journal of Consulting and Clinical Psychology, 55,* 3–9.

Luhrmann, T. M. (2000). *Of two minds: The growing disorder in American psychiatry.* New York: Knopf.

Luria, A. (1961). *The role of speech in the regulation of normal and abnormal behavior.* New York: Pergamon Press.

Luria, A. (1966). *Higher cortical functions in man.* New York: Basic Books.

Lykken, D. T. (1957). A study of anxiety in the sociopathic personality. *Journal of Abnormal and Social Psychology, 55,* 6–10.

Maes, B., Fryns, J. P., Van Walleghem, M., & Van den Berghe, H. (1993). Fragile X syndrome and autism: A prevalent association or a misinterpreted connection? *Genetic Counseling, 4*(4), 245–263.

Mahler, M. (1952). On child psychosis and schizophrenia: Autistic and symbiotic infantile psychosis. *Psychoanalytic Study of the Child, 7,* 286–305.

Mahurin, R. K. (1998). Neural network modeling of basal ganglia function in Parkinson's disease and related disorders. In R. W. Parks, D. S. Levine, & D. L. Long (Eds.), *Fundamentals of neural network modeling: Neuropsychology and cognitive neuroscience* (pp. 331–355). Cambridge, MA: MIT Press.

Malizia, A. L., Cunningham, V. J., Bell, C. J., Liddle, P. F., Jones, T., & Nutt, D. J. (1998). Decreased brain GABA$_A$ benzodiazepine receptor binding in panic disorder. *Archives of General Psychiatry, 55,* 715–720.

Mangan, P. A. (1992). *Spatial memory abilities and abnormal development of the hippocamal formation in Down syndrome.* Unpublished doctoral dissertation, University of Arizona, Tucson.

Mangan, P., & Nadel, L. (1992). Spatial memory development and development of the hippocampal formation in Down syndrome [Abstract]. *International Journal of Psychology, 27,* 129.

Manis, F. R., Seidenberg, M. S., Doi, L. M., McBride-Chang, C., & Petersen, A. (1996). On the bases of two subtypes of developmental dyslexia. *Cognition, 58,* 157–195.

Manuck, S. B., Flory, J. D., Ferrell, R. E., Dent, K. M., Mann, J. J., & Muldoon, M. F. (1999). Aggression and anger-related traits associated with a polymorphism of the tryptophan hydroxylase gene. *Biological Psychiatry, 45*(5), 603–614.

Manuck, S. B., Flory, J. D., Ferrell, R. E., Dent, K. M., Mann, J. J., & Muldoon, M. F. (1998). Aggression, impulsivity, and central nervous system serontonergic responsivity in a nonpatient sample. *Neuropsychopharmacology, 19*(4), 287–299.

Marcell, M. M., & Weeks, S. L. (1988). Short-term memory difficulties and Down's syndrome. *Journal of Mental Deficiency Research, 32,* 153–162.

Marenco, S., & Weinberger, D. R. (2000). The neurodevelopmental hypothesis of schizophrenia: Following a trail of evidence from cradle to grave. *Development and Psychopathology, 12*(3), 501–527.

Marks, I. (1977). Phobias and obsessions: Clinical phenomena in search of laboratory models. In J. D. Maser & M. E. P. Seligman (Eds.), *Psychopathology: Experimental models* (pp. 174–213). San Francisco: Freeman.

Marshall, J. C., & Newcombe, F. (1966). Syntactic and semantic errors in paralexia. *Neuropsychologia, 4,* 169–176.

Mataro, M., Garcia-Sanchez, C., Junque, C., Estevez-Gonzales, A., & Pujol, J. (1997). Magnetic resonance imaging measurement of the caudate nucleus in adolescents with attention-deficit hyperactivity disorder and its relationship with neuropsychological and behavioral measures. *Archives of Neurology, 54,* 963–968.

Mattes, J. A. (1989). The role of frontal lobe dysfunction in childhood hyperkinesis. *Comprehensive Psychiatry, 21,* 358–369.

Mattingly, I. G. (1972). Reading, the linguistic process, and linguistic awareness. In J. F. Kavanaugh & I. G. Mattingly (Eds.), *Language by ear and by eye: The relationship between speech and reading* (pp. 131–147). Cambridge, MA: MIT Press.

Mayr, E. (2000). Darwin's influence on modern thought. *Scientific American, 283,* 78–83.

Mazzanti, C. M., Lappalainen, J., Long, J. C., Bengel, D., Naukkarinen, H., Eggert, M.,

Virkkunen, M., Linnoila, M., & Goldman, D. (1998). Role of the serotonin transporter promoter polymorphism in anxiety-related traits. *Archives of General Psychiatry, 55,* 936–940.

Mazzocco, M. M. M., Hagerman, R. J., Cronister-Silverman, A., & Pennington, B. F. (1992). Specific frontal lobe deficits in women with the fragile X gene. *Journal of the American Academy of Child and Adolescent Psychiatry, 31,* 1141–1148.

Mazzocco, M. M. M., Pennington, B. F., & Hagerman, R. J. (1993). The neurocognitive phenotype of females carriers of fragile X: Additional evidence for specificity. *Journal of Developmental and Behavioral Pediatrics, 14,* 328–335.

McEachin, J. J., Smith, T., & Lovaas, O. I. (1993). Long-term outcome for children with autism who received early intensive behavioral treatment. *American Journal on Mental Retardation, 97,* 359–372.

McGee, R., Feehan, M., Williams, S., & Anderson, J. C. (1992). DSM-III disorders from age 11 to age 15 years. *Journal of the American Academy of Child and Adolescent Psychiatry, 31,* 932–940.

McGuffin, P., & Huckle, P. (1990). Simulation of Mendelism revisited: The recessive gene for attending medical school. *American Journal of Human Genetics, 46,* 994–999.

McNally, R. J. (1999). Posttraumatic stress disorder. In T. Millon, P. H. Blaney, & R. D. Davis (Eds.), *Oxford textbook of psychopathology* (pp. 144–165). New York: Oxford University Press.

Meaney, J. J., Diorio, J., Francis, D., Widdowson, J., LaPlante, P., Caldji, C., Sharma, S., Seckl, J. R., & Plotsky, P. M. (1996). Early environmental regulation of forebrain glucocorticoid receptor gene expression: Implications for adrenocortical response to stress. *Developmental Neuroscience, 18,* 49–72.

Mednick, S. A., Gabrielli, W. F., & Hutchings, B. (1983). Genetic influences in criminal behavior: Some evidence from an adoption cohort. In K. T. VanDusen & S. A. Mednick (Eds.), *Prospective studies of crime and delinquency* (pp. 39–56). Hingham, MA: Martinus Nyhoff.

Meehl, P. E. (1973). Schizotaxia, schizotypy, schizophrenia. *American Psychology, 17,* 827–838.

Meltzoff, A. N. (1995). Understanding the intentions of others: Re-enactment of intended acts by 18-month-old children. *Developmental Psychology, 31,* 1–16.

Meltzoff, A. N., & Gopnik, A. (1993). The role of imitation in understanding persons and developing a theory of mind. In S. Baron-Cohen, H. Tager-Flusberg, & D. J. Cohen (Eds), *Understanding other minds* (pp. 335–366). Oxford, UK: Oxford University Press.

Merikangas, K. R., & Kupfer, D. F. (1995). Mood disorders: Genetic aspects. In H. I. Kaplan & B. J. Sadock (Eds.), *Comprehensive textbook of psychiatry* (6th ed., pp. 1102–1116). Baltimore: Williams & Wilkins.

Mervis, C. B. (1999). The Williams syndrome cognitive profile: Strengths, weaknesses, and interrelations among auditory short term memory, language, and visuospatial constructive cognition. In R. Fivush, W. Hirst, & E. Winograd (Eds.), *Essays in honor of Ulric Neisser* (pp. 193–227). Mahwah, NJ: Erlbaum.

Mervis, C. B., & Bertrand, J. (1997). Developmental relations between cognition and language: Evidence from Williams syndrome. In L. B. Adamson & M. A. Rornski (Eds.), *Research on communication and language acquisition: Discoveries from atypical development* (pp. 75–106). New York: Brookes.

Mervis, C. B., & Klein-Tasman, B. P. (2000). Williams syndrome: Cognition, personality, and adaptive behavior. *Mental Retardation and Developmental Disabilities Research Reviews, 6,* 148–158.

Mervis, C. B., Morris, C. A., Bertrand, J., & Robinson, B. F. (1999). Williams syndrome:

Findings from an integrated program of research. In H. Tager-Flusberg (Ed.), *Neurodevelopmental disorders* (pp. 65–110). Cambridge, MA: MIT Press.

Miezejeski, C. M., Jenkins, E. C., Hill, A. L., Wisniewski, K., French, J. H., & Brown, W. T. (1986). A profile of cognitive deficit in females from fragile X families. *Neuropsychology, 24,* 405–409.

Miklowitz, D. J., & Goldstein, M. J. (1990). Behavioral family treatment for patients with bipolar affective disorder. *Behavior Modification, 14,* 457–489.

Miller, J. N., & Ozonoff, S. (1997). Did Asperger's cases have Asperger disorder?: A research note. *Journal of Child Psychology and Psychiatry, 38,* 247–251.

Miller, K. D., Keller, J. B., & Stryker, M. P. (1989). Ocular dominance column development: Analysis and simulation. *Science, 245,* 605–615.

Mineka, S., Gunnar, M., & Champoux, M. (1986). Control and early socioemotional development: Infant rhesus monkeys reared in controllable versus uncontrollable environments. *Child Development, 57,* 1241–1256.

Moffitt, T. E. (1993). Adolescence-limited and life-course-persistent antisocial behavior: A developmental taxonomy. *Psychological Review, 100,* 674–701.

Molenaar, P. C. M., Boomsma, D. I., & Dolan, C. V. (1993). A third source of developmental differences, *Behavior Genetics, 23,* 519–524.

Monroe, S. M., & Depue, R. A. (1991). Life stress and depression. In J. Becker & A. Kleinman (Eds.), *Psychosocial aspects of depression* (pp. 101–130). Hillsdale, NJ: Erlbaum.

Morais, J., Cary, L., Algeria, J., & Bertelson, P. (1979). Does awareness of speech as a sequence of phonemes arise spontaneously? *Cognition, 7,* 323–331.

Morgan, T. H. (1917). The theory of the gene. *The American Naturalist, LL,* 513–545.

Moore, D. G., Hobson, R. P., & Lee, A. (1997). Components of person perception: An investigation with autistic, non-autistic retarded and typically developing children and adolescents. *British Journal of Developmental Psychology, 15,* 401–423.

Morris, R. (1984, February). *Multivariate methods for neuropsychology: Techniques for classification, identification, and prediction research.* Paper presented at the meeting of the International Neuropsychological Society, Houston, TX.

Morton, J., & Frith, U. (1995). Causal modeling: A structural approach to developmental psychopathology. In D. Cicchetti & D. J. Cohen (Eds.), *Developmental psychopathology: Vol. 1. Theory and methods* (pp. 357–390). New York: Wiley.

Mowrer, O. H. (1939). Stimulus response theory of anxiety. *Psychological Review, 46,* 553–565.

MTA Cooperative Group. (1999). A 14-month randomized clinical trial of treatment strategies for attention-deficit/hyperactivity disorder. *Archives of General Psychiatry, 56,* 1073–1086.

Mukherjee, S., Sackeim, H. A., & Schnur, D. B. (1994). Electroconvulsive therapy of acute manic episodes: A review of 50 years' experience. *American Journal of Psychiatry, 151,* 169–176.

Mundy, P., & Neal, R. (2000). Neural plasticity, joint attention, and a transactional social-orienting model of autism. *International Review of Research in Mental Retardation, 20,* 139–168.

Mundy, P., & Sigman, M. (1989). Specifying the nature of the social impairment in autism. In G. Dawson (Ed.), *Autism: Nature, diagnosis, and treatment* (pp. 3–21). New York: Guilford Press.

Mundy, P., Sigman, M., Ungerer, J., & Sherman, T. (1986). Defining the social deficits of autism: The contribution of nonverbal communication measures. *Journal of Child Psychology and Psychiatry, 27,* 657–669.

Murray, C. J., & Lopez, A. D. (1997). Global mortality, disability, and the contribution of risk factors: Global Burden of Disease Study. *Lancet, 349,* 1436–1442.

Nadder, T. S., Silberg, J. L., Eaves, L. J., Maes, H. H., & Meyer, J. M. (1998). Genetic effects on ADHD symptomatology in 7– to 13–year-old twins: Results from a telephone survey. *Behavior Genetics, 28*, 83–99.

Nadel, L. (1986). Down syndrome in neurobiological perspective. In C. J. Epstein (Ed.), *The neurobiology of Down syndrome* (pp. 239–251). New York: Raven Press.

Nadel, L. (1999). Down syndrome in cognitive neuroscience perspective. In H. Tager-Flushberg (Ed.), *Neurodevelopmental disorders* (pp. 197–221). Cambridge, MA: MIT Press.

Neale M. C., & Kendler, K. S. (1995). Models of comorbidity for multifactorial disorders. *Journal of Human Genetics, 57*, 935–953.

Nemeroff, C. B. (1998). The neurobiology of depression. *Scientific American, 278*, 42–49.

Neville, H. J. (1990). Intermodal competition and compensation in development: Evidence from studies of the visual system in congenitally deaf adults. In A. Diamond (Ed.), The development and neural bases of higher cognitive functions. *Annals of the New York Academy of Sciences, 608*, 71–91.

Nichols, P. L. (1984). Twin studies of ability, personality, and interests. *Behavior Genetics, 14*, 161–170.

Nielsen, D. A., Goldman, D., Virkunnen, M., Tokola, R., Rawlings, R., & Linnoila, M. (1994). Suicidality and 5–hydroxyindoleactic acid concentration associated with a tryptophan hydroxylase polymorphism. *Archives of General Psychiatry, 51*(1), 34–38.

Nietzel, M. T., Speltz, M. L., McCauley, E. A., & Bernstein, D. A. (1998). *Abnormal psychology.* Boston: Allyn & Bacon.

Nigg, J. T. (1999). The ADHD response inhibition deficit as measured by the Stop Task: Replication with DSM-IV combined type, extension, and qualification. *Journal of Abnormal Child Psychology, 27*, 391–400.

Nigg, J. T. (2000). On inhibition/disinhibition in developmental psychopathology: Views from cognitive and personality psychology and a working inhibition taxonomy. *Psychological Bulletin, 126*, 1–27.

Nigg, J. T., Hinshaw, S. P., Carte, E., & Treuting, J. (1998). Neuropsychological correlates of childhood attention deficit hyperactivity disorder: Explainable by comorbid disruptive behavior or reading problems? *Journal of Abnormal Psychology, 107*, 468–480.

Nöthan, M. M., Schulte-Körne, G., Grimm, T., Cichon, S., Vogt, I. R., Müller-Myhsok, B., Propping, P., & Remschmidt, H. (1999). Genetic linkage analysis with dyslexia: Evidence for linkage of spelling disability to chromosome 15. *European Child and Adolescent Psychiatry, 8*, 56–59.

Nowakowski, R. S. (1987). Basic concepts of CNS development. *Child Development, 58*, 568–595.

Nurnberger, J. I., & Gershon, E. S. (1992). Genetics. In E. S. Paykel (Ed.), *Handbook of affective disorders* (pp. 126–145). New York: Guilford Press.

Nye, C., Foster, S., & Seaman, D. (1987). Effectiveness of language intervention with the language/learning disabled. *Journal of Speech and Hearing Disorders, 52*, 348–357.

Oades, R. D. (1987). Attention deficit disorder with hyperactivity: The contribution of catecholaminergic activity. *Progress in Neurobiology, 29*, 365–391.

Offord, D. R., Alder, R. J., & Boyle, M. H. (1986). Prevalence and sociodemographic correlates of conduct disorder. *American Journal of Social Psychiatry, 4*, 272–278.

Ohara, K., Suzuki, Y., Ochiai, M., Tsukamoto, T., Tani, K., & Ohara, K. (1999). A variable number tandem repeat of the serotonin transporter gene and anxiety disorders. *Progress in Neuropsychopharmacology and Biological Psychiatry, 23*, 55–65.

Öhman, A. (2000). Fear and anxiety: Evolutionary, cognitive, and clinical perspectives. In M. Lewis & J. M. Haviland-Jones (Eds.), *Handbook of emotions* (2nd ed., pp. 573–593). New York: Guilford Press.

Olds, D., Henderson, C. R., Jr., Cole, R., Eckenrode, J., Kitzman, H., Luckey, D., Pettitt, L., Sidora, K., Morris, P., & Powers, J. (1998). Long-term effects of nurse home visitation on children's criminal and antisocial behavior: 15-year follow-up of a randomized controlled trial. *Journal of the American Medical Association, 280,* 1238–1244.

Oliver, A., Johnson, M. H., Karmiloff-Smith, A., & Pennington, B. (2000). Deviations in the emergence of representations: A neuroconstructivist framework for analyzing developmental disorders. *Developmental Science, 3,* 1–40.

Oosterlaan, J., & Sergeant, J. A. (1998). Response inhibition in ADHD, CD, comorbid ADHD + CD, anxious and normal children: A meta-analysis of studies with the stop task. *Journal of Child Psychology and Psychiatry, 39,* 411–426.

O'Regan, K. (1979). Moment to moment control of eye saccades as a function of textual parameters in reading. In P. A. Kolers, M. E. Wrolstad, & H. Bouma (Eds.), *Processing of visible language, I* (pp. 49–60). New York: Plenum Press.

O'Reilly, R. C., & Munakata, Y. (2000). *Computational explorations in cognitive neuroscience: Understanding the mind by simulating the brain.* Cambridge, MA: MIT Press.

Orton, S. T. (1925). "Word-blindness" in school children. *Archives of Neurology and Psychiatry, 14,* 582–615.

Orton, S. T. (1937). *Reading, writing, and speech problems in children.* New York: Norton.

Osterling, J., & Dawson, G. (1994). Early recognition of children with autism: A study of first birthday home videotapes. *Journal of Autism and Developmental Disorders, 24,* 247–257.

Oyama, S. (1999). Locating development: Locating developmental systems. In E. K. Scholnick & K. Nelson (Eds.), *Conceptual development: Piaget's legacy* (pp. 185–208). Mahwah, NJ: Erlbaum.

Ozonoff, S., & Cathcart, K. (1998). Effectiveness of a home program intervention for young children with autism. *Journal of Autism and Developmental Disorders, 28,* 25–32.

Ozonoff, S., Pennington, B. F., & Rogers, S. (1990). Are there emotion perception deficits in young autistic children? *Journal of Child Psychology and Psychiatry, 31*(3), 343–361.

Ozonoff, S., Pennington, B. F., & Rogers, S. J. (1991). Executive function deficits in high-functioning autistic individuals: Relationship to theory of mind. *Journal of Child Psychology and Psychiatry, 32*(7), 1081–1105.

Ozonoff, S. Strayer, D. L., McMahon, W. M., & Filloux, F. (1998). Inhibitory deficits in Tourette syndrome: A function of comorbidity and symptom severity. *Journal of Child Psychiatry, 39,* 1109–1118.

Palfrey, J. S., Levine, M. D., Walker, D. K., & Sullivan, M. (1985). The emergence of attention deficits in early childhood: A prospective study. *Journal of Developmental and Behavioral Pediatrics, 6,* 339–348.

Panksepp, J. (1998). *Affective neuroscience: The foundations of human and animal emotions.* New York: Oxford University Press.

Park, S., & Holzman, P. (1992). Schizophrenics show spatial working memory deficits. *Archives of General Psychiatry, 49,* 975–982.

Patrick, C. J., Cuthbert, B. N., & Lang, P. J. (1994). Emotion in the criminal psychopath: Fear image processing. *Journal of Abnormal Psychology, 103,* 523–534.

Patterson, K. E., Marshall, J. C., & Coltheart, M. (1985). *Surface dyslexia.* Hillsdale, NJ: Erlbaum.

Patzer, D. K., & Volkmar, R. R. (1999). The neurobiology of autism and the pervasive developmental disorders. In D. S. Charney, E. J., Nestler, & B. S. Bunney (Eds.), *Neurobiology of mental illness* (pp. 761–778). New York: Oxford University Press.

Paulesu, E., Frith, U., Snowling, M., Gallagher, A., Morton, J., Frackowiak, R. S., &

Frith, C. D. (1996). Is developmental dyslexia a disconnection syndrome? Evidence from PET scanning. *Brain, 119*, 143–157.

Pauls, D. L., Alsobrook, J. P., Goodman, W., Rasmussen, S., & Leckman, J. F. (1995). A family study of obsessive–compulsive disorder. *American Journal of Psychiatry, 152*, 76–84.

Pauls, D. L., Hurst, C. R., Kruger, S. D., Leckman, J. F., Kidd, K. K., & Cohen, D. J. (1986a). Gilles de la Tourette's syndrome and attention deficit disorder with hyperactivity. *Archives of General Psychiatry, 43*, 1177–1179.

Pauls, D. L., & Leckman, J. F. (1986). The inheritance of Gilles de la Tourette's syndrome and associated behaviors. *New England Journal of Medicine, 315*, 993–997.

Pauls, D. L., Towbin, K. E., Leckman, J. F., Zahner, G. E. P., & Cohen, D. J. (1986b). Gilles de la Tourette's syndrome and obsessive-compulsive disorder. *Archives of General Psychiatry, 43*, 1180–1182.

Pelham, W. E., Jr., Wheeler, T., & Chronis, A. (1998). Empirically supported psychosocial treatments for attention deficit hyperactivity disorder. *Journal of Clinical Child Psychology, 27*, 190–205.

Pennington, B. F. (1991). *Diagnosing learning disorders: A neuropsychological framework.* New York: Guilford Press.

Pennington, B. F. (1994). The working memory function of the prefrontal cortices: Implications for developmental and individual differences in cognition. In M. M. Haith, J. Benson, R. Roberts, & B. F. Pennington (Eds.), *The development of future oriented processes* (pp. 243–289). Chicago: University of Chicago Press.

Pennington, B. F. (1997). Using genetics to dissect cognition [Invited editorial]. *American Journal of Human Genetics, 60*, 13–16.

Pennington, B. F., & Bennetto, L. (1998). Toward a neuropsychology of mental retardation. In J. A. Burack, R. M. Hodapp, & E. Zigler (Eds.), *Handbook of mental retardation and development* (pp. 210–248). Cambridge, UK: Cambridge University Press.

Pennington, B. F., & Bennetto, L. (1993). Main effects or transactions in the neuropsychology of conduct disorder?: Commentary on "the neuropsychology of conduct disorder. " *Development and Psychopathology, 5*, 151–164.

Pennington, B. F., Filipek, P. A., Lefly, D., Churchwell, J., Kennedy, D. N., Simon, J. H., Filley, C. M., Galaburda, A., Alarcon, M., & DeFries, J. C. (1999). Brain morphometry in reading-disabled twins. *Neurology, 53*, 723–729.

Pennington, B. F., Grossier, D., & Welsh, M. C. (1993). Contrasting cognitive deficits in attention deficit hyperactivity disorder versus reading disability. *Developmental Psychology, 29*, 511–523.

Pennington, B. F., & Lefly, D. L. (2001). Early reading development in children at family risk for dyslexia. *Child Development, 72*, 816–833.

Pennington, B. F., Moon, J., Edgin, J., Stedron, J., & Nadel, L. (2001). *The neuropsychology of Down syndrome: Evidence for hippocampal dysfunction.* Manuscript submitted for publication.

Pennington, B. F., & Ozonoff, S. (1991). A neuroscientific perspective on continuity and discontinuity in developmental psychopathology. In D. Cicchetti (Ed.), *Rochester Symposium on Developmental Psychopathology* (Vol. III, pp. 117–159). Rochester, NY: University of Rochester Press.

Pennington, B. F., & Ozonoff, S. (1996). Executive functions and developmental psychopathology. *Journal of Child Psychology and Psychiatry, 37*, 51–87.

Pennington, B. F., Smith, S. D., Kimberling, W. J., Green, P. A., & Haith, M. M. (1987). Left-handedness and immune disorders in familial dyslexics. *Archives of Neurology, 44*, 634–639.

Pennington, B. F., Van Orden, G. C., Smith, S. D., Green, P. A., & Haith, M. M. (1990).

Phonological processing skills and deficits in adult dyslexics. *Child Development,* 61(6), 1753–1778.

Pennington, B. F., & Welsh, M. C. (1995). Neuropsychology and developmental psychopathology. In D. Cicchetti & D. J. Cohen (Eds.), *Manual of developmental psychopathology* (Vol. I, pp. 254–290). New York: Wiley.

Perfetti, C. A. (1985). *Reading ability.* New York: Oxford University Press.

Perfetti, C. A, & Lesgold, A. M. (1979). Coding and comprehension in skilled reading and implications for reading instruction. In L. B. Resnick & P. A. Weaver (Eds.), *Theory and practice of early reading, Volume 1* (pp. 57–84). Hillsdale, NJ: Erlbaum.

Persico, A. M., D'Agruma, L., Mauirano, N., Totaro, A., Militerni, R., Bravaccio, C., Wassink, T. H., Schneider, C., Melmed, R., Trillo, S., Montecchi, F., Palermo, M., Pascucci, T., Puglisi-Allegra, S., Reichelt, K. L., Conciatori, M., Marino, R., Quattrocchi, C. C., Baldi, A., Zelante, L., Gasparin, P., Keller, F., & Collaborative Linkage Study of Autism. (2001). Reelin gene alleles and haplotypes as a factor predisposing to autistic disorder. *Molecular Psychiatry, 6,* 150–159.

Pert, C. B. (1997). *Molecules of emotion.* New York: Scribner's.

Peterson, B. S., Leckman, J. F., & Cohen, D. J. (1995). Tourette's syndrome: A genetically predisposed and an environmentally specified developmental psychopathology. In D. Cicchetti & D. J. Cohen (Eds.), *Developmental psychopathology* (pp. 213–242). New York: Wiley.

Petryshen, T. L., Kaplan, B. J., & Field, L. (1999). Evidence for a susceptibility locus for phonological coding dyslexia on chromosome 6q13–q16.2. *American Journal of Human Genetics, 65,* A32.

Petryshen, T. L., Kaplan, B. J., Liu, M. F., & Field, L. L. (2000). Absence of significant linkage between phonological coding dyslexia and chromosome 6p23–21.3, as determined by use of quantitative-trait methods: Confirmation of qualitative analyses. *American Journal of Human Genetics, 66*(2), 708–714.

Piven, J., Arndt, S., Bailey, J., Havercamp., S., Andreasen, N., & Palmer, P. (1995). An MRI study of brain size in autism. *American Journal of Psychiatry, 152,* 1145–1149.

Plante, E., Swisher, L., Vance, R., & Rapcsak, S. (1991). MRI findings in boys with specific language impairment. *Brain and Language, 41,* 52–66.

Plaut, D. (1995). Double dissociation without modularity: Evidence from connectionist neuropsychology. *Journal of Clinical and Experimental Neuropsychology, 17,* 291–321.

Plaut, D., McClelland, J. L., Seidenberg, M. S., & Patterson, K. E. (1996). Visual word recognition: Are two routes really necessary? *Psychological Review, 103,* 56–115.

Plomin, R. (1990). The role of inheritance in behavior. *Science, 248,* 183–188.

Plomin, R., DeFries, J. C. McClearn, G. E., & Rutter, M. (1997). *Behavioral genetics.* New York: Freeman.

Plomin, R., Lichtenstein, P., Pedersen, N., McClearn, G. E., & Nesselroade, J. R. (1990). Genetic influences on life events during the last half of the life span. *Psychology of Aging, 5,* 25–30.

Plomin, R., & Rutter, M. (1998). Child development, molecular genetics, and what to do with genes once they are found. *Child Development, 69,* 1223–1242.

Pontius, A. A. (1973). Dysfunctional patterns analogous to frontal lobe system and caudate nucleus syndromes in some groups of minimal brain dysfunction. *Journal of American Medical Women Association, 28,* 285–292.

Popper, C., & West, S. A. (1999). Disorders usually first diagnosed in infancy, childhood, or adolescence. In R. E. Hales, S. C. Yudofsky, & J. A. Talbott (Eds.), *Textbook of psychiatry* (3rd ed., pp. 825–954). Washington, DC: American Psychiatric Press.

Post, R. (1992). Transduction of psychosocial stress into the neurobiology of recurrent affective disorder. *American Journal of Psychiatry, 149,* 999–1010.

Post, R., Rubinow, D., & Ballenger, J. (1986). Conditioning and sensitization in the longitudinal course of affective illness. *British Journal of Psychiatry, 149,* 191–201.

Poulton, K., Holmes, J., Hever, T., Trumper, A., Fitzpatrick, H., McGufin, P., Owen, M., Worthington, J., Ollier, W., Harrington, R., & Thapar, A. (1998). A molecular genetic study of hyperkinetic disorder/attention deficit hyperactivity disorder. *American Journal of Medical Genetics, 81,* 458.

Prange, A., Wilson, I., Lynn, C., Alltop, L., & Stikeleather, R. (1974). L-trytophan in mania: Contribution to a permissive hypothesis of affective disorders [Abstract]. *Archives of General Psychiatry, 30,* 56–62.

Pringle-Morgan, W. P. (1896). A case of congenital word-blindness (inability to learn to read). *British Medical Journal, 2,* 1543–1544.

Prouty, L. A., Rogers, R. C., Stevenson, R. E., Dean, J. H., Palmer, K. K., Simensen, R. J., Coston, G. N., & Schwartz, C. E. (1988). Fragile X syndrome: Growth development and intellectual function. *American Journal of Medical Genetics, 30,* 123–142.

Pueschel, S. M., Gallagher, P. L., Zartler, A. S., & Pezzullo, J. C. (1987). Cognitive and learning processes in children with Down syndrome. *Research in Developmental Disabilities, 8,* 21–37.

Rack, J., Snowling, M., & Olson, R. (1992). The nonword reading deficit in developmental dyslexia: A review. *Reading Research Quarterly, 27,* 28–53.

Raine, A. (1993). *The psychopathology of crime.* New York: Academic Press.

Raine, A., Brennan, P., & Mednick, S. A. (1997). Interaction between birth complications and early maternal rejection in predisposing individuals to adult violence: Specificity to serious, early-onset violence. *American Journal of Psychiatry, 154*(9), 1265–1271.

Raine, A., & Jones, F. (1987). Attention, autonomic arousal, and personality in behaviorally disordered children. *Journal of Abnormal Child Psychology, 15,* 583–599.

Raine, A., Venebles, P. H., & Williams, M. (1990). Relationships between central and autonomic measures of arousal at age 15 years and criminality at age 24 years. *Archives of General Psychiatry, 47,* 1003–1007.

Raleigh, M. J., McGuire, M. T., Brammer, G. L., & Yuwiler, A. (1984). Social and environmental influence on blood serotonin concentrations in monkeys. *Archives of General Psychiatry, 47,* 405–410.

Ramey, C. T., & Campbell, F. A. (1984). Preventive education for high-risk children: Cognitive consequence of the Carolina Abecedarian Project. *American Journal on Mental Deficiency, 88,* 515–523.

Rapin, I. (1987). Searching for the cause of autism: A neurologic perspective. In D. J. Cohen & A. M. Donnellan (Eds.), *Handbook of autism and pervasive developmental disorders* (pp. 710–717). New York: Wiley.

Rauch, S. L., van der Kolk, B. A., Fisler, R. E., Alpert, N. M., Ort, S. P., Savage, C. R., Fischman, A. J., Jenike, M. A., & Pitman, R. K. (1996). A symptom provocation study of posttraumatic stress disorder using positron emission tomography and script-driven imagery. *Archives of General Psychiatry, 53,* 380–387.

Rayner, K., & Pollatesek, A. (1989). *The psychology of reading.* Englewood Cliffs, NJ: Prentice-Hall.

Raz, N., Torres, I. J., Briggs, S. D., Spencer, W. D., Thornton, A. E., Loken, W. J., Gunning, F. M., McQuain, J. D., Driesen, N. R., & Acker, J. D. (1995). Selective neuroanatomical abnormalities in Down syndrome and their cognitive correlates: Evidence from MRI morphometry. *Neurology, 45,* 356–366.

Reed, E. W., & Reed, S. C. (1965). *Mental retardation: A family study.* Philadelphia: Saunders.

Reeves, R. H., Baxter, L. L., & Richtsmeir, J. T. (2001). Too much of a good thing: Mechanisms of gene action in Down syndrome. *Trends in Genetics, 17,* 83–88.

Reiss, A. L., Aylward, E., Freund, L. S., Joshi, P. K., & Bryan, R. N. (1991). Neuroanatomy of the fragile X syndrome: The posterior fossa. *Annals of Neurology, 29,* 26–32.

Reiss, A. L., & Freund, L. S. (1991). Behavioral phenotype of fragile X syndrome: DSM-III-R autistic behavior in male children. *American Journal of Medical Genetics, 43,* 35–46.

Rende, R., & Plomin, R. (1995). Nature, nurture, and the development of psychopathology. In D. Cicchetti & D. J. Cohen (Eds.), *Developmental psychopathology, Vol 1: Theory and methods* (pp. 291–314). New York: Wiley.

Rende, R. D., Plomin, R., Reiss, D., & Hetherington, E. M. (1993). Genetic and environmental influences on depressive symptomatology in adolescence: Individual differences and extreme scores. *Journal of Child Psychology and Psychiatry, 8,* 1387–1398.

Resick, P., & Schnicke, M. (1992). Cognitive processing therapy for sexual assault victims. *Journal of Consulting and Clinical Psychology, 60,* 748–756.

Rice, M., & Oetting, J. (1993). Morphological deficits in children with SLI: Evaluation of number marking and agreement. *Journal of Speech and Hearing Research, 36,* 1249–1257.

Ricketts, M. H., Hamer, R. M., Sage, J. L., Manowitz, P., Feng, F., & Menza, M. A. (1998). Association of a serotonin transporter gene promoter polymorphism with harm avoidance behavior in an elderly population. *Psychiatric Genetics, 8,* 41–44.

Rimland, B. (1964). *Infantile autism.* New York: Meredith.

Risch, N., & Merikangas, K. (1996). The future of genetic studies of complex human diseases. *Science, 272,* 1516–1517.

Roberts, R. J., & Pennington, B. F. (1996). An interactive framework for examining prefrontal cognitive processes. *Developmental Neuropsychology, 12,* 105–126.

Robertson, M. M., & Stern, J. S. (1998). Tic disorders: New developments in Tourette syndrome and related disorders. *Current Opinions in Neurology, 11,* 373–380.

Robins, L. (1966). *Deviant children grown up.* Baltimore: Williams & Wilkins.

Robins, L. N. (1991). Conduct disorder. *Journal of Child Psychology and Psychiatry, 32*(1), 193–212.

Rodier, P. M. (2000). The early origins of autism. *Scientific American, 282,* 56–63.

Rogers, S. J., & Pennington, B. F. (1991). A theoretical approach to the deficits in infantile autism. *Development and Psychopathology, 3,* 137–163.

Rogers, S. J. (1998). Empirically supported comprehensive treatments of young children with autism. *Journal of Clinical Child Psychology, 27,* 168–179.

Rogers, S. I., Wehner, B, & Pennington, B. F. (2002). *Joint attention and understanding intentions in young children with autism.* Manuscript in preparation.

Rolls, E. T. (1999). *The brain and emotion.* New York: Oxford University Press.

Rondal, J. A. (1993). Exceptional cases of language development in mental retardation: The relative autonomy of language as a cognitive system. In H. Tager-Flusberg (Ed.), *Constraints on language acquisition* (pp. 155–174). Hillsdale, NJ: Erlbaum.

Rosenbaum, J. F., Biederman, J., Gersten, M., Hirshfeld, D. R., Meminger, S. R., Herman, J. B., Kagan, J., Reznick, J. S., & Snidman, N. (1988). Behavioral inhibition in children of parents with panic disorder and agoraphobia: A controlled study. *Archives of General Psychiatry, 45,* 463–470.

Rosenbaum, J. F., Biederman, J., Hirschfeld, D. R., Bolduc, E. A., & Chaloff, J. (1991a). Behavioral inhibition in children: A possible, precursor to panic disorder or social phobia. *Journal of Clinical Psychiatry, 52*(Suppl. 5), 5–9.

Rosenbaum, J. F., Biederman, J., Hirschfeld, D. R., Bolduc, E. A., Faraone, S. V., Kagan, J., Snidman, N., & Reznick, J. S. (1991b). Further evidence of an association between behavioral inhibition and anxiety disorders: Results from a family study of children from a non-clinical sample. *Journal of Psychiatric Research, 25,* 49–65.

Rosenthal, R. H., & Allen, T. W. (1978). An examination of attention, arousal and learning dysfunctions of hyperkinetic children. *Psychological Bulletin, 85,* 689–715.

Rowe, D. C., Stever, C., Gard, J. M. C., Cleveland, H. H., Sander, M. L., Abramowitz, A., Kozol, S. T., Mohr, J. H., Sherman, S. L., & Waldman, I. D. (1998). The relation of the dopamine transporter gene (DAT1) to symptoms of internalizing disorders in children. *Behavior Genetics, 28,* 215–225.

Rowe, D. C., Stever, G., Giedinghagen, L. N., Gard, J. M., Cleveland, H. H., Terris, S. T., Hohr, J. H., Sherman, S., Abramowitz, A., & Waldman, I. D. (1998). Dopamine DRD4 receptor polymorphism and attention deficit hyperactivity disorder. *Molecular Psychiatry, 3,* 419–426.

Rozin, P., Haidt, J., & McCauley, C. R. (2000). Disgust. In M. Lewis & J. M. Haviland-Jones (Eds.), *Handbook of emotions* (pp. 637–653). New York: Guilford Press.

Rumsey, J. M. (1996). Neuroimaging in developmental dyslexia: A review and conceptualization. In G. R. Lyon & J. M. Rumsey (Eds.), *Neuroimaging* (pp. 57–77). Baltimore: Brookes.

Rumsey, J. M., Donohue, B. C., Brady, D. R., Nace, K., Giedd, J. N., & Andreason, P. (1997). A magnetic resonance imaging study of planum temporale asymmetry in men with developmental dyslexia. *Archives of Neurology, 54,* 1481–1489.

Rumsey, J. M., Horwitz, B., Donohue, B. C., Nace, K., Maisog, J. M., & Andreason, P. (1997). Phonologic and orthographic components of word recognition: A PET-rCBF study. *Brain, 120,* 739–759.

Rumsey, J. M., Nace, K., Donohue, B., Wise, D., Maisog, J. M., & Andreason, P. (1997). A PET study of impaired word recognition and phonological processing in dyslexic men. *Archives of Neurology, 54,* 562–578.

Russell, A. T., Bott, L., & Sammons, C. (1989). The phenomenology of schizophrenia occurring in childhood. *Journal of the American Academy of Child and Adolescent Psychiatry, 28,* 399–407.

Russell, J. (1996). *Agency.* London: Taylor & Francis.

Russell, J. (1997). *Autism as an executive disorder.* New York: Oxford University Press.

Russell, J., & Hill, E. L. (2001). Action-monitoring and intention reporting in children with autism. *Journal of Child Psychology and Psychiatry, 42*(3), 317–328.

Russo, J., Vitaliano, P. P., Brewer, D. D., Katon, W., & Becker, J. (1995). Psychiatric disorders in spouse caregivers of care recipients with Alzheimer's disease and matched controls: A diathesis-stress model of psychopathology. *Journal of Abnormal Psychology, 104*(1), 197–204.

Rutter, M. L. (1997). Nature–nurture integration: The example of antisocial behavior. *American Psychologist, 52,* 390–398.

Rutter, M. (2000). Genetic studies of autism: From the 1970s into the millennium. *Journal of Abnormal Child Psychology, 28,* 3–14.

Rutter, M. (2001, April). *Nature, nurture, and development: From evangelism through science towards policy and practice.* Presidential address presented to the Society for Research and Child Development, Minneapolis, MN.

Rutter, M., Andersen-Wood, L., Beckett, C., Bredenkamp, D., Castle, J., Groothues, C., Kreppner, J., Keaveney, L., Lord, C., O'Connor, T. G., & English and Romanian Adoptee (ERA) Study Team. (1999). Quasi-autistic patterns following severe early global privation. *Journal of Child Psychology and Psychiatry, 40,* 537–549.

Rutter, M., & Mahwood, L. (1991). The long-term psychosocial sequelae of specific developmental disorders of speech and language. In M. Rutter & P. Casaer (Eds.), *Biological risk factors for psychosocial disorders* (pp. 233–259). Cambridge, UK: Cambridge University Press.

Rutter, M., & Quinton, D. (1977). Psychiatric disorders: Ecological factors and concepts of causation. In H. McGurk (Ed.), *Ecological factors in human development* (pp. 173–187). Amsterdam: North-Holland.

Rutter, M., & Quinton, D. (1984). Parental psychiatric disorder: Effects on children. *Psychological Medicine, 14,* 853–880.

Sachar, E. J. (1981). Psychobiology of affective disorders. In E. R. Kandel & J. H. Schwartz (Eds.), *Principles of neural science* (pp. 611–619). New York: Elsevier/ North-Holland.

Sameroff, A., & Chandler, M. I. (1975). Reproductive risk and the continuum of caretaking causality. In F. D. Horowitz, M. Hetherington, S. Scarr-Salapatek, & G. Siegel (Eds.), *Review of child development research* (Vol. 4, pp. 187–244). Chicago: University of Chicago Press.

Sanchez, M. M., Ladd, C. O., & Plotsky, P. M. (2001). Early adverse experience as a developmental risk factor for later psychopathology: Evidence from rodent and primate models. *Development and Psychopathology, 13,* 419–449.

Sanders, A. F. (1983). Towards a model of stress and performance. *Acta Psychologica, 53,* 61–97.

Sanderson, W., Rapee, R., & Barlow, D. (1989). The influence of perceived control on panic attacks induced via inhalation of 5.5% CO_2-enriched air. *Archives of General Psychiatry, 46,* 157–162.

Sapolsky, R. M. (1994). *Why zebras don't get ulcers: A guide to stress, stress related diseases, and coping.* New York: Freeman.

Sapolsky, R. M. (1996). Why stress is bad for your brain. *Science, 273,* 749–750.

Sarter, M., Bernston, G. G., & Cacioppo, J. T. (1996). Brain imaging and cognitive neuroscience. *American Psychologist, 51,* 13–21.

Satcher, D. (1999). *Mental health: A report of the surgeon general* [Online]. Available: http: //www. mentalhealth.org/specials/surgeongeneralreport

Saykin, A. J., Gur, R. C., Gur, R. E., Mozley, P. D., Mozley, L. H., Resnick, S. M., Kester, D. B., & Stafiniak, P. (1991). Neuropsychological function in schizophrenia: Selective impairment in memory and learning. *Archives of General Psychiatry, 48,* 618–624.

Scarr, S. (1992). Developmental theories for the 1990's: Development and individual differences. *Child Development, 63,* 1–19.

Scarr, S., & Salapatek, P. (1970). Patterns of fear development during infancy. *Merrill–Palmer Quarterly, 16,* 53–90.

Scazufca, M., & Kuipers, E. (1998). Stability of expressed emotion in relatives of those with schizophrenia and its relationship with burden of care and perception of patients: Social functioning. *Psychological Medicine, 28,* 453–461.

Schachar, R. J., Tannock, R., & Logan, G. (1993). Inhibitory control, impulsiveness, and attention deficit hyperactivity disorder. *Clinical Psychology Review, 13,* 721–739.

Schain, R., & Yannet, H. (1960). Infantile autism: An analysis of 50 cases and a consideration of certain relevant neurophysiological concepts. *Journal of Pediatrics, 57,* 550–567.

Scheuffgen, K., Happé, F. Anderson, M., & Frith, U. (2000). High "intelligence," low "IQ"?: Speed of processing and measured IQ in children with autism. *Development and Psychopathology, 12,* 83–90.

Schildkraut, J. (1965). The catecholamine hypothesis of affective disorders: A review of supporting evidence. *American Journal of Psychiatry, 122,* 509–522.

Schmidt-Sidor, B., Wisniewski, K. E, Shepard, T. H., & Serson, E. A. (1990). Brain growth in Down syndrome subjects 15 to 22 weeks of gestational age and birth to 60 months. *Clinical Neuropathology, 9*(4), 181–190.

Schmidt, N. B., Storey, J., Greenberg, B. D., Santiago, H. T., Li, Q., & Murphy, D. L.

(2000). Evaluating gene x psychological risk factor effects in the pathogenesis of anxiety: A new model approach. *Journal of Abnormal Psychology, 109*(2), 308–320.

Schultz, R. R., Cho, N. K., Staib, L. H., Kier, L., & Fletcher, J. (1994). Brain morphology in normal and dyslexic children: The influence of sex and age. *Annals of Neurology, 35*, 732–742.

Schultz, R. T., Gauthier, I., Klin, A., Fulbright, R. K., Anderson, A. W., Volkmar, F., Skudlarski, P., Lacadie, C., Cohen, D. J., & Gore, J. C. (2000). Abnormal ventral temporal cortical activity during face discrimination among individuals with autism and Asperger syndrome. *Archives of General Psychiatry, 57*, 331–340.

Schwartz, J. M., Stoessel, P. W., Baxter, L. R., Jr., Martin, K. M., & Phelps, M. E. (1996). Systematic changes in cerebral glucose metabolic rate after successful behavioral modification treatment of obsessive–compulsive disorder. *Archives of General Psychiatry, 53*, 109–113.

Seaman, M. I., Fisher, J. B., Chang, F., & Kidd, K. K. (1999). Tandem duplication polymorphism upstream of the dopamine D4 receptor gene (DRD4). *American Journal of Medical Genetics, 88*(6), 705–709.

Seidenberg, M. S., & McClelland, J. L. (1989). A distributed developmental model of word recognition and naming. *Psychological Review, 96*, 447–452.

Seligman, M. E. P. (1975). *Helplessness: On depression, development, and death.* San Francisco: Freeman.

Seligman, M. E. P., Walker, E. F., & Rosenhan, D. L. (2001). *Abnormal psychology* (4th ed.). New York: Norton.

Semrud-Clikeman, M., Filipek, P. A., Biederman, J., Steingard, R., Kennedy, D., Renshaw, P., & Bekken, K. (1994). Attention-deficit hyperactivity disorder: Magnetic resonance imaging morphometric analysis of the corpus callosum. *Journal of the American Academy of Child and Adolescent Psychiatry, 33*, 875–881.

Sergeant, J. A., & van der Meere, J. J. (1990). Convergence of approaches in localizing the hyperactivity deficit. In B. B. Lahey & A. E. Kazdin (Eds.), *Advancements in clinical child psychology* (Vol. 13, pp. 207–245). New York: Plenum Press.

Shalev, A. Y., Peri, T., Canetti, L., & Schreiber, S. (1996). Predictors of PTSD in injured trauma survivors: A prospective study. *American Journal of Psychiatry, 153*, 219–225.

Shallice, T. (1988). *From neuropsychology to mental structure.* New York: Cambridge University Press.

Share, D. L., & Stanovich, K. E. (1995). Cognitive processes in early reading development: Accommodating individual differences into a model of acquisition. *Issues in Education: Contributions from Educational Psychology, 1*, 1–57.

Shaywitz, B. A., Cohen, D. J., & Bowers, M. B. (1977). CSF monoamine metabolites in children with minimal brain dysfunction: Evidence for alteration of brain dopamine. *Journal of Pediatrics, 90*, 6771.

Shaywitz, S. E., Shaywitz, B. A., Cohen, D. J., & Young, J. G. (1983). Monoaminegic mechanisms in hyperactivity. In M. Rutter (Ed.), *Developmental neuropsychiatry* (pp. 330–347). New York: Guilford Press.

Shaywitz, S. E., Shaywitz, B. A., Fletcher, J. M., & Escobar, M. D. (1990). Prevalence of reading disability in boys and girls. *Journal of the American Medical Association, 264*, 998–1002.

Sherman, D., Iacono, W., & McGue, M. (1997). Attention-deficit/hyperactivity disorder dimensions: A twin study of inattention and impulsivity/hyperactivity. *Journal of the American Academy of Child and Adolescent Psychiatry, 36*, 745–753.

Sherman, J. (1998). Effects of psychotherapeutic treatments for PTSD: A meta-analysis of controlled clinical trials. *Journal of Traumatic Stress, 11*(3), 413–435.

Sherman, S. (1996). Epidemiology. In R. Hagerman & A. Cronister (Eds.), *Fragile X syndrome* (pp. 165–192). Baltimore: Johns Hopkins University Press.

Shin, L. M., Kosslyn, S. M., McNally, R. J., Alpert, N. M., Thompson, W. L., Rauch, S. L., Macklin, M. L., & Pitman, R. K. (1997). Visual imagery and perception in posttraumatic stress disorder: A positron emission tomographic investigation. *Archives of General Psychiatry, 54*, 233–241.

Shin, L. M., McNally, R. J., Kosslyn, S. M., Thompson, W. L., Rauch, S. L., Alpert, N. M., Metzger, L. J., Lasko, N. B., Orr, S. P., & Pitman, R. K. (1999). Regional cerebral blood flow during script-driven imagery in childhood sexual abuse-related posttraumatic stress disorder: A positron emission tomographic investigation. *American Journal of Psychiatry, 156*(4), 575–584.

Shonkoff, J. P., & Phillips, D. A. (2000). *From neurons to neighborhoods: The science of early childhood development.* Washington, DC: National Academy Press.

Shriberg, L. D., Tomblin, J. B., & McSweeny, J. L. (1999). Prevalence of speech delay in 6–year-old children and comorbidity with language impairment. *Journal of Speech, Language, and Hearing Research, 42*, 1461–1481.

Silberg, J., Rutter, M., Meyer, J., Maes, H., Hewitt, J., Simonoff, E., Pickles, A., Loeber, R., & Eaves, L. (1996). Genetic and environmental influences on the covariation between hyperactivity and conduct disturbance in juvenile twins. *Journal of Child Psychology and Psychiatry, 37*, 803–816.

Silver, L. B. (1995). Controversial therapies. *Journal of Child Neurology, 10*, S96–S100.

Silverstein, A. B., Legutski, G., Friedman, S. L., & Tayakama, D. L. (1982). Performance of Down syndrome individuals on the Stanford–Binet intelligence scale. *American Journal of Mental Deficiency, 86*, 548–551.

Simon, J. A., Keenan, J. M., Pennington, B. F., Taylor, A. K., & Hagerman, R. J. (2001). Discourse processing in women with Fragile X syndrome: Evidence for a deficit establishing coherence. *Cognitive Neuropsychology, 18*, 1–18.

Simonoff, E., Bolton, P., & Rutter, M. (1998). Genetic perspectives on mental retardation. In J. A. Burack, R. M. Hodapp, & E. Zigler (Eds.), *Handbook of mental retardation and development* (pp. 41–79). Cambridge, UK: Cambridge University Press.

Singer, H. S., Reiss, A. L., Brown, J. E., Aylward, E. H., Shih, B., Chee, E., Harris, E. L., Reader, M. J., Chase, G. A., Bryan, R. N., & Denckla, M. B. (1993). Volumetric MRI changes in basal ganglia of children with Tourette's syndrome. *Neurology, 43*, 950–956.

Skre, I., Onstad, S., & Torgersen, S., Lygren, S., & Kringlen, E. (1993). A twin study of DSM-III-R (1987), anxiety disorders. *Acta Psychiatrica Scandinavia, 88*, 85–92.

Skuse, D. H. (1997). Genetic factors in the etiology of child psychiatric disorders. *Current Opinion in Pediatrics, 9*, 354–360.

Skuse, D. H. (2000). Behavioral neuroscience and child psychopathology: Insights from model systems. *Journal of Child Psychology and Psychiatry and Allied Disciplines, 41*(1), 3–31.

Smalley, S. L., Bailey, J. N., Palmer, G. G., Cantwell, D. P., McGough, J. J., Del'Homme, M. A., Asarnow, J. R., Woodward, J. A., Ramsey, C., & Nelson, S. F. (1998). Evidence that the dopamine D4 receptor is a susceptibility gene in attention deficit hyperactivity disorder. *Molecular Psychiatry, 3*, 427–430.

Smith, A., & Weissman, M. M. (1992). Epidemiology. In E. S. Paykel (Ed.), *Handbook of affective disorders* (2nd ed., pp. 111–129). New York: Guilford Press.

Smith, S. D., Gilger, J. W., & Pennington, B. F. (in press). Dyslexia and other specific learning disorders. In D. L. Rimoin, J. M. Conner, & R. E. Pyeritz (Eds.), *Emery and Rimoin's principles and practice of medical genetics* (4th ed.). New York: Churchill Livingstone.

Snow, C. P. (1947). *The light and the dark.* New York: Scribner's.

Snowling, M. J. (1981). Phonemic deficits in developmental dyslexia. *Psychological Research, 43*(2), 219–234.

Snowling, M. J., Bishop, D. V. M., & Stothard, S. E. (2000). Is preschool language impairment a risk factor for dyslexia in adolescence? *Journal of Child Psychology and Psychiatry and Allied Disciplines, 41*(5), 587–600.

Sobesky, W. E., Hull, C. E., & Hagerman, R. J. (1994). Symptoms of schizotypal personality disorder in fragile X females. *Journal of the American Academy of Child and Adolescent Psychiatry, 33*(2), 247–255.

Sonuga-Barke, E. J. S., Taylor, E., Sembi, S., & Smith, J. (1992). Hyperactivity and Delay Aversion: I. The effect of delay on choice. *Journal of Child Psychology and Psychiatry, 33,* 387–398.

Sparrow, S. S., Balla, D. A., & Cicchetti, D. V. (1984). *Vineland adaptive behavior scales.* Circle Pines, MN: American Guidance Service.

Spielman, R. S., McGinnis, R. E., & Ewens, W. J. (1993). Transmission test of linkage disequilibrium: The insulin gene region and insulin-dependent diabetes mellitus (IDDM). *American Journal of Human Genetics, 52,* 506–516.

Spreen, O., Tupper, D., Risser, A., Tuckko, H., & Edgell, D. (1984). *Human developmental neuropsychology.* New York: Oxford University Press.

Sprenger, J. (1948). *Malleus maleficarum* (M. Summers, Trans.) London: Puskin. (Original work published 1489)

Staley, L. W., Hull, C. E., Mazzocco, M. M., Thibodeau, S. N., Snow, K., Wilson, V. L., Taylor, A., McGavran, L., Weiner, D., & Riddle, J. (1993). Molecular-clinical correlations in children and adults with fragile X syndrome. *American Journal Disorders of Children, 147,* 723–726.

Stamm, J. S., & Kreder, S. V. (1979). Minimal brain dysfunction: Psychological and neuropsychological disorders in hyperkinetic children. In M. S. Gazzaniga (Ed.), *Handbook of behavioral neurology: Vol. 2. Neuropsychology* (pp. 119–150). New York: Plenum Press.

Stanovich, K. E., Siegel, L. S., & Gottardo, A. (in press). Converging evidence for phonological and surface subtypes of reading disability. *Journal of Educational Psychology.*

Steffenburg, S., Gillberg, C., Hellgren, L., Andersson, L., Gillberg, I., Jakobson, G., & Bohman, M. (1989). A twin study of autism in Denmark, Finland, Iceland, Norway and Sweden. *Journal of Child Psychology and Psychiatry, 30,* 405–416.

Stern, D. N. (1985). *The interpersonal world of the infant: A view from psychoanalysis and developmental psychology.* New York: Basic Books.

Stevenson, J. (1992). Evidence for a genetic etiology in hyperactivity in children. *Behavior Genetics, 22,* 337–344.

Stevenson, J., Batten, N., & Cherner, M. (1992). Fears and fearfulness in children and adolescents: A genetic analysis of twin data. *Journal of Child Psychology and Psychiatry, 33,* 977–985.

Still, G. F. (1902). Some abnormal psychiacal conditions in children. *Lancet, 1,* 1008–1012, 1077–1082, 1163–1168.

Stone, E. A. (1975). Stress and catecholamines. In A. J. Fredhoff (Ed.), *Catecholamines and behavior.* (pp. 31–72). New York: Plenum Press.

Strauss, A., & Lehtinen, L. (1947). *Psychopathology and education of the brain-injured child.* New York: Grune & Stratton.

Stuss, D. T., & Benson, D. F. (1986). *The frontal lobes.* New York: Raven Press.

Styron, W. (1990). *Darkness visible: A memoir of madness.* New York: Random House.

Sudhalter, V. (1987, December). *Speech and language characteristics and intervention strategies with fragile X patients.* Paper presented at the First National Fragile X Conference, Denver, CO.

Sudhalter, V., Cohen, I. L., Silverman, W. P., & Wolf-Schein, E. G. (1990). Conversational analyses of males with fragile X, Down syndrome, and autism: A comparison of the emergence of deviant language. *American Journal of Mental Retardation, 94,* 431–441.

Sudhalter, V., Scarborough, H. S., & Cohen, I. C. (1991). Syntactic delay and pragmatic deviance in the language of fragile X males. *American Journal of Medical Genetics, 38,* 493–497.

Suomi, S. J. (1991). Early stress and adult emotional reactivity in rhesus monkeys. *CIBA Foundation Symposium, 156,* 171–183.

Swanson, J., Oosterlaan, J., Murias, M., Shuck, S., Flodman, P., Spence, A., Wasdell, M., Ding, Y., Chi, H., Smith, M., Mann, M., Carlson, C., Kennedy, J. L., Sergeant, J. A., Leung, P., Zhang, Y., Sadeh, A., Chen, C., Whalen, C. K., Babb, K. A., Moyzis, R., & Posner, M. I. (2000). Attention deficit/hyperactivity disorder in children with a 7–repeat allele of the dopamine receptor D4 gene have extreme behavior but normal performance on critical neuropsychological tests of attention. *Proceedings of the National Academy of Sciences of the United States of America, 97,* 4754–4759.

Swanson, J., Sunhora, G. A., Kennedy, J. L., Regino, R., Fineberg, E., Wigal, T., Lerner, M., Williams, L., LaHoste, G. J., & Wigal, S. (1998). Association of the dopamine receptor D4 (DRD4) gene with a refined phenotype of attention deficit hyperactivity disorder (ADHD): A family based approach. *Molecular Psychiatry, 3,* 38–41.

Swedo, S. E. (1994). Sydenham's chorea: A model for childhood autoimmune neuropsychiatric disorders. *Journal of the American Medical Association, 272,* 1788–1791.

Swedo, S. E., Leonard, H. L., Garvey, M., Mittleman, B., Allen, A. J., Perlmutter, S., Lougee, L., Dow, S., Zamkoff, J., & Dubbert, B. K. (1998). Pediatric autoimmune neuropsychiatric disorders associated with streptococcal infections: Clinical description of the first 50 cases. *American Journal of Psychiatry, 154,* 264–271.

Swerdlow, N. R., & Koob, G. F. (1987). Dopamine, schizophrenia, mania, and depression: Toward a unified hypothesis of cortico–strito–pallido–thalamic function. *Behavioral and Brain Science, 10,* 197–245.

Szatmari, P., Offord, D. R., & Boyle, M. (1989). Correlates, associated impairments, and patterns of service utilization of children with attention deficit disorders: Findings from the Ontario Child Health Study. *Journal of Child Psychology and Psychiatry, 30,* 205–217.

Tager-Flusberg, H. (in press). A re-examination of the theory of mind hypothesis of autism. To appear in J. Burack, T. Charman, N. Yirmiya, & P. Zelazo (Eds.), *The development of autism: Perspectives from theory and research.* Mahwah, NJ: Erlbaum.

Tager-Flusberg, H., Boshart, J., & Baron-Cohen, S. (1998). Reading the windows to the soul: Evidence of domain-specific sparing in Williams syndrome. *Journal of Cognitive Neuroscience, 10,* 631–639.

Tager-Flusberg, M., & Sullivan, K. (1998). Early language development in children with mental retardation. In J. A. Burack, R. M. Hodapp, & E. Zigler (Eds.), *Handbook of mental retardation and development* (pp. 208–239). Cambridge, UK: Cambridge University Press.

Tager-Flusberg, H., & Sullivan, K. (2000). A componential view of theory of mind: Evidence from Williams syndrome. *Cognition, 76(1),* 59–90.

Tager-Flusberg, H., Sullivan, K., & Boshart, J. (1997). Executive functions and performance on false belief tasks. *Developmental Neuropsychology, 13,* 487–493.

Tallal, P., Stark, R. E., & Mellits, E. D. (1985). Identification of language impaired children on the basis of rapid perception and production skill. *Brain and Language, 25,* 314–322.

Teicher, M. H., Polcari, A., English, C. D., Anderson, C. M., Anderson, S. L., Glod, C. A., & Renshaw, P. (1996). Dose-dependent effects of methylphenidate on activity, attention, and magnetic resonance imaging measures in children with ADHD [Abstract]. *Society for Neuroscience Abstracts, 22,* 1191.

Temple, C. M. (1985). Surface dyslexia and the development of reading. In K. E. Patterson, J. C. Marshall, & M. Coltheart (Eds.), *Surface dyslexia: Neuropsychological and cognitive studies of phonological reading* (pp. 261–288). Hillsdale, NJ: Erlbaum.

Temple, C. M., & Marshall, J. C. (1983). A case study of developmental phonological dyslexia. *British Journal of Psychology, 74,* 517–533.

Terwilliger, J. D., & Ott, J. (1992). A haplotype-based "haplotype relative risk" approach to detecting allelic associations. *Human Heredity, 42*(6), 337–346.

Thapar, A., Harold, G., & McGuffin, P. (1998). Life events and depressive symptoms in childhood—shared genes or shared adversity?: A research note. *Journal of Child Psychology and Psychiatry and Allied Disciplines, 39,* 1153–1158.

Thapar, A., Hervas, A., & McGuffin, P. (1995). Childhood hyperactivity scores are highly heritable and show sibling competition effects: Twin study evidence. *Behavior Genetics, 25,* 537–544.

Thapar, A., & McGuffin, P. (1995). Are anxiety symptoms in childhood heritable? *Journal of Child Psychology and Psychiatry, 36,* 439–447.

Thapar, A., & McGuffin, P. (1997). Anxiety and depressive symptoms in childhood: A genetic study of comorbidity. *Journal of Child Psychology and Psychiatry, 38,* 651–656.

Theobold, T., Hay, D., & Judge, C. (1987). Individual variation and specific cognitive deficits in the fra(X) syndrome. *American Journal of Medical Genetics, 28,* 1–11.

Thomas, M., & Karmiloff-Smith, A. (2002). *Are developmental disorders like cases of adult brain damage? Implications from connectionist modelling.* Manuscript submitted for publication.

Todd, R. D., Neuman, R., Geller, B., Fox, L. W., & Hickok, J. (1993). Genetic studies of affective disorders: Should we be starting with childhood onset probands? *Journal of the American Academy of Child and Adolescent Psychiatry, 32,* 1164–1171.

Tomblin, J. B., & Buckwalter, P. R. (1998). Heritability of poor language achievement among twins. *Journal of Speech, Language and Hearing Research, 41*(1), 188–199.

Topolski, T. D., Hewitt, J. K., Eaves, L. J., Silberg, J. L., Meyer, J. M., Rutter, M., Pickles, A., & Simonoff, E. (1997). Genetic and environmental influences on child reports of manifest anxiety and symptoms of separation anxiety and overanxious disorders: A community-based twin study. *Behavior Genetics, 27,* 15–28.

Torgesen, J. K. (1997). The prevention and remediation of reading disabilities: Evaluating what we know from research. *American Language Therapy, 1,* 11–47.

Tourette Syndrome Association International Consortium for Genetics. (1999). A complete genome screen in sib pairs affected by Gilles de la Tourette Syndrome. *American Journal of Human Genetics, 65,* 1428–1436.

Trevarthen, C. (1979). Communication and cooperation in early infancy: A description of primary intersubjectivity. In M. Bullowa (Ed.), *Before speech: The beginning of human communication* (pp. 321–347). London: Cambridge University Press.

True, W. R., Rice, J., Eisen, S. A., Heather, A. C., Goldberg, J., Lyons, J. J., & Nowak, J. (1993). A twin study of genetic and environmental contributions to liability for posttraumatic stress symptoms. *Archives of General Psychiatry, 50,* 257–264.

van der Kolk, B. A., & Greenberg, M. S. (1987). The psychobiology of the trauma response: Hyperarousal, constriction, and addiction to traumatic reexposure. In B. A. van der Kolk (Ed.), *Psychological trauma* (pp. 63–87). Washington, DC: American Psychiatric Press.

van der Lely, H. (1994). Canonical linking rules: Forward versus reverse linking in normally developing and specifically language-impaired children. *Cognition, 51,* 29–72.

Van Orden, G. C., & Paap, K. R. (1997). Functional neuroimages fail to discover pieces of mind in the parts of the brain. *Philosophy of Science, 64,* S85–S94.

Van Orden, G. C., Pennington, B. F., & Stone, G. O. (1990). Word identification in reading and the promise of subsymbolic psycholinguistics. *Psychological Review, 97*(4), 488–522.

Van Orden, G. C., Pennington, B. F., & Stone, G. O. (2001). What do double dissociations prove? *Cognitive Science, 25,* 111–172.

Varga-Khadem, F., Gadian, D. G., Watkins, K. E., Connelly, A., van Paesschen, W., & Mishkin, M. (1997). Differential effects of early hippocampal pathology on episodic and semantic memory. *Science, 277,* 376–380.

Vazquez, D. M., & Lopez, E. M. (2001, April). *Low cortisol levels and failure to terminate the stress response in psychosocial dwarfism: A mechanism for growth failure.* Paper presented at the Society for Research in Child Development, Minneapolis, MN.

Vellutino, F. R. (1979). *Dyslexia: Theory and research.* Cambridge, MA: MIT Press.

Verkerk, A. J., Pieretti, M., Sutcliffe, J. S., Fu, Y. H., Kuhl, D. P., Pizzuti, A., Reiner, O., Richards, S., Victoria, M. F., Zhang, F. P., Eussen, B. E., VanOmmen, G. J. B., Blonden, L. A. J., Riggins, G. J., Chastain, J. L., Kunst, C. B., Galjaard, H., Caskey, T. C., Nelson, D. L., Oostra, B. A., & Warren, S. T. (1991). Identification of a gene (FMR-1) containing a CGG repeat coincident with a breakpoint cluster region exhibiting length variation in fragile X syndrome. *Cell, 65,* 904–914.

Vicente, A. M., Macciardi, F., Verga, M., Bassett, A. S., Honer, W. G., Bean, G., & Kennedy, J. L. (1997). NCAM and schizophrenia: Genetic studies. *Molecular Psychiatry, 2*(1), 65–69.

Wadsworth, S. J., DeFries, J. C., Stevenson, J., Gilger, J. W., & Pennington, B. F. (1992). Gender ratios among reading-disabled children and their siblings as a function of parental impairment. *Journal of Child Psychology and Psychiatry, 33,* 1229–1239.

Wagner, R. K., & Torgesen, J. K. (1987). The nature of phonological processing and its causal role in the acquisition of reading skills. *Psychological Bulletin, 101,* 192–212.

Waldman, I., Rhee, S. H., Levy, F., & Hay, D. A. (2001). Causes of the overlap among symptoms of ADHD, oppositional defiant disorder, and conduct disorder. In F. Levy & D. A. Hay (Eds.), *Attention, genes, and ADHD* (pp. 115–138). East Sussex, UK: Brunner-Routledge.

Waldman, I. D., Rowe, D. C., Abramowitz, A., Kozel, S., Mohr, J., Sherman, S. L., Cleveland, H. H., Sanders, M. L., & Stever, C. (1996). Association of the dopamine transporter gene (DAT1) and attention deficit hyperactivity disorder in children. *American Journal of Human Genetics, 59,* A25.

Wallach, M. A., & Wallach, L. (1983). *Psychology's sanction for selfishness: The error of egoism in theory and therapy.* San Francisco: Freeman.

Walsh, B. T. (1998). *Child psychopharmacology.* Washington, DC: American Psychiatric Press.

Wang, P. P., & Bellugi, U. (1994). Evidence from two genetic syndromes for a dissociation between verbal and visual–spatial short-term memory. *Journal of Clinical and Experimental Neuropsychology, 16,* 317–322.

Wang, P. P., Doherty, S., Rourke, S. B., & Bellugi, U. (1995). Unique profile of visuoperceptual skills in a genetic syndrome. *Brain and Cognition, 29,* 54–65.

Weiss, S. (1991). Morphometry and magnetic resonance imaging of the brain in normal controls and Down's syndrome. *Anatomical Record, 231,* 593–598.

Weissman, M. M., Gershon, E. S., & Kidd, K. K. (1984). Psychiatric disorders in the relatives of probands with affective disorders: The Yale University National Institute of Mental Health Collaborative Study. *Archives of General Psychiatry, 41,* 13–21.

Welsh, M. C., Pennington, B. F., Ozonoff, S., Rouse, B., & McCabe, E. R. B. (1990). Neuropsychology of early-treated phenylketonuria: Specific executive function deficits. *Child Development, 61,* 1697–1713.

Willcutt, E. G., & Pennington, B. F. (1997). *Symptoms of anxiety and depression in children: Common genetic influence on both dimensions.* Unpublished manuscript.

Willcutt, E. G., & Pennington, B. F. (2000). Psychiatric comorbidity in children and adolescents with reading disability. *Journal of Child Psychology and Psychiatry, 41,* 1039–1048.

Willcutt, E. G., Pennington, B. F., & DeFries, J. C. (2000a). Etiology of inattention and hyperactivity/impulsivity in a community sample of twins with learning difficulties. *Journal of Abnormal Child Psychology, 28,* 149–159.

Willcutt, E. G., Pennington, B. F., DeFries, J. C. (2000b). A twin study of the etiology of comorbidity between reading disability and attention-deficit /hyperactivity disorder. *American Journal of Medical Genetics (Neuropsychiatric Genetics), 96,* 293–301.

Willcutt, E. G., Pennington, B. F., Smith, S. D., Cardon, L. R., Gayan, J., Knopik, V. S., Olson, R. K., & DeFries, J. C. (in press). Quantitative trait locus for reading disability on chromosome 6p is pleiotropic for ADHD. *Neuropsychiatric Genetics.*

Willerman, L. (1973). Activity level and hyperactivity in twins. *Child Development, 44,* 288–293.

Wing, L. (1991). The relationship between Asperger's syndrome and Kanner's autism. In U. Frith (Ed.), *Autism and Asperger syndrome* (pp. 93–121). New York: Cambridge University Press.

Wisniewski, K. E., Segan, S. M., Miezejeski, C. M., Sersen, E. A., & Rudelli, R. D. (1991). The fragile X syndrome: Neurological, electrophysiological and neuropathological abnormalities. *American Journal of Medical Genetics, 38,* 476–480.

Witt, R. M., Kaspar, B. K., Brazelton, A. D., Comery, T. A., Craig, A. M., Weiler, I. J., & Greenough, W. T. (1995). Developmental localization of fragile X mRNA in rat brain [Abstract]. *Society for Neuroscience Abstracts, 21,* 734.

Wright, S. (1920). The relative importance of heredity and environment in determining the piebald pattern of guinea pigs. *Proceedings of the National Academy of Sciences of the United States of America, 6,* 321–332.

Zametkin, A. J., Liebenauer, L. L., Fitzgerald, G. A., King, A. C., Minkunas, D. V., Herscovitch, P., Yamada, E. M., & Cohen, R. M. (1993). Brain metabolism in teenagers with attention-deficit hyperactivity disorder. *Archives of General Psychiatry, 50,* 333–340.

Zametkin, A. J., Nordahl, T. E., Gross, M., King, A. C., Semple, W. E., Rumsey, J., Hamburger, S., & Cohen, R. M. (1990). Cerebral glucose metabolism in adults with hyperactivity of childhood onset. *New England Journal of Medicine, 323,* 1361–1366.

Zametkin, A. J., & Rapoport, J. L. (1986). The pathophysiology of attention deficit disorders. In B. B. Lahey & A. E. Kazdin (Eds.), *Advances in clinical child psychology* (pp. 177–216). New York: Plenum Press.

Zeaman, D., & House, B. (1963). The role of attention in retardate discriminant learning. In N. R. Ellis (Ed.), *Handbook of mental deficiency psychological theory and research* (pp. 159–223). New York: McGraw-Hill.

Zigler, E. (1969). Developmental versus difference theories of mental retardation and the problem of motivation. *American Journal of Mental Deficiency, 73,* 536–556.

Index